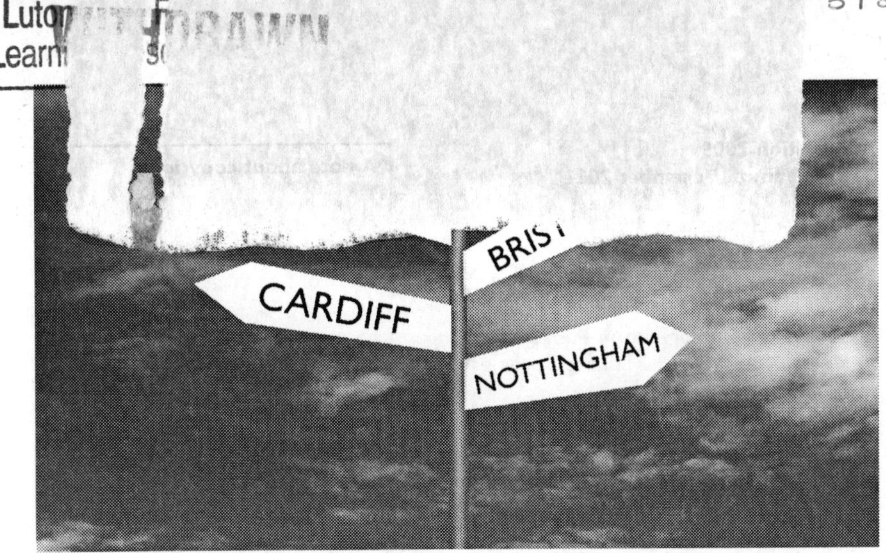

Choosing a Medical School

An essential guide to UK medical schools

Second Edition

Alexander Young, Alexander Aquilina, William Dougal, Thomas Judd & Matt Green

First edition 2009
Second edition December 2011

ISBN 9781 4453 8150 3
Previous ISBN 9781 9068 3911 6
e-ISBN 9781 4453 8568 6

British Library Cataloguing-in-Publication Data
A catalogue record for this book is available from the British Library

Published by
BPP Learning Media Ltd
BPP House, Aldine Place
London W12 8AA

www.bpp.com/health

Typeset by Replika Press Pvt Ltd, India
Printed in the United Kingdom

Your learning materials, published by BPP Learning Media Ltd, are printed on paper sourced from sustainable, managed forests.

The views expressed in this book are those of BPP Learning Media and not those of the NHS. BPP Learning Media are in no way associated with or endorsed by the NHS.

The contents of this book are intended as a guide and not professional advice. Although every effort has been made to ensure that the contents of this book are correct at the time of going to press, BPP Learning Media, the Editor and the Author make no warranty that the information in this book is accurate or complete and accept no liability for any loss or damage suffered by any person acting or refraining from acting as a result of the material in this book.

Every effort has been made to contact the copyright holders of any material reproduced within this publication. If any have been inadvertently overlooked, BPP Learning Media will be pleased to make the appropriate credits in any subsequent reprints or editions.

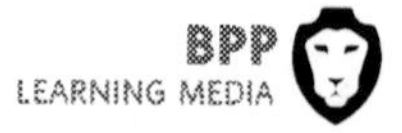

Contents

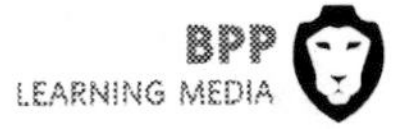

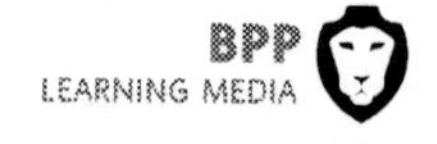
BPP
LEARNING MEDIA

About the Publisher

BPP Learning Media is dedicated to supporting aspiring professionals with top quality learning material. BPP Learning Media's commitment to success is shown by our record of quality, innovation and market leadership in paper-based and e-learning materials. BPP Learning Media's study materials are written by professionally-qualified specialists who know from personal experience the importance of top quality materials for success.

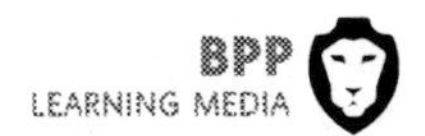

Reaching your Goal

The process of applying to medical school can be a somewhat long and arduous process but the rewards of a career within Medicine are infinite. BPP Learning Media and BPP University College School of Health are committed to supporting aspiring and current doctors to progress their career through our comprehensive range of books, personal development courses and degree programmes. I often say there is no other vocation that provides such breadth and depth of career options for the individual to follow and specialise in. Whether it is the fast paced nature of the A&E department or the measured environment of Pathology, there is something for everyone.

There is no greater privilege than being responsible for leading the treatment of patients and sharing in their recovery. There are few other careers that provide such diversity on a daily basis. A passion for helping others, clear communication skills especially empathy, excellent team working and leadership qualities as well as the ability to strike a work-life balance are all skills that an accomplished doctor should possess.

The decision to follow a career in Medicine is something that should not be taken lightly and you should undertake careful research to ensure it really is for you. A career in Medicine is not for everyone and I would urge readers to ensure they have undertaken sufficient work experience to gain a balanced insight into what becoming a doctor really entails.

I first began mentoring aspiring medical students seven years ago when it was clear that many individuals were not gaining access to the help and support they required to successfully apply to medical school. It was with this in mind that I embarked on publishing our *Entry to Medical School Series* to provide a clear insight into the various facets of successfully getting into medical school. Whether it is help with choosing the right medical school, how to prepare an outstanding personal statement or how to succeed in your medical school interview, our comprehensive range of books provide the advice that is so often hard to find.

I would like to take this opportunity to wish you the very best of luck with applying to medical school and hope that you pass on some of the gems of wisdom that you acquire along the way to other aspiring medics.

Matt Green
Series Editor – Entry to Medical School
Medical Publishing Director

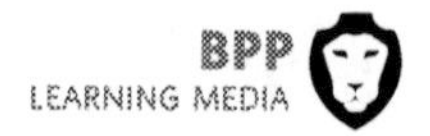

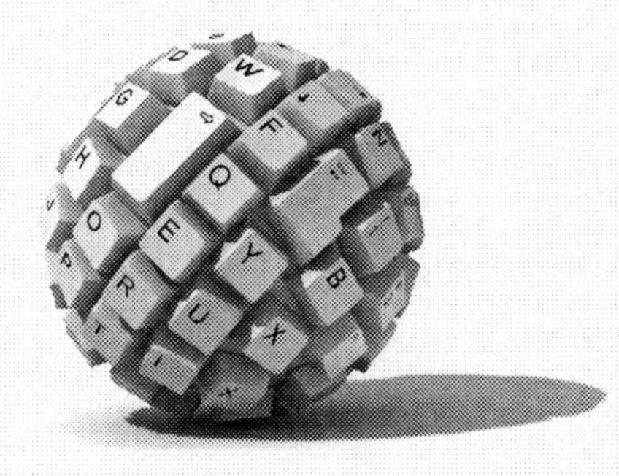

Free Companion Material

Readers can access an interactive map, with links to each UK medical school, for free online.

To access the above companion material please visit **www.bpp.com/freehealthresources**

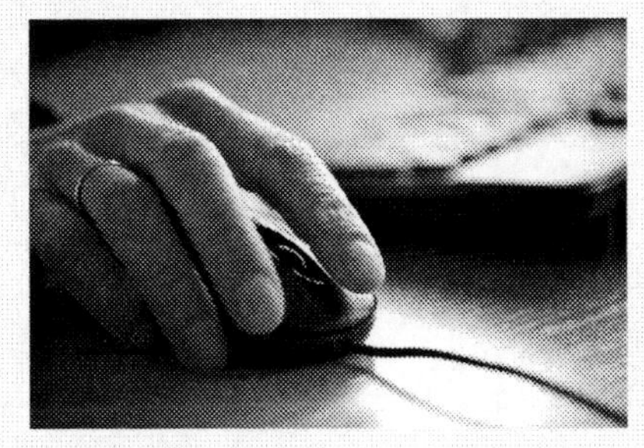

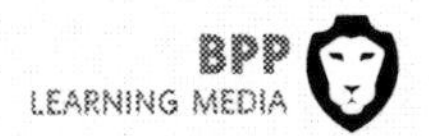

Acknowledgements

The authors would like to thank all of the contributors who helped to provide the latest, most pertinent information about life at their respective medical schools.

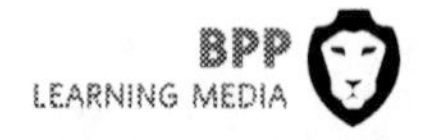

Contributors

Gregory Young
Phillip Lucas
Charlotte Adams
John Paul
Miles Gandolfi
Rosie Ives
Andy Mahon
Oliver Reed
James Thomson
Louise O'Reilly
Raphael Rogans-Watson
Harsimran Singh
Matthew Kuet
Bnar Talabani
Amy Ruffle
Claire Farrington
Kenneth Mackenzie
Mairi Crawford
Emma Scott
Arma Patel
Laura Woodhead
Steve Knight
Lopa Patel
Perryhan Hiotis
Louise Merchison
Rosie Utton
Paul Healy
David Gabrera
Laura Wark
Arvinder Sood
Kapil Sugand
Ghanshyam Kacha
Patrick Haslam
David Clarke
Max Kamath
Harpreet Sood
Hew Torrance
Nicholas Boxall
Anthony Howard
Tiffany Berrington
Lucie Pearce
Annette Haines
Tim Robbins
Tom Barge
Jack Pottle
Daniel Djemal
Tom Hannan
Sarah Weldon
Caroline Tait
Jamie A'Court
Niel Gordon
Nick Gallop
Ian King
Davina Mehta
Varun Dravid
Jamie-Anne Gilmour
Andrew Burgess
Simon Lammy
Jack Artley
Johan Fox
Tim Hughes
Preshan Jeevaratnam
Tom Hutchinson
Aiden Plant
Kar-Hung Kuet
Oscar Rhylah
Richard Booth
Rahul Neelamkavil
Fay Meakin
Ed Klaber
Alexandra Smith
Carrie Broughton
Laura Walker
Timothy Alce
Herjit Sidu
Steve Dauncey
David Clark
Lucy Aquilina

Abbreviations

BMA British Medical Association

BMAT Biomedical Admissions Test

BMJ British Medical Journal

BSc Bachelor of Science

CAL Computer Assisted Learning

CT 1/2 Core Trainee Year 1/2

DGH District General Hospital

DR Dissection Room

EMQ Extended Matching Questions

FY1/FY2 Foundation Year 1/2

GAMSAT Graduate Medical School Admissions Test

GMC General Medical Council

HCA Health Care Assistant

MBChB Bachelor of Medicine, Bachelor of Chirgurie

MBBS Bachelor of Medicine, Bachelor of Surgery

MCQ Multiple Choice Questions

MDU Medical Defence Union

MMC Modernising Medical Careers

MPS Medical Protection Society

MRCS Member of the Royal College of Surgeons

MRCP Member of the Royal College of Physicians

MSc Master of Science

MTAS Medical Training Application Service

NHS National Health Service

OSLER Objective Structured Long Examination Record

OSCE Observed Skills and Clinical Examination

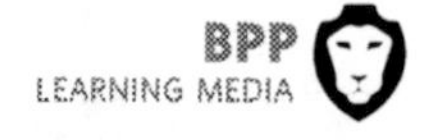

PBL Problem-Based Learning

PRHO Pre-Registration House Officer

RCS Royal College of Surgeons

SBA Single Best Answer

SHO Senior House Officer

SpR Specialist Registrar

SSC/SSM/SSU Student Selected Component/Module/Unit

ST1/2 Specialist Trainee Year 1/2

UCAS University and College Admissions Service

UKCAT UK Clinical Aptitude Test

Preface to Second Edition

When visiting a new city a guidebook is essential if you wish to experience all that the city has to offer. When choosing a medical school it is vital that you weigh up all that the city, university and medical school have to offer before reaching a final decision.

At its core Medicine is the recognition, treatment and prevention of disease. A medical career will blend problem-solving and recognition skills with communication and practical skills. Though study and life working in hospitals can be intense the practical nature of the job together with the knowledge that you are helping others makes Medicine a fantastic career choice.

By picking up this book you have already shown that you have an interest in a medical career whether this is the result of clinical experiences, a desire to help others or due to advice from school or parents.

The second edition of this book aims to give more focus on student opinions and the differences between the medical schools.

The book is best paired with *Becoming a Doctor*, which guides the reader through the process of applying to and securing a place at medical school.

This book divides each UK medical school into sections covering the medical school itself, the city and the university. Factors such as intercalation, foreign travel and distance of clinical placements, that you may not have considered, are all covered together with details of individual courses and facilities. Each chapter includes opinions from UK medical students studying at the medical school to give a feeling of what life is like in the early and later years.

This guide distils what it is like being a medic at each UK medical school and provides you with pertinent insight into the positives and negatives of each city, university and medical school before you come to a final decision.

Good luck for the future.

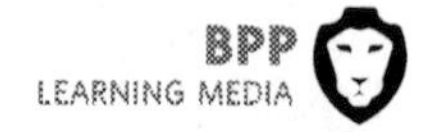

Foreword by Sir Liam Donaldson

Medicine is a unique and challenging career. Choosing to apply to medical school is the first step on a long journey. It is not a decision to be taken lightly. Your time as a medical student will be challenging. There will be the intellectual challenge of learning the subject, and you will spend many long hours studying. But you will also face emotional challenges, perhaps being confronted with stories or events that upset you. In return, you can expect a fulfilling career offering variety, stimulation and the opportunity to help others.

Your days as a medical student are the foundation for your medical career. It is not only the opportunity to learn the basic skills and knowledge necessary for a career in Medicine, but it is also when life-long habits of learning and professional attitudes are developed. University is an exciting time, and for many, the first long period away from home. New friendships are formed, some, of which last a lifetime. Many opportunities exist to develop new interests or build on existing ones.

I would encourage you to take time to consider if Medicine is right for you, and where is best for you to study. There is an increasing number of medical schools with different strengths and opportunities. Over recent years, post-graduate courses have blossomed and open up the opportunity to study Medicine to a wider range of individuals. The university town is also where you will live for the best part of five or six years, with many students staying on longer to complete their foundation year training in the same area. The different university towns and their regions may have very different living costs, as well as offering different opportunities for things to do in your spare time. It is worth reflecting on all of these options and carefully considering what would suit you. This book provides a wealth of information, not only about individual medical schools and their differences, but also the university and its town.

Applying to university and medical school is an exciting time, which opens the door to a student life and career of opportunity. I am sure you will find this book helpful in making the right choices, and I hope you find your university career enjoyable and fulfilling.

Sir Liam Donaldson
Chief Medial Officer for England

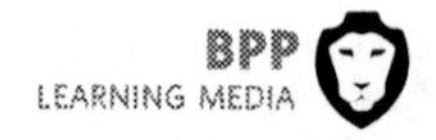

Foreword by Professor Ian Gilmore

This is a 'no holds barred' long hard look at the rocky road to becoming a doctor and the reader will be getting the information straight from students who have recently walked that road. The detail is enormous and will add to the information out there for prospective medical students, who will realise that changes occur so fast that the more sources of facts the better.

It is tough to get there but an enormously rewarding career to look forward to. Doctors remain the most trusted sector of society (trusted by more than 90% of the population and more than 50 points ahead of politicians and journalists!). But with that trust comes the responsibility to earn it. The Royal College of Physicians has found it enormously positive to engage with medical students recently on issues of professionalism and to find that tomorrow's doctors understand and value their unique position in society. I hope this book serves as guide to help you reach that exciting future.

Professor Ian Gilmore
President Royal College of Physicians

Foreword by John Black and Professor Mike Larvin

It is a pleasure to see a group of medical students drawing on their personal experience to assist potential applicants to medical schools. Doctors who went through the application process some time ago will have forgotten the stresses and strains involved, and their advice may not be helpful to today's applicants who face a more rigorous admissions process. The authors are closer to the action here, and have drawn on a large number of contributors to provide comprehensive coverage across our UK medical schools.

Readers should not skip the first chapter, which helps manage expectations of what a career in Medicine really involves and 'how to get in', or the second chapter, which explains life at medical school and beyond. Whilst no amount of coaching will help an unsuitable applicant to gain entry into medical school, the fact is that we turn down many good potential doctors every year as demand considerably exceeds supply. A well-informed applicant is more likely to succeed, having entered the process in a better-informed and prepared position.

The book contains up to date details for each UK medical school with web links for further reading. Ideally each school's section should be read as you have many choices to make over course type and location. It is nice to see history valued, as it was to read about our own medical schools – how things have changed! Of particular note was information on clinical teaching sites located away from the main campuses, with travel times. This is important, now that expansion has led to most clinical teaching being provided off site from traditional teaching centres, instead taking place at district hospitals and in the community. The views of students themselves provide the human touch that statistics and facts alone cannot. There are also additional useful notes for international applicants, for whom this book will be all the more valuable.

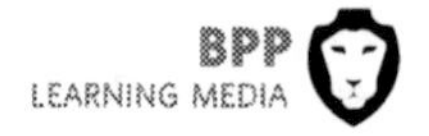

We feel sure that you will find this book useful, and that it will inspire you to follow in the footsteps of its authors.

John Black PRCS President
Mike Larvin FRCS Director of Education *(Admissions Tutor, University of Nottingham 2005–8)*
The Royal College of Surgeons of England

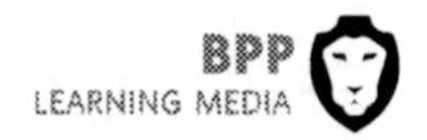

Chapter 1

Choosing Medicine

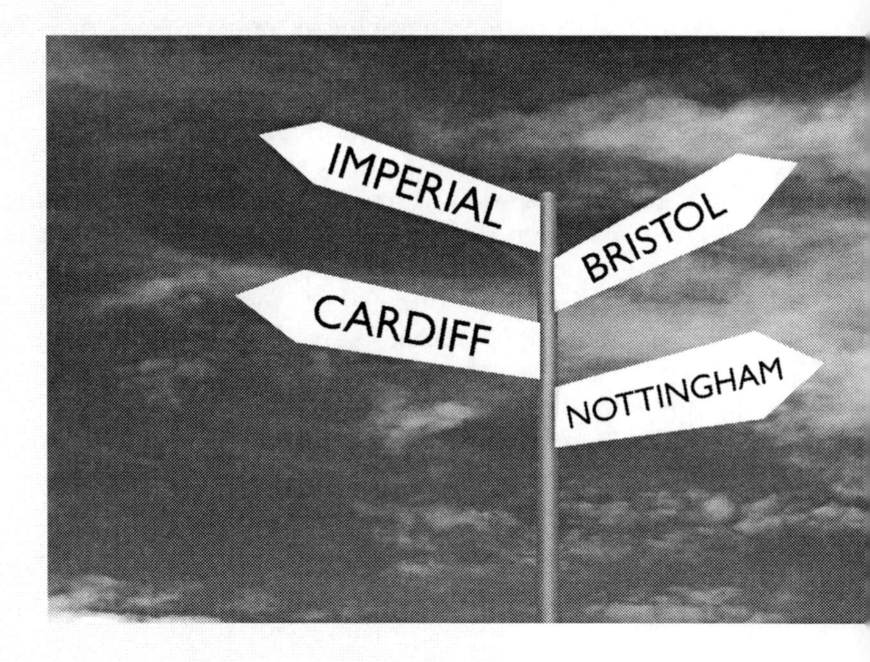

Choosing Medicine

Is Medicine the right choice?

Medicine is one of the oldest professions on the planet and the importance of an individual's health and wellbeing has made the role of the doctor one of the most respected in any society. Traditionally doctors were trained as apprentices and medical students were expected to live and work under experienced Physicians or Surgeons in order to recognise and understand common diseases. Today Medicine is taught through lectures, exposure to patients in hospitals and through modern teaching methods such as simulation suites and online tutorials.

The course

In the United Kingdom 32 medical schools offer medical degrees to students wishing to embark on a career in Medicine. While most degree courses require three years of study at university before graduating and starting work Medicine requires at least four years split between learning theory in lecture theatres and spending time in hospitals developing communication and practical skills.

Medicine on television

Choosing a career in Medicine is not a decision to be taken lightly.

While television and the media depict Medicine as a well-paid and attractive profession there is also a lot of hard work, study and discipline required to reach the end of medical training and achieve Consultant status. Selection into a medical degree course is fierce and only students demonstrating both academic ability and a determination to pursue both medical and extra-curricular achievements will be offered places.

It is unlikely that even as a qualified doctor you will be making diagnoses in the style of *House* or dealing with the drama depicted in *Grey's Anatomy*.

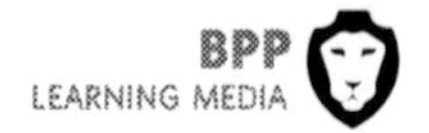

Applying is just the beginning

Once you have been offered a place at medical school it is important not to become complacent. At the end of the medical course there is competition for foundation doctor posts and it is the students that have displayed outstanding academic and extra-curricular achievements that receive the highest scores and pick of hospital placements.

As a medical student and, following graduation, as a doctor you will be expected to uphold a high level of probity and maintain your practice to the highest standards to ensure that patients receive the best possible care. With this responsibility comes pressure and it is important to realise that while Medicine is an extremely rewarding profession it is also a high-pressure environment and it is important to have interests outside of work.

The General Medical Council regulates UK doctors and ensures good medical practice. The GMC outlines what constitutes a good doctor in its publication *Tomorrow's Doctors*. This is certainly a vital read if you are interested in Medicine and is essential reading for those fortunate enough to be called to interview at a UK medical institution.

Examinations

As a medical student you will be continually examined to maintain a high standard of clinical and scientific knowledge. Examinations continue following graduation from university and post-grad exams can cost over £500 to sit. Exams can be tough and disciplined, self-directed learning is the only way to pass comfortably to the next stage of medical education.

Finance

Financing your way through medical school can also prove costly. Following the introduction of top-up fees expect to graduate with debts in excess of £20,000 and medical textbooks and equipment can be very expensive.

Having spent five years as a student, and with friends on three-year courses already earning, the prospect of receiving your first pay cheque can often seem a long way away. Foundation doctors can expect to earn between £22,000 – £28,000 per year rising to upwards of £100,000 as a GP, Consultant Surgeon or Physician.

Work-life balance

A junior doctor traditionally worked upwards of 80 hours per week and it was not uncommon to be working over 24 hours straight during night shifts and over weekends. Recent reforms in medical education together with the implementation of the European Working Time Directive mean that doctors in training should be working a maximum of 48 hours per week in order to reduce mistakes due to tiredness and to maintain patient safety. The downside of limiting working time is that time spent in training is also reduced and while doctors used to be able to accumulate many hours of practice in hospital identifying conditions and performing practical procedures this time has now been significantly reduced. This means that time spent on the wards in medical school is even more important and prospective doctors should take every opportunity to practise their craft while in hospitals.

Make sure before you apply

Before making a final decision make sure that you understand what it is like being a medical student or junior doctor on the wards. Try to spend time gaining work experience in your local hospital, speak with friends who are doctors and attend lectures of interest at local hospitals or societies.

Despite the competitive nature of the medical degree course and constant examinations the moment that you receive your medical diploma and the title Dr before your name is something that is difficult to equal.

You can refer to Chapter 1 in *Becoming a Doctor,* which is also part of the *Entry to Medical School Series* published by BPP Learning Media for further tips on whether Medicine is the right career for you.

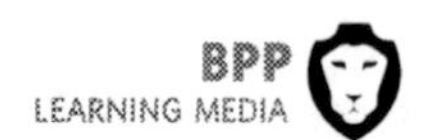

Choosing a medical school: things to consider

Once you have decided on a career in Medicine choosing a medical school can be an extremely difficult decision. It is important that you know as much about the course and host institution as possible before making your choice and beginning the long period of study required to become a doctor. While factors such as location, peer recommendation and reputation of the medical school play a vital role in the decision-making process it can be difficult to think of other important aspects to consider.

Do your homework

Individual decisions may be influenced by a number of factors ranging from sports facilities at the university to size of the city and number of surrounding hospitals.

To facilitate your decision-making process this book provides readers with key facts and student opinions from all 32 UK medical schools. While the contents of the book provide a comprehensive overview of UK medical schools it is important to visit the institutions themselves on open days and to check the university websites for the latest and most up-to-date admission criteria.

Location

Studying in an environment that you enjoy is extremely important. Together with distance from home and the city itself it is important to make sure that you are happy with the student accommodation in both first and later years, the location of clinical attachments and student activities in the city. While Medicine is an extremely competitive degree course, make sure that you are happy with your choice of city and university prior to applying.

Types of course

Although each UK medical school aims to award students with a medical degree the teaching, experiences and opportunities that each school provides can be quite different. Important differences include length of the course, entry requirements and whether the medical school offers a traditional or problem-based approach to teaching.

Traditional courses: These are divided into two years of pre-clinical, lecture-based teaching covering topics such as biochemistry, physiology and basic medical sciences followed by three years of clinical teaching in surrounding hospitals when students interact with patients and build upon their existing knowledge.

Problem-based learning courses: Adopted by a number of institutions, PBL aims to stimulate self-directed learning through the use of case-based group discussions and scenarios.

Integrated courses: Feature early clinical attachments with teaching integrated into placements.

Each UK medical school provides students with teaching and clinical experiences designed to produce the safest, most proficient junior doctors possible. Despite each medical school having this same goal each institution takes slightly different approaches to undergraduate teaching and it is important that you select the medical school that best suits your learning style and interests.

Exams

Although the majority of medical exams take the form of single best answer and extended matching questions together with clinical examinations, the timing and number of exams differs between medical schools.

League tables

University and medical school league tables are published annually in *The Times*, *The Guardian* and *The Complete University Guide*. These tables rank universities based on data relating to UCAS entry score, student satisfaction, class of degree, quality of research, staff expenditure and employability.

It is the authors' opinions that these should be viewed with caution and a healthy dose of cynicism. While it may be easy to select a 'top' medical school based on rankings tables it is important to remember that rankings will not affect employability of doctors. Far more important are the above factors relating to the medical course, the university and the city.

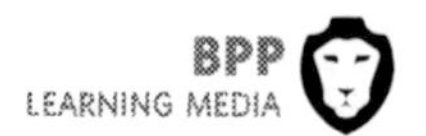

Have a Plan-B

Medicine is an extremely competitive degree course and not everyone will have the luxury of being accepted by their first choice medical school. The best way to maximise your selection choice is to work hard during GCSE and A level years and to demonstrate your aptitude for Medicine through your UCAS personal statement and university interviews.

Take the whole application process as a learning experience and do not be disheartened if you are not offered your first choice.

Getting in

> *'By medicine life may be prolonged, yet death will seize the doctor too.'*
>
> (William Shakespeare)

Once you are sure that Medicine is the career for you the next step is attaining a place at medical school. Selection is competitive and a high academic standard is required with science subjects taking precedent in GCSEs and A levels. Medicine is not just about an outstanding academic record. Application is through UCAS and it is important to have a strong personal statement submitted early to maximise your chances of being selected for interview. UCAS opens from mid-September so try to plan to have a completed form ready for early submission.

Personal statement

The selection panel are looking for your personal statement to reflect an understanding of the commitment needed for a career in Medicine. In addition you will need to show that you are sufficiently motivated to undertake the long period of study required to qualify.

Work experience: While it is unlikely that your role will involve more than 'shadowing' a medical professional, gaining insight into what day-to-day life is like for a doctor is extremely important. Due to the numerous medical subspecialties there are lots of different jobs to gain experience in. Many hospitals offer a 'shadowing' programme for sixth form students to follow junior doctors at work. This is a great opportunity to not only see what they do but also to pick their brain on application advice.

Don't be put off if your local hospital doesn't offer 'shadowing'. Try phoning the postgraduate centre or arranging a placement through your school.

Voluntary work: Gaining voluntary experience in a hospital or hospice environment is a great way to show commitment to helping people and is a necessity on many university admission panels. Working at a youth centre, nursing home, or as a healthcare assistant are all excellent ways to demonstrate a desire to help others.

Extra-curricular activities: Owing to the intense nature of medical education and pressures of being a doctor it is vital to demonstrate interests outside of Medicine whether this be through sport, music or other interests. If you have pursued your interests outside of Medicine to a high standard this also demonstrates your determination and dedication.

Courses and prizes: Local hospitals and societies such as The Royal Society of Medicine in London and MedLink in Nottingham often hold events aimed at prospective medical students. Attending these events not only increases your medical knowledge and skills but also shows your commitment to Medicine. A number of societies also offer medical essay prizes for sixth form students which is, again, an excellent way to help you stand out from the crowd.

Reading

In order to maximise your knowledge of Medicine for both the personal statement and interviews it is prudent to read as much medical literature as possible and it is wise to have knowledge of in vogue topics such as reforms to training or breakthroughs in disease management. The *Student BMJ* and *New Scientist* are a good start and books such as this one will offer tips for applying.

Admissions tests

Certain medical schools also require entrance exams such as BMAT (BioMedical Admissions Test) or UKCAT (UK Clinical Aptitude Test) for undergraduates or the GAMSAT (Graduate Medical School

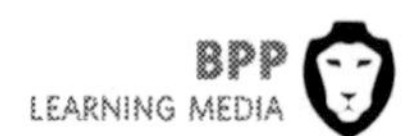

Admissions Test) for graduate entry medics. These exams aim to supplement GCSE and A level results.

The best way to prepare for these is to practise as many questions as possible prior to sitting the exam.

UKCAT

The UKCAT is a two-hour multiple choice written paper testing perceived non-academic qualities including verbal reasoning, quantitive reasoning, abstract reasoning, decision analysis and non-cognitive analysis. Registration opens in early May and testing takes place in July. The registration fee in 2011 was £65 for EU applicants and £100 for non-EU applicants, and bursaries are available for those with maintenance loans.

Further information about the UKCAT can be found at www.ukcat.ac.uk.

BMAT

The BMAT is a two-hour written paper required by Cambridge, Imperial, Oxford and UCL medical schools. The test is split into two multiple-choice sections (aptitude and skills and scientific knowledge and application) and an essay question. Applications for entries open in September and the test itself takes place in November with results announced in December. Registration cost £42.50 for EU candidates and £72.50 for non-EU candidates in 2011.

Further information can be found at www.admissionstests.cambridgeassessment.org.uk.

GAMSAT

The GAMSAT is required for four-year graduate-entry courses at St George's, Keele, Nottingham, Peninsula and Swansea. Registration opens in June and the test happens in September. The registration fee in 2011 was £195 and results are announced in November.

The exam itself requires a full day with a five and a half hour exam with a one-hour recess. The test is divided into three sections:

Reasoning in Humanities and Social Sciences, Written Communication and Reasoning in Biological and Physical Sciences.

Further information can be found at www.gamsatuk.org.

University medical admission examinations

Medical School	UKCAT	BMAT	GAMSAT
Aberdeen	Yes	No	No
Belfast	Yes	No	No
Birmingham	No	No	No
Brighton Sussex	Yes	No	No
Bristol	No	No	No
Cambridge	No	Yes	No
Cardiff	Yes	No	No
Dundee	Yes	No	No
Durham	Yes	No	No
East Anglia	Yes	No	No
Edinburgh	Yes	No	No
Glasgow	Yes	No	No
Hull York	Yes	No	No
Keele	Yes	No	Yes
Leeds	Yes	No	No
Leicester	Yes	No	No
Liverpool	No	No	No
London: Barts	Yes	No	No
London: Imperial	Yes (Graduate Entry)	Yes	No
London: King's	Yes	No	No
London: UCL	No	Yes	No
London: St George's	Yes	No	Yes
Manchester	Yes	No	No
Newcastle upon Tyne	Yes	No	No
Nottingham	Yes	No	Yes (Derby)

Medical School	UKCAT	BMAT	GAMSAT
Oxford	Yes (Graduate Entry)	Yes	No
Peninsula	Yes	No	Yes
Sheffield	Yes	No	No
Southampton	Yes	No	No
St Andrews	Yes	No	No
Swansea	No	No	Yes
Warwick	Yes (Graduate Entry)	No	No

Interviews

Having submitted an application through UCAS you may then face a long wait before receiving confirmation of an offer or interview. It is important not to be disheartened if you are not short-listed for interview. Stay positive and focus on things that you can influence such as your A2 subjects and extra-curricular commitments.

Medical interviews occur at different times of the year and vary between medical schools. Interview panels usually consist of faculty members, doctors and senior medical students. The interview is a chance to convey your personality to the interviewers and to demonstrate both your communication skills and your ability to cope under pressure.

There are a number of what might be described as standard medical interview questions:

> 'Why do you want to study Medicine?'
> 'Can you talk about any recent medical news?'
> 'Can you tell me about some of your recent voluntary experiences?'

Most if not all of the questions will be related to your personal statement, so make sure you know it inside out before you step into the interview room.

It is not uncommon to be presented with an ethical dilemma to solve such as a fellow student or fellow doctor being inebriated on the wards and how you would deal with this. In a case like this, generally the safest answer world be to suggest rather than whistle blowing or concealing a friend's actions.

If possible try to attend practice interviews with local doctors or through your school to maximise your chances.

See Chapters 2 and 3 of *Becoming a Doctor*, which is also part of the *Entry to Medical School Series* published by BPP Learning Media for further tips on getting in.

Pre-medical/foundation and access courses

> *'Medicine is the only profession that labours incessantly to destroy the reason for its own existence.'*
>
> (James Bryce)

Although many decide early to go directly from school to a university medical course others may decide later to pursue a career in Medicine.

For those that chose non-science subjects before deciding upon a career in Medicine several medical schools offer pre-medical/ foundation courses or access courses.

Pre-medical/foundation courses

These extend the undergraduate course by an extra year and aim to give students a firm grounding in Biology and Chemistry before commencing the formal medical programme. Foundation courses are aimed at students who did not study science subjects at A level but wish to pursue a career in medicine.

Students apply for the pre-med / foundation course through UCAS and following one year of full time study at the university students are guaranteed a place on the undergraduate medical course.

Pre-med/foundation courses

Bristol (p. 95)
Cardiff (p. 120)
Dundee (p. 136)
Keele (p. 216)

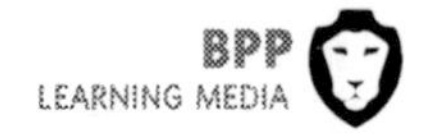

London: King's (p. 307)
London: St George's (p. 334)
Manchester (p. 350)
Nottingham (p. 377)
Sheffield (p. 421)
Southampton (p. 434)

Access courses

Some institutions that do not have a medical school run medical access courses. These are primarily designed for mature students to demonstrate recent academic activity, though some can help to augment those who received poor A level grades.

Many medical schools do not recognise access courses and no place at a medical school is guaranteed following their completion (unlike foundation courses). Medical schools that do accept students with access degrees will likely require high scoring applicants. It is advisable to check with both the access course institution and desired medical school to see whether the course is eligible for application to an undergraduate medical course.

Access courses

City & Islington College, London
City College Norwich, Norfolk
College of West Anglia, Norfolk (Linked with UEA Medical School)
Lambeth College, London
The Manchester College, Manchester
St Martin's College, Lancashire
Sussex Downs College, East Sussex (Linked with Brighton & Sussex Medical School)
University of Bradford (Linked with Leeds Medical School)

Graduate entry courses

For those who decided upon Medicine after completing a prior degree course there are also a number of graduate entry programmes.

Graduate Entry Medicine programmes (GEMs) are often condensed to fast-tack, four-year courses and it can prove challenging studying for multiple examinations and attending multiple lectures in order to fit five years into a four-year course. Graduate entry courses assume well-developed learning skills and prior scientific knowledge.

Graduates are also eligible to apply for the regular undergraduate courses if they choose.

Choosing GEM

Choosing to undertake a four- or five-year degree course after completing a previous degree can be a difficult decision. Not only do graduate entry students face another lengthy period of study, they must also deal with the financial and social implications of returning to university.

Graduate entry medics do have the advantage of knowing the amount of work required to do well at university and, having already experienced the highs of freshers' week and first year, may be keen to get down to work from the outset.

Eligibility

The entry criteria for graduate entry programmes vary between medical schools and it is advisable to check the medical school admissions website to make sure that you have the necessary degree and A levels. The corresponding admissions tests are summarised below.

Getting in to graduate entry programmes

Most universities require applicants for graduate-entry courses to have at least a 2:1 degree in a science-based subject. In general your postgraduate degree counts for more than your A level results.

Some graduate entry programmes require applicants to sit the GAMSAT or UKCAT admissions test prior to application (see below).

The courses

GEM courses vary between medical schools in both their sizes and workload required. In general the same decisions regarding the medical school, university and city in which you will be studying apply. The insider views of graduate entry medics have been highlighted in the corresponding chapters.

Medical schools offering graduate entry courses

Medical school	Degree	Admissions test	Page
Birmingham	1st	None	67
Bristol	2:1	None	95
Cambridge	2:1	BMAT	108
Keele	2:1	GAMSAT	216
Leicester	2:1	UKCAT	246
Liverpool	2:1	None	261
London: Barts	2:1	UKCAT	277
London: Imperial	2:1	UKCAT	291
London: King's	2:1	UKCAT	307
London: St George's	2:2	GAMSAT	334
Newcastle	2:1	UKCAT	363
Nottingham	2:2	GAMSAT	377
Oxford	2:1	UKCAT	391
Southampton	2:1	None	434
Swansea	2:1	GAMSAT	458
Warwick	2:1	UKCAT	468

International students and mature students

Just as there are places for graduate entry medics and pre-medics not every one in the lecture theatre will be fresh from school. A number of medical school places are available for mature students and international students.

Potential medics may also have to weigh-up undertaking a lengthily degree course while supporting families and children.

Other commitments such as a blossoming sporting career or working in the armed forces can also be juggled around a medical career.

International students

While the majority of medical students are from the UK a growing number of applicants are from Europe, Asia, Africa or the Middle East. International medics face the added difficulties of adjusting to the British lifestyle and weather together with learning Medicine in a foreign language and the high cost of studying in the UK. Despite these barriers the quality of medical education in UK medical schools and the prestige of being awarded a UK medical degree make studying in the UK extremely appealing. It is advisable to contact the medical school directly and to sort out visa and student permits early to find out what is involved.

Although expenses can be high some universities offer bursaries for international students.

Student's view: being an international medic

'Having grown up in Hong Kong with both parents as doctors it was likely that I would follow in their footsteps. Deciding to study in the UK was a big decision. While medical programmes in the East are very good I felt that I wanted a new challenge and attaining a medical degree at a university in the UK is seen as very prestigious. My family and friends were very supportive and helped me with the application process that can seem scary. It can be difficult finding out exactly what grades UK medical schools require of international applicants, however, I found that the best way to find out information was to phone the medical school directly to discuss how they cater to international students. By doing this I also learned of a bursary scheme that I would not otherwise have known about.

The biggest problem for international applicants are the high fees charged by universities. I was lucky that my parents were happy to support me, however, many will be unable to study abroad due to the high costs for international students. The other problem can be the language. I was lucky as my English was good having been to British school in Hong Kong, however, others may find it difficult being taught in a foreign language.

Having been offered a place it was scary to be leaving my home to study in England. I lived in halls of residence and also joined a society for international students that helped me to fit in and get to know lots of

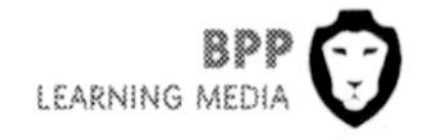

people. The medical lectures were very well taught and I would definitely recommend studying in the UK.'

Mature students and medics with families

Like postgraduate students, mature medics may find it difficult returning to study surrounded by younger students. Established relationships, young children or caring for a loved one can make studying for a medical degree seem impossible. A number of medical students do manage to juggle these commitments and most medical schools will go out of their way to help medics with family commitments. It is worth speaking to the admissions department directly prior to applying to find out if they will offer help to those with families and this also gives you a good feel for how welcoming the medical school is.

It is important to keep in mind that even after medical school a medical career may require you to move around the country in search of jobs and that working over holiday periods can be detrimental to family life. There are always ways around difficulties with rotas or placements and most work colleagues will go out of their way to help you out when it comes to family life.

Student's view: balancing family life

'Be in no doubt, being a parent and a medical student is hard. There is a constant tussle between study and family. When I started med school, I had a 3-year-old boy and 10-month-old girl. I was fortunate; my wife didn't work and looked after the children.

Being an older student, I worried that the learning would be tough after so long out of education. There was no need, it was like getting fit for a marathon – it hurt for a few weeks and then it all began to slot in place. Being older is also a help in that you are better at focusing on what information was important and disregarding the less relevant stuff.

The medical school really helped in placements, putting me near the family and that made a huge difference. The hardest thing is that during exams most students can go to their rooms, lock the door and study constantly. With a family you have a role and place in society; there are letters to open, calls to make, family to look after and a house to maintain. These things can't be put on hold. I found myself taking risks in the learning, skirting over some aspects in order to focus on more important material in order to make time. One thing I did throughout the course without exception, for the sake of the family was to make every Sunday Medicine-free, 9.00am Monday exam or not. I would recommend to anyone with the family to consider doing similar – it helps give you energy for the rest of the week.'

Other commitments

It is extremely important to have a balanced life while studying medicine and those wishing to pursue sporting commitments or active interests outside of work may need to balance these with time spent studying. High level achievements in sport are encouraged by most medical schools and there will always be ways to attain your medical degree between training sessions and attending competitions and events.

Choosing to be a medic in the armed forces is an extremely worthwhile pursuit and the army, RAF and navy reward trainees with bursaries that can help to offset high levels of debt incurred as an undergraduate. Further information on medicine in the forces can be found through the respective forces' websites.

Student's view: working in the forces

'If you like to work hard and play hard, then it is well worth considering the forces; you can go and find out about it all without having to sign your life away and there is plenty of careers information out there to let you make an informed choice.

Commitment during studies depends on which service you go for, but expect to spend an evening a week with the forces plus a few weeks on Summer Camp. This is not a drag though as there are plenty of socials and activities that you would struggle to do elsewhere. You get to socialise with students that are not involved with Medicine, which can be a breath of fresh air once a week. There is the chance to organise good electives and visits to military sites, both at home and overseas.

Once you graduate you'll have to do your Foundation work at a hospital that has military people there; there are several around the country. The upside is that you don't have to go through the Foundation application process and the rotations are generally pretty good.

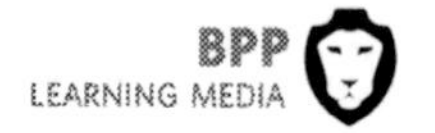

Once you have graduated you are committed for a certain number of years working for the forces. Be aware of current operations that you are likely to be involved in one way or another once you are fully qualified. That will be many years down the road from now, but may inspire you or put you off. If it puts you off then it may be worth staying away but if you are inspired then the sky's the limit!'

Chapter 2

Life at medical school

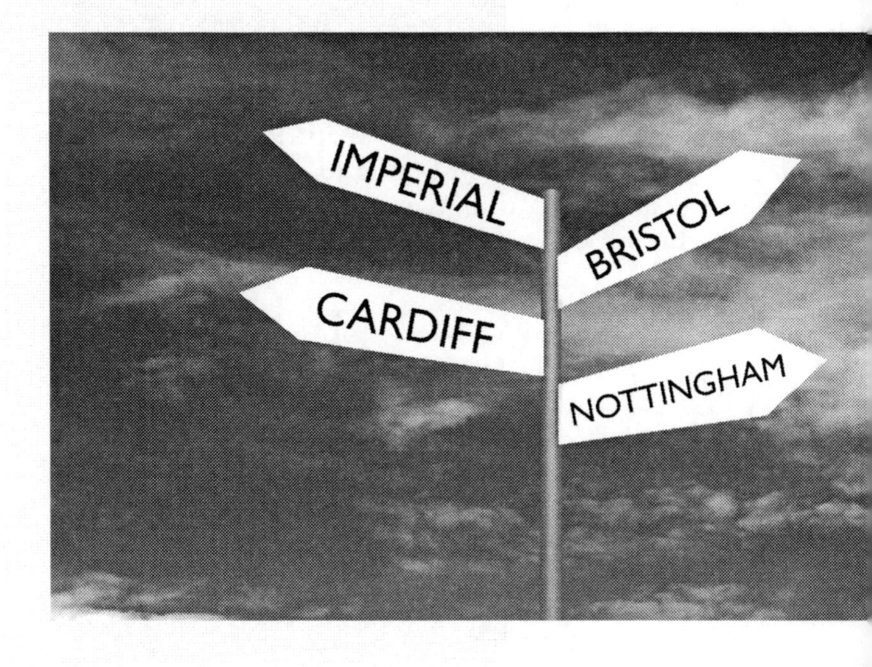

Life at medical school

What to expect

> *'They do certainly give very strange, and newfangled, names to diseases.'*
>
> (Plato)

No matter who you are or what you have done prior to commencing your medical degree walking into the lecture theatre on the first day will be one of the scariest experiences of your university life. It is, however, also one of the best as all the work that you have put in during school and A levels will have come to fruition and you will be on your way to becoming a doctor. It is important to remember that everyone is feeling the same as you, and the atmosphere in the lecture hall will have a very different buzz to normal, due to everyone's excitement and expectations.

Your first day

The best thing to do is to find a seat and start chatting. It would be a good idea to get there a little early so that you get a chance to speak to the person you choose to sit next to for a bit before the lecture starts. And remember to keep a look out for your future wife/husband, as they are probably sitting somewhere in that room!

Meeting new people is what students tend to worry about most when they first arrive at university. Everyone is looking to make new friends and the best thing to do is to get involved in all the actives going on during your freshers' week, and other activities that run throughout the first term.

Lectures

Lectures normally last between 45 minutes and an hour. There will tend to be a lot of information covered during each lecture and you will usually be provided with a handout with all the basic information, which you can then annotate. Coloured pens can help to make good notes. It is also useful to copy up these notes into a neat form to help you with revision. Handouts also

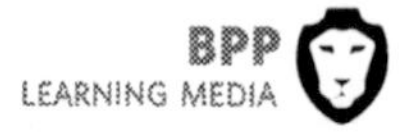

tend to be available on the Internet, should you wish to look over them again.

Self-directed learning

Studying at university is a stark contrast to school. Learning is much more self-directed and it is important to put aside enough time to read around topics and to prepare in advance for tutorials and group teaching. You will need to read through the lecture material as you are taught it to make sure you understand it all. Most medical schools also use online tutorials and questions to help test your understanding of the material you have been taught. Buying or loaning books to help you with topics is also a good idea. The medical school will normally provide you with a reading list prior to commencing the course but if they do not there are a few popular suggestions listed at the end of this book.

Using libraries

Each medical school will have a library especially for medical students. A library induction session will normally take place in the first few weeks so that you are familiar with how to search for and take out books from the library. You will also learn how to use online databases to search for articles in medical journals. This is one of the most important things you will learn in your first term at university, as finding and utilising appropriate journal articles will prove vital for study projects and future research.

University libraries are also vital when it comes to revising for examinations. They offer a quiet retreat away from the distractions of your halls of residence and noisy flatmates. Indeed it is important to factor in enough time to revise as lecture notes tend to pile up during term time.

Sports and social activities

Thankfully medical school is not just about libraries and revision. There will be a medical society at your medical school and you must join! Not only do you then get a chance to be involved in sports teams but this is also a great chance to meet more senior medical students who can advise you on textbooks, housing and nights out.

Medical career structure

> *'The doctor of the future will give no medicine but will interest his patients in the care of the human frame, in diet and in the cause and prevention of disease.'*
>
> (Thomas Edison)

Although it may seem like a long way off, in your final year of medical school you will be asked to apply for your first job as a doctor.

Foundation years (FY1–2)

The first year after graduating is spent as a Foundation year one (F1) doctor. This was originally known as the junior house officer from the days when doctors were required to live in the hospital. F1 doctors have provisional registration with the General Medical Council and must complete the first year, meeting a set criteria before achieving full registration as a Foundation year two (F2) doctor. F1 posts usually comprise four months' surgery, four months' Medicine and four months' in another specialty. During this year the Foundation doctor will spend their time on the wards performing ward jobs such as taking blood, delivering imaging requests and updating inpatient lists.

The application process for F1 doctors consists of a written component and interviews in a similar style to medical school applications. Applicants are scored on a set criteria with the highest scoring applicants getting first pick of the jobs.

Specialty training (CT/ST 1–2 + 3–6)

During medical school and F1/2 years it is hoped that you will have developed an interest in a particular field of Medicine such as surgery, medicine, anaesthetics or general practice. In January of the F2 year applications are opened for specialist jobs.

Specialist training position selection is very competitive. Postgraduate exams can be taken during F1 or F2. These might include the first parts of the Membership of Royal College of Physicians or Surgeons (MRCP/MRCS).

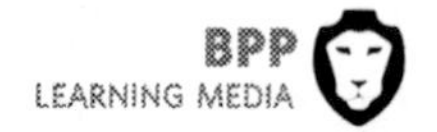

Once selected on to a training programme expect to spend at least seven further years in training before achieving a certificate of completion of training and a consultant post.

Consultant post

Following completion of specialist training and exit examinations you will apply for a consultant post in your chosen specialty.

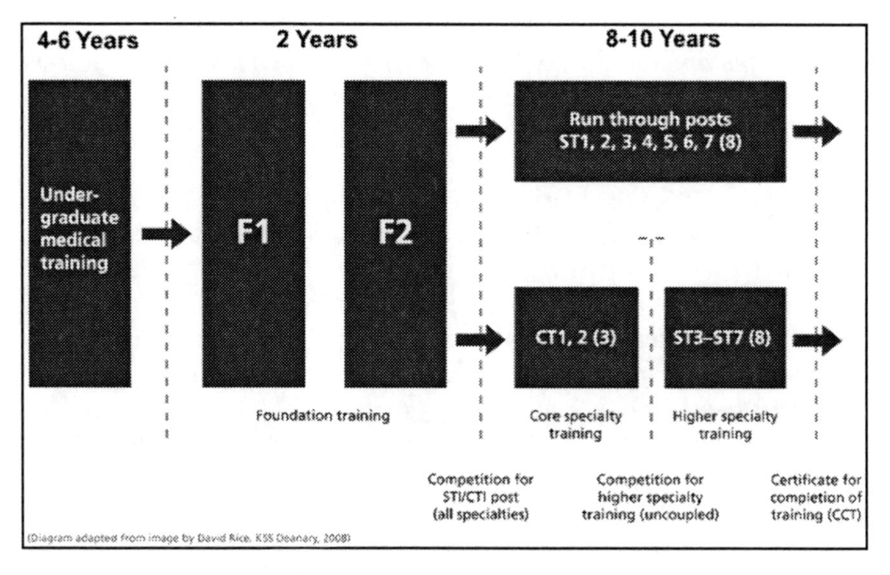

Figure 2.1 Overview of medical career structure (diagram adapted from image by David Rice, KSS Deanery, 2008)

An example day

Example pre-clinical timetable

	Monday	Tuesday	Wednesday	Thursday	Friday
Morning	Anatomy	Lectures	Seminars/ tutorials	Lectures	Lectures
	Lunch	*Lunch*	*Lunch*	*Lunch*	*Lunch*
Afternoon	Lectures	GP clinical attachment	FREE for sport	Practical	SSC

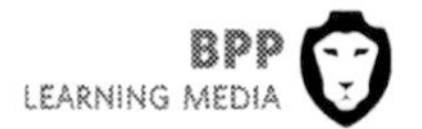

A day in the life of a pre-clinical student

'A pre-clinical day will normally start off with you feeling hungover!

Once you manage to get showered and have your breakfast you will walk to the lecture theatre for a 9.00am start. Lectures last around 50 minutes and there will be between two and four lectures in the morning. There is normally a break for lunch between 1.00–2.00pm and then you will return for more teaching. The days that drag on have another three lectures in the afternoon. The more interesting days have a couple of hours of anatomy or a practical workshop in the afternoon followed by sport or socialising in the evening or maybe with an hour's work if you are so inclined.

The lecture material can be quite scientific and seem not too relevant to Medicine, especially in the first year. The second year material becomes much more medically based, and as you get your first real taste of clinical medicine the lecture material becomes far more relevant. Pre-clinical medicine, in particular the first year, is not as fun as the clinical years in terms of teaching. However you must remember that the first year should be spent enjoying university life, and making sure you get the work: play balance. You do not need to spend three hours a night doing more work. You should do any "homework" that is set and make sure you keep on top of the work, but this will only require a few hours a week outside of the "classroom".'

Example clinical timetable

	Monday	Tuesday	Wednesday	Thursday	Friday
Morning	Ward round	Tutorials	Clinical skills	Ward work	Clinic and tutorials
	Lunch	*Lunch*	*Lunch*	*Lunch*	*Lunch*
Afternoon	Clinic	Theatre	Clinic	GP attachment	Ward work

A day in the life of a clinical student

'By the time you are a clinical student, you will have to take things more seriously. There is no waking up hung-over on week days, but fortunately what you get to do during the day has you far more enthused to attend teaching.

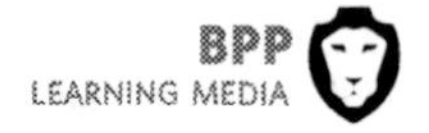

You get to the hospital for 8.30am to go on the morning ward round, or go to the trauma meeting. (A meeting for the Orthopaedic surgeons discussing how to deal with the trauma cases that came overnight.) Once the ward round is over you can go and take a history from and/or examine some of the interesting patient cases that you saw on the ward round. Then you may have a small (three to six people) group tutorial for an hour before lunch. Lunch is not quite in the timetable as in the pre-clinical years. Often you may have teaching, clinics or theatre to get to for 1.30pm.

In the afternoon you may choose to go to theatre, go talk to some more patients or go to a clinic. Hopefully what has come across is that you have much more autonomy during a clinical day than a pre-clinical day. There is some timetabled teaching but it is up to you which clinic to attend or when to go to theatre. You therefore can go into much more detail in areas that you have a real passion for. Try not to slip into the trap of never going to clinics in specialties you do not care for as they will still come up in exams!'

Clinical placements

During the clinical years of your medical school training you will be taught in hospitals. You will be placed in both large teaching hospitals and in District General Hospitals (DGHs).

Accommodation

When at a local hospital you will live in your student house, but you will be provided with accommodation when your placement is further afield. The accommodation varies quite significantly but if you expect to be back in a halls of residence standard of accommodation you will not be disappointed. If you like to keep fit some of the hospitals have gyms for the students, but if not, you can often use the physiotherapists' gym in the hospital or nearby facilities.

Being in hospital

When you go to your first clinical placement it can be quite a daunting experience. You are out of the comfort of lecture theatres and into the big world of hospitals where you may feel like a small fish in a big pond. You have to remember that all your fellow students are in the same situation and that quite quickly things will become more familiar.

Not only are you in this foreign world of hospitals, but also you may not be with your best friends from medical school. You are randomly allocated into groups and so again, like halls, find yourself living with people you barely know. However for most this is very rewarding as you get to know more of your fellow students. Serendipity may work its magic and you could find a new boyfriend/girlfriend who you never knew simply because you used to sit at different sides of the lecture theatre.

Learning during clinical placements

Clinical attachments are the way you learn clinical medicine so you need to embrace them, and if you do you will get much more out of the experience. If you look at it positively it is a chance to meet new people and make more friends.

You will find that the hospital staff have more time for you in the DGHs, furthermore they all want to be the best teaching DGH so that competition drives them forwards. The big hospitals tend to have more varied patients and specialist units, however the staff often have less time to teach you. Both have their pros and cons, and you will be placed in both during your clinical training so get the opportunity to experience the best of both worlds.

When you get to the hospitals the style of learning is different from the lecture-based teaching in the pre-clinical years. You have to be much more self-directed. There are still small group teaching sessions, but the onus is put onto you to get the experience. The old cliché of what you put in you get out applies strongly to academy learning. It is very easy to get left behind as the doctors and nurses get on with their busy lives, however if you are enthusiastic they will reciprocate and teach you enthusiastically. All of a sudden you will be taking arterial blood gases, suturing in theatre and getting that buzz that you are a doctor in training! Make sure you ask though, or else you will only get to hear about these stories, rather than featuring in one.

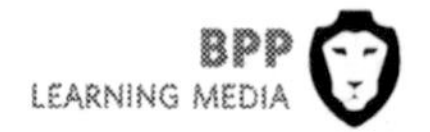

Students on the ward

Essential equipment

Before you begin life on the wards it is useful to buy a quick reference guide such as the *Oxford Handbook of Clinical Medicine*.

The only other essential item is a stethoscope. A Littmann classic is more than adequate but if you want to hear those more subtle murmurs then there are more expensive stethoscopes, though a standard stethoscope will be adequate for most students.

Other equipment that probably should be bought is a tendon hammer and a pen torch. There is no requirement to purchase a sphygmanometer (blood pressure cuff), opthalmoscope or otoscope.

Ward rounds

A ward round is when the doctor and his team (junior doctors, nurses, physiotherapists, medical students) go around the ward reviewing the patients under his/her care. They can last between half an hour and four hours, and happen in the morning and afternoon.

As a medical student ward rounds can sometimes be overwhelming. A lot of information can go above your head, and sometimes you can feel you are more of a hindrance. However it is a good opportunity to see/hear a lot of different pathologies in patients in a short period of time.

Make sure you go on at least one ward round in each speciality to meet the team, and the patients on the ward.

Remember, every time you go onto the ward wash your hands and introduce yourself to the nursing staff so they know who you are.

Clinic

Clinics take place either in the morning or the afternoon and are when the doctor sees outpatients under his/her care. The doctors are more than happy to have you to sit in the clinic with them. As you will find out when you get into clinical medicine time constraints can often make teaching difficult. Sometimes clinics are so busy that the doctor will not be able to take too much time to explain what is going on. Do not be afraid to ask questions though. Most of the time the doctors love explaining what is going on and getting you involved.

If you are lucky the doctor will let you run the clinic under his supervision and you get to feel like you are doctor. Walking out into the waiting room and calling in Mr/Mrs Bloggs to the consultation room gives you a massive thrill.

Clinics, like ward rounds, are a good way to see lots of different patients in a relatively short period of time and can be more useful than ward rounds.

Theatre

Theatre is the place most medical students cannot wait to get in to. As a medical student theatres can be a variable experience. If you are enthusiastic and hang around long enough you may get the opportunity to suture, or even do some minor surgery. However the reality can often be less exciting. If there is a Consultant, Registrar and several theatre nurses around the patient, your view of what is going on can be severely reduced and you can feel like you have spent two hours of your morning learning very little.

Intercalating

What is 'intercalation'?

Intercalation is an option available to many medical students and requires a year out from medicine to study for and attain a degree in another subject. This is usually a BSc (Bachelor of Science) or BA (Bachelor of Arts) degree and can be taken in a large variety of different subjects, some of which are directly relevant to Medicine and some of which are less so. The idea of intercalation is to broaden your knowledge in a specific subject area, gain new experiences that will further your learning and gain a qualification that will enhance your CV.

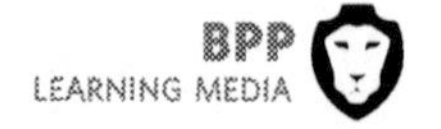

When you're applying to medical school, the decision of whether or not you want to intercalate may seem quite far off. A few people may know from the outset whether they want to intercalate or not, but most people make the choice as they go along. There are many options available to medical students who are considering intercalating – including which subject to study, at which university, and even when the intercalated year will take place.

Advantages of intercalation

Many students relish the challenge that intercalation presents. It is an opportunity to study a subject that interests you – be it Physiology or Ethics – in great depth and gain a broad range of skills that will be transferable to your medical studies and subsequent career. Specific advantages of intercalating include:

- A degree qualification that will be recognised in your future career and will contribute to your application to be an F1/F2 doctor, as well as applications for more senior posts later on
- A chance to study a particular subject area in detail
- The opportunity to gain laboratory-based research experience if desired
- Development of your personal and professional skills such as communication skills, presenting your ideas to an audience and searching for relevant literature
- A year out of medicine in which to do something a little bit different
- If you are thinking of an academic career, intercalation is a good step in the right direction
- Depending upon the projects undertaken during your intercalated year, you may be fortunate enough to get a publication or present your work at a conference
- You may find that a year studying something different reignites the excitement you feel about medicine and the skills you acquire may prepare you better for the remainder of the course

Disadvantages of intercalation

Intercalation is not an easy option and is not suitable for everyone. Possible downsides to intercalation are:

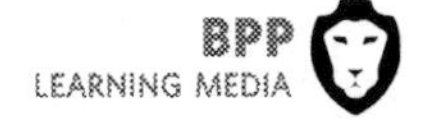

- It adds another year to a course that is already five years long – some people just want to get on with it!
- The financial implications of being at university for another year need to be considered
- Many students find the year a difficult one – although the majority of people find their subject interesting as they have chosen it, the workload is often high. Depending upon where you study medicine and where you intercalate, there may be more deadlines, more essays and perhaps a dissertation, so careful time management is crucial
- At some medical schools the option to intercalate is not open to everyone as places are limited – therefore acceptance to a programme can be competitive and examination grades in the first few years may be taken into consideration, as well as application forms
- Having a year out may make you anxious about recommencing Medicine

Where can I intercalate?

Most medical schools offer the option to intercalate in various different subjects. At some medical schools, intercalation is incorporated into a six-year medicine programme and therefore all students must intercalate. At other universities only a small proportion of the year group intercalates and students either join a specific intercalation programme for medical students or join the third year of a BSc or BA course. There is also the possibility of undertaking intercalation at a medical school other than your own if the course you want to do is not offered at your current school.

What subject can I study?

The subjects open to you to study very much depends upon the medical school. Some common science intercalation subjects are: Physiological Sciences, Pharmacology, Neuroscience, Medical Sciences and Anatomy. Many students decide that they want a break from science and opt for a course such as Ethics or Sociology. There is a possibility to attend a different medical school to carry out your intercalated degree if another medical school is offering a subject you would particularly like to study.

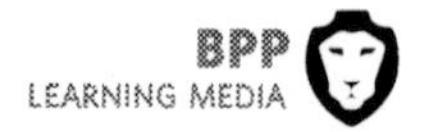

When can I intercalate?

Again this varies from medical school to medical school. It is common at some medical schools to intercalate between the second and third year – in between the pre-clinical and clinical years. Many students think this makes sense as it seems like a natural break. Other students would prefer to intercalate between third and fourth year or even fourth and fifth year, and different medical schools have different policies on this.

Student's opinion

'I intercalated in Physiological Sciences at the University of Bristol between my second and third years of Medicine. I chose to intercalate for a number of reasons – I wanted to be able to explore a subject in depth and felt that intercalation would enable me to do this while also achieving a BSc degree which I believed would be beneficial to me in my future career. At my medical school most people intercalate between the second and third year and so I followed this plan. At Bristol I joined the final year Physiology students. It was rather strange joining a different degree programme at first, and early on I felt rather out of my depth at times. The workload was very different to Medicine – we had a lot more essays and assessed work. Personally, I believe I gained a great deal from intercalating and am pleased to have a BSc under my belt!

My favourite part of the year was undertaking my research project which I found very interesting and it was fascinating to experience working in a lab and see what goes on in Medicine behind the scenes. I felt a great sense of achievement on completing my dissertation and the skills I gained during it will prove very useful later on. I now feel very confident presenting my work – a skill I honed when studying Physiology and which is integral to practising Medicine. Presenting at a national conference was something I would not have had the opportunity to do if I had not intercalated. On the downside, intercalation was by no means a 'year off' and was very hard work. I had a lot of deadlines and work to do, but in my case I would say that the challenge was worth it.

It is important to remember that intercalation is not for everybody. Most of my friends who also intercalated feel better prepared for the third year and clinical school and are very glad they intercalated, but a lot of my friends who didn't intercalate know that they would have hated it and are glad they didn't! It's a personal choice.

Although intercalation is something to consider now, as it is important to keep your options open, the decision to intercalate does not need to be made until you are at medical school and you have a better understanding of what the process involves. As explained there are advantages and disadvantages to carrying out an intercalated degree, which must be weighed up by the individual. The possibility of intercalation is just one aspect to consider when choosing a medical school; the teaching style and opportunities available also vary greatly from place to place and therefore it is important that you choose carefully which medical school would suit you best.'

Finances

> *'My doctor gave me six months to live, but when I couldn't pay the bill he gave me six months more.'*
>
> (Dick Wilson)

Paying for a five-year course can be extremely demanding on both individuals and families. Tuition fees are on the rise with students who start university after 1 September 2012 paying up to £9,000 in tuition fees. Factor in costs for living and accommodation and it is easy to see why some individuals may be put off from higher education.

There are a number of financial support options available to help fund students through medical school.

Student loan

The first is a student loan. A loan covers tuition fees and can be paid back once the student is earning more than £21,000. In practical terms this means that a portion of your monthly salary, once you qualify, will go towards repaying the loan each month.

A maintenance grant is income-assessed meaning that students from households with lower annual incomes are eligible for larger, non-repayable grants. This can equate to around £5,500 per year for students from lower income households.

Student loans are distributed through the Student Loans Company together with your local education authority. In order to make sure your loan reaches your account in time for the start of each

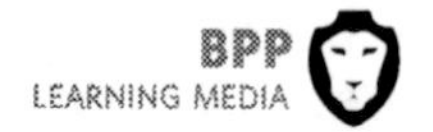

semester be sure to complete and return the required forms as early as possible.

Bursaries

Scholarships and bursaries from individual universities are often offered to students from lower income households or to students showing particular sporting or academic prowess. It is worth checking the university finance homepage to see whether you qualify for any bursaries.

Prizes

Throughout each year student bodies, medical societies and organisations run various essay and presentation prizes. These prizes not only look excellent on your CV but also often come with cash prizes ranging from £250-£1,000. A list of medical societies can be found in the appendix of this book.

Travel expenses

Travel expenses between hospital placements and accommodation can often be reclaimed from the university or through the hospital trust. It is worth spending some time researching whether you are entitled to reclaim travel expenses before deciding to commute to work.

Travel abroad and, in particular, medical electives are another potential financial drain. Various organisations offer elective bursaries and these, again, look excellent on your CV.

Travel

There are many opportunities to travel abroad in Medicine, from a couple of weeks to a few months.

The elective

The most commonly known opportunity to travel abroad is the elective. This is normally an eight-week period either at the beginning or end of the fifth year where you study Medicine outside of where you have been training. There is no obligation to leave the UK, but most medical students these days relish the opportunity to go and explore a completely different country. The possible destinations are almost limitless. You will not be allowed to go to countries that the Foreign and Commonwealth Office deems too dangerous to travel too, or that the WHO has declared is at risk for SARS. You may need to explain your decision if going to an area that has very high levels of HIV / Aids. This aside, as long as there is a hospital, and they will take you, you can go anywhere. Common destinations range from first world countries like Australia and USA to third world countries in Africa and Asia.

The idea of the elective is to study Medicine in a different culture; however it is also an amazing opportunity to travel to your favourite destinations. When speaking to many people who have done their elective, the advice is to go to a destination you want to travel to. Often the elective is at either end of the summer holiday and thus it is not unknown to be away for three months.

There are pros and cons regarding electives in the west and in developing countries. The big advantage of western electives is that the practice you will see will be similar to the NHS. The surgical techniques, drugs used and diseases presenting will be more familiar. Therefore it gives you more experience with the type of Medicine you will practise in your career. Second, if you want to see the world's leading treatments for cancer or surgery you will have to go to modern, industrialised countries. One big disadvantage is that it will make your elective far more expensive. The best aspect about doing an elective in the developing world is the complete contrast that you will see. In one afternoon there will be a clinic with 200 patients. (Compared to a 'busy' NHS clinic with 15–20 patients).

The type of diseases that present will be very different, and anecdotally one gets far more hands on experience doing electives in developing countries. There are stories of the doctors going on holiday and leaving the medical student in charge of the ward. Obviously it will be much cheaper. Travel guides say you can live on £10 / day in India compared with £35 / day in Australia. Certainly an elective in a developing nation will make for wonderful dinner party stories, but may not be of much relevance to your future career.

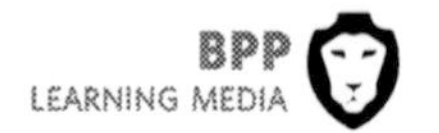

Student Selected Components/Modules

Throughout medical school you will have to carry out SSCs/SSM. An SSC is a Student Selected Component/Module where you have the autonomy to choose a certain amount of what you study each year. This is a big part of what makes up the GMC's *Tomorrow's Doctors*. As long as you have the self-motivation to sort something out yourself and can justify it to the medical school, there is opportunity to travel in some of the SSCs. For example a medical student from Bristol went to New York in their third year SSC to look at robotic surgery.

Erasmus

Some medical schools offer the Erasmus scheme. This is where you go to study Medicine in another (commonly) European country. Often it will be in the third year when you are starting clinical medicine. It is an exchange-like system. Therefore the places you can go to depend on which cities/universities your medical school has contacts with. France, Spain and Germany are common destinations for Erasmus. Speaking the language of the country you go to is a help, however you do not need an A level in the language to go. You are away for half of the teaching year usually, so about four months. The feedback from students who go on Erasmus is very positive. Your knowledge of the medical topics covered when out there may suffer for various reasons; however most students love the opportunity to live in another country for a sustained period of time. Imagine being in Grenoble and going skiing after lectures.

Holidays

Finally one must remember that the first two years of medical school run on the same term times as other students. Therefore the summer holidays after the first and second year will be a good three months and allow plenty of time to do some travelling with your friends.

Beyond medical school

After you have graduated from medical school, if the travelling bug is still itching at you, there are opportunities to travel. Many

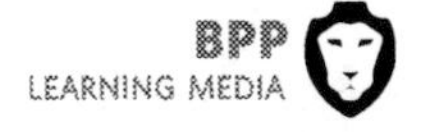

doctors choose to do their F2 year abroad in Australia and have an amazing time. Others go into 'Medicins Sans Frontieres', and provide emergency aid to people affected by armed conflict, epidemics, healthcare exclusion and natural disasters. Often it will be that person's elective in a developing country that made them realise 'Medicins Sans Frontieres' was for them.

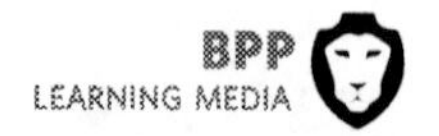

Chapter 3–34

The guide to UK medical schools

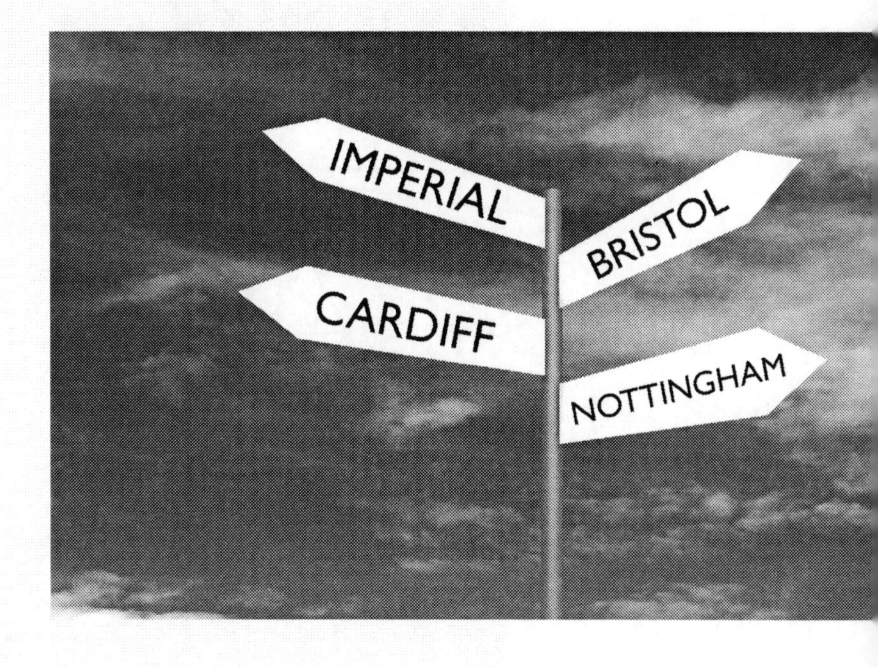

Chapters 3–34 The guide to UK medical schools

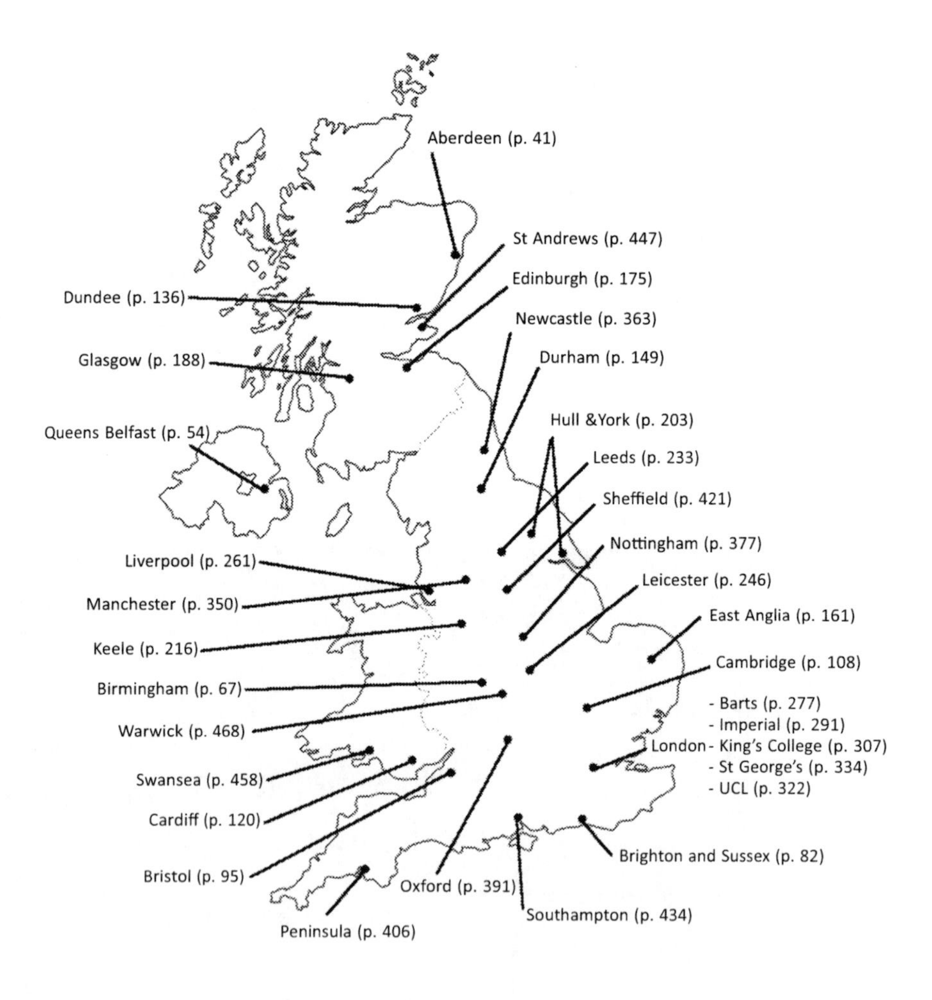

Aberdeen

Aberdeen School of Medicine and Dentistry
3rd Floor
Polwarth Building
Foresterhill
Aberdeen
AB25 2ZD

www.abdn.ac.uk/medicine-dentistry

Aberdeen is a buzzing city, rich with thick accents from all across the globe. It provides a taste of city life as well as offering beautiful beaches and hills to the west, a bike ride away. The University of Aberdeen was founded in 1495 by William Elphinstone, making it the UK's fifth oldest university. It is a small but beautifully preserved university, with a student population of approximately 11,000.

The medical school is over 500 years old and is situated in the compact Foresterhill campus, one of the largest medical campuses in Europe, allowing students to cross from one corner to another in 10 minutes. A revised medical curriculum has recently commenced in the new Suttie Centre, a purpose-built teaching centre for healthcare professionals that provides an environment for achieving clinical excellence in a building hoped to inspire the minds of those who use it.

The medical course

Key facts

Course Type	Traditional	Degree Awarded	MBChB
Basic Entry Requirements	AAA	Entrance Exams	UKCAT
Year Size	175	Open Days	Late Aug/Sept
Admissions Website	www.abdn.ac.uk/medicine/prospective/admissions/requirements/		

Getting in – student tips

The beauty of Aberdeen is their intention of finding students who truly want to create a vocation in Medicine. Demonstrating that you are keen to do this is key to getting through the application process. Evidence of enthusiasm, drive, determination, creativity and team working will help you in this process. Reflect on your experiences and use them to illustrate what makes you tick and why you could be a good doctor. 25% of entry weighting is on your grades, the rest is UKCAT and you.

No student will be offered a place without an interview. There will be a minimum of two interviewers on the panel who may be medical school staff or doctors from primary or secondary care. Each interview will last approximately 20 minutes.

Course details

Foundation/ Pre-Med	No	Graduate	No
Student Population	Male: female ratio: 40:60	Term Length	Pre-clinical: 12 weeks Clinical: variable
Erasmus/ Foreign Exchange	N/A	Elective Period	Year 5 – 8 weeks

Intercalation

Stage	Between year 3 and 4 or year 4 and 5	Degree Awarded	BScMedSci (Hons)
Requirements	40 places available, depends on academic achievements	Subjects	Medical Sciences

Anatomy teaching

Anatomy is taught over years 1–3 with relevance to the system being studied. Cadaveric prosections prepared by trained anatomy demonstrators are the mainstay of the teaching along with dry sessions focussing on histology and embryology and focused radiology tutorials. The Suttie Centre offers new state of the art 3D anatomy software, based upon CT / MRI projections, to supplement anatomy teaching. For students keen to do their own dissection there is the option to undertake this as part of medical humanities.

Pre-clinical/Years 1–2	
Topics	***Year 1:*** Foundations of medical science and disease (basic anatomy, physiology, biochemistry and pathology). Respiratory and cardiovascular systems along with the corresponding anatomy and clinical skills teaching. The Community Course accommodating General Practice, Public Health, Occupational and Environmental medicine, Medicine for the elderly and Paediatrics runs concurrently throughout years 1–3. ***Year 2:*** Alimentary, Urinary, Nervous and Musculoskeletal systems, Diabetes/Endocrine, ENT/Max-fax and Dermatology, anatomy and clinical skills. Community Course.
Teaching	The teaching comprises mainly lectures and small group tutorials. Students will be divided into groups for anatomy and clinical skills sessions, case based tutorials and the community course sessions.
SSC periods	There is an SSC period in each of the three pre-clinical years as well as the Medical Humanities module. The first year SSC takes place after the Easter break and introduces group work and research skills. The second year SSC is entitled molecular mechanisms in disease and aims to build on these skills.
Exams	Short answer questions and Extended Matching Questions. Examinations in the first and second year take place in January and June. Anatomy and clinical skills assessment occurs throughout the years 1–3 in conjunction with the appropriate system.

Clinical/Years 3–5	
Topics	***Year 3:*** Lecture based teaching in O+G, Breast, Psychiatry, Paediatrics, Dermatology, Haematology, ENT, Anaesthetics, Forensics, Genetics, Infection. Weekly GP attachment and hospital-based teaching. ***Year 4:*** Weekly rotations in single specialties, split up into blocks of five weeks eg one week Breast, one week gynae clinics, one week gynae surgery, one week labour wards and theatre, one paediatrics. ***Year 5:*** Four eight-week rotations, one surgery, one medicine, one elective and one GP/Mental Health block. At the end of the year there is a six-week professional practice block, which takes you through GMC registration, guidelines, regulations and paperwork such as filling in death certificates.
SSC periods	***Year 3:*** Medical Humanities block ***Year 4:*** Epidemiological-based project
Exams	***Year 3:*** March, these are not too difficult if you work continually through the year. ***Year 4:*** Mock finals in December and finals late June. This is very daunting but only ~10 students fail. Four exams, two Modified Essay Question (MEQs) papers, one Extended Matching Question (EMQ) paper and one Multiple Choice Question (MCQs) paper. There is one day of clinical assessment, OSCE. ***Year 5:*** Two days of clinical exams (OSCEs) at the end of the year. (The theory exams are therefore only in fourth year.)

Hospital placements/academies

In the fourth year you can apply to do Remote and Rural (R+R), which will see you staying in Inverness for the whole year at Raigmore Hospital. This option was created to allow students to learn about providing Medicine to a small population scattered over a large distance and the students will have time to visit the western isles, Fort William's Belford Hospital and Wick and Thurso and the Orkney and Shetland islands. Everyone in the fourth year must do at least five weeks at Raigmore. You are allocated a room in a flat, which has been recently renovated and is comfortable to live in. The best part of this is you share with other healthcare professionals, not only students but also working professionals and this always provides essential work hard, play hard banter. There are 18 R+R students and ~36 other fourth years up at Inverness at any one time. The five-week GP block can see you staying anywhere within Aberdeen or Inverness and in the surrounding areas, the furthest placement being in Gairloch! You are provided with B+B or hotel accommodation.

The fifth year allows you to continue the experience of learning Medicine away from Aberdeen and Inverness in places such as Elgin, Stornoway in Skye, Orkney, Shetland and Fort William. You are always provided with accommodation. It is important to know that as an Aberdeen medical student you will be travelling a lot and although you are reimbursed for essential travel trips you will find you will end up paying for some travelling.

Hospitals and Travel Time from University	
Royal Cornhill Hospital	5 minutes
Foresterhill	7 minutes
Woodend	15 minutes

 *The medical school*

Work	●	●	●			Good work life balance
Facilities	●	●	●	●		Three-storey medical library, located on the Foresterhill site with easy access for all students
Support	●	●	●	●		The medical secretaries are like surrogate mothers. Clinical tutors are ready and willing to give extra tuition
Feedback	●	●	●			Year ranking after exams

Facilities

Polwarth building holds two lecture theatres, the medical library, IT suites and the Ref, a comfortable place to eat tasty food and meet folk. The new clinical skills centre has three floors dedicated to teaching students, the anatomy department, and clinical suites with simulation areas including SimMan and the first UK SimBaby. It is the perfect environment to get to grips with difficult clinical scenarios before you have to deal with them on the wards. Inverness boasts a new clinical skills centre as well providing excellent facilities for teaching.

Student support

Aberdeen is fantastic because it has the means to teach and care for a relatively small class size. Attendance both good and bad does not go unnoticed and you will find wherever you go there will be somebody willing to help you. During the course of the degree you will meet Margaret Moir, Jill Davey, Morag Simpson, Fiona Petrie and Penny Linneman (Student Support Officer), who are all at hand if ever you get confused.

At the beginning of the degree you are assigned a regent who will support you throughout your entire degree. Each regent has a medical background so they have an appreciation of what Medicine expects from you. TIP: If you're nice to them they may take you out for dinner!

The adoption party takes place in the first semester where first years are allocated two second year parents and a brother or sister. The success of the family depends on those in it! (They are often a great resource for past papers.)

Medical societies

MedSoc (Aberdeen Medical Society) is run by the fourth years and always creates amazing activities including beerinteerin. Everyone gets involved with MedSoc as it organises the famous not-to-be-missed MedSoc Ball, The Review and lots more.

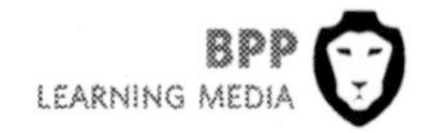

Highlights include:

- SNIMS – Scottish and Northern Ireland Medical Sports weekend in association with MedSoc.
- The Ogston Society – for those interested in pursuing a surgical career, gives extra tuition.
- Movies and Medicine – Watching films with your friends along with a slice or two of pizza and throw in someone knowledgeable to discuss the topics addressed in the film.

Finance

Further info: www.abdn.ac.uk/undergraduate/finance
See scholarships: www.abdn.ac.uk/undergraduate/scholarships
There are hardship funds available: www.abdn.ac.uk/students/financial-services.php

Student opinion

'Aberdeen is brilliant because it is small enough to get to know students, staff, nurses, doctors and the patients and you really feel a sense of community when you wander through the hospital. You are taught by some of the best doctors in the country who treat you with respect (most of the time!). The school caters for everyone and if there is something you're not happy with be sure to know they will ask you to evaluate it. Having the opportunity to work out of Aberdeen allows you to discover what much of Grampian and the Highlands have to offer. From first hand experience I can confidently say if you have any problems, whether they are professional, personal or financial, the university will support you and there will always be someone in whom to confide.'

The university

Accommodation	Hillhead Halls and Crombie/Johnston halls of residence
Further info	www.abdn.ac.uk/accommodation/living-in-halls/

Accommodation

Hillhead, the largest site of the halls, is a 15-minute walk from the university campus and a 40-minute walk from the medical school. Crombie/Johnston is 30 minutes from the medical school but sits on the university campus. All the halls offer an array of accommodation, single rooms, en-suite, 4-7 bedrooms arranged in flats, self-catering and catered. Hector Boece is renowned for mischief and mayhem and is nicknamed The Ghetto, Crombie/Johnston is considered 'posh' by Hillhead students and Elphinstone is reserved for the mature undergraduate or postgraduate students.

Most students would suggest staying in halls as you meet lots of people. As a medic, it allows you to meet non-medics as soon as you arrive.

Study facilities

The Queen Mother Library (QML) is the main university library at the centre of King's college campus. It is on six floors and covers Social Sciences, Science and Engineering, Arts, Humanities and Divinity, and other services such as reprographics. There is also the Taylor (Law) library. Medical students predominantly use these libraries during SSC periods. There are 50 computers at QML; however the Edward Wright building acts as the main computer classroom containing 270 computers. There is WiFi internet throughout libraries, teaching areas and university accommodation.

University sports and students' union

In partnership with Aberdeen City Council and Sport Scotland, AUSA (Aberdeen University Student Association) Sport opened the Aberdeen Sports Village. This new building includes a fully equipped gym, sports hall, full size FIFA approved indoor football pitch, athletics stadium etc. King's pavilion and playing fields are located at the centre of the King's College campus and there are also grass and synthetic pitches at Hillhead.

The AUSA (Aberdeen University Student Association) is housed in The Hub. It contains a food hall, a café, 16 computers plus WiFi internet and several quiet rooms. With regard to nights out, the students take over night clubs The Shack and Capitol, and Liquid,

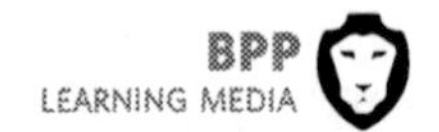

throughout the week as well as lots of other venues throughout the city.

Student opinion

'I would suggest living near the university campus while you begin your degree because whatever degree you are studying your experience of student life is shaped by the environment and the people you meet. Life as a medical student can often segregate you from the student population anyway as the medical school is sited 30 minutes away. Take up all the opportunities on offer and don't worry about making a fool of yourself, it's what we do.'

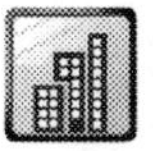

The city

Safety						Aberdeen is one of the safer cities in Scotland
Nightlife						Union street and its side-streets and Belmont Street for clubs bars and pubs
Transport						Parking is limited at Foresterhill though plentiful in the city, bus service will suffice in years 1-3, car may be needed in year 4
Cost of Living						Rent in private flats cost around £300 per month, a taxi to Belmont street £7

Things to do

The granite city boasts a number of stunning buildings and attractions. Marischal college, owned by Aberdeen University currently housing Marischal Museum, is the second largest granite building in the world, and was also claimed to be Adolf Hitler's favourite building in the UK.

Union Square is the best place to shop and also boasts the biggest cinema complex in Aberdeen. Union Street has a wide range of shops, restaurants, bars and clubs as well as the Aberdeen music

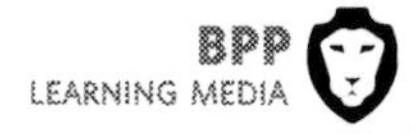

hall. Aberdeen Exhibition and Concert Centre (AECC) acts as the main venue for headline acts and His Majesty's Theatre has a busy and impressive programme. For any football fans Aberdeen FC play their home matches in the SPL and the occasional European adventure at Pittodrie.

Places to go		
Place	**Brief Description**	**Entry Fee/Opening Time**
Liquid	Popular club off Bridge Street	£4; Mon, Wed-Sun 10.00pm-3.00am
Tiger Tiger	Club on Shiprow, bottom end of Union Street	£5; Mon & Sat 10.00pm-3.00am
Snafu Tunnels	Electro bar/club located on Union Street Cool underground club with live music	£3; Mon-Sat 10.00pm-3.00am £4; Wed-Sun 8.00pm-3.00am
The Bobbin	Student pub with live sport on King Street	£Free; all week 11.00am-12.00pm

Student opinion

'Everything is going on in Aberdeen, whether you're into clubbing, sport, shopping, live music, culture or taking it easy in beautiful surroundings, Aberdeen is the city for you.'

Student's view

Pre-clinical

'I chose to do medicine at Aberdeen as I liked the sound of the traditional lecture style course and how all the teaching took place on the Foresterhill campus as well as Aberdeen's reputation as an excellent university in a busy student city. The pre-clinical years at Aberdeen for me were about striking the right balance between work and everything else the medical school and university has to offer. I feel like I achieved this with doing the necessary amount of work at less busy times of my week and making the most of the time available for sport and the odd night out.

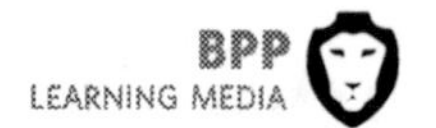

A typical day meant getting to the medical school for the 9.00am lecture, usually by bus or on foot. In advance of morning lectures printing off the lecture notes from the online Medical Resource Centre allowed me to note down anything else mentioned in the lecture that, as it turned out, often turned up in exams. Lunch is available at the Ref on the second floor of the Polwarth building, which was always bustling with students, as well as the reasonably priced Phase II canteen in the hospital and a café on the ground floor of the Suttie Centre.

I would encourage students while in years 1-3 to make sure they keep up as much as possible with friends from their year in halls of residence, as like at any university medics can become a tight knit group, and to make the most of their sporting interests or other societies. Making sure you stay on top of things work wise is also very important as it makes revising for exams much more about revision than learning at the last minute under pressure.

My best memories of these years were winning BUSA in second year as part of the Aberdeen University Golf Team, the annual Sports Ball and Medsoc Ball, as well as two great MSF Pimms On Pitches football tournaments.'

Clinical

'With the early introduction to ward life in years 2 and 3 you manage to adopt a role on the ward, and rather than get under everyone's feet you see where you could be utilised, even if it's tying up someone's hair into a bobble as they hurl vomit on your shoes.

With the opportunity to do night shift in A&E, O&G, Paediatrics and anything you might be mad enough to try, every day is different. You could be holding a retractor in theatre for five hours, sitting in on the medical clinics or on a ward round which hopefully won't take more than two hours. Some lovely nurse allocates you the job of Spirogel squirter as there is a hand-washing audit taking place and the beady eye is watching over you. This gives you a job to focus on, mark my words. You could be in just for a morning or for ten hours, the variety and constant change is exciting, often overwhelming but also exhausting!

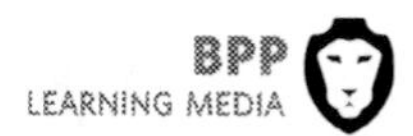

I enjoy the freedom of working within my own limitations, being encouraged to put into practice what has been heard across the auditorium and feel exceptionally privileged to share patient's experiences, good and bad, with them and their families.

With the long hours and moving from Aberdeen to Inverness and back again hockey has taken a back seat but I think it's worth it.'

Once you get in...

The first thing to sort out will be accommodation. The AUSA accommodation office will send you information on halls of residence etc as soon as you have accepted your place and you will be asked to rank your top four choices in order.

Once September approaches the AUSA will send you a freshers' pack containing lots of goodies but importantly your freshers' guide. This contains information about the university itself, the AUSA, clubs and societies, where to go and the nightlife in Aberdeen, a freshers' week programme and other useful advice. There will also be an application form to join MedSoc, a must to save hassle when you arrive, and a freshers' week timetable from the medical school, comprising a few introductory sessions dealing with paper work as well as opportunities to get to know other medical students before term starts.

The Best Thing	Excellent new facilities and regular contact with staff
The Worst Thing	Cold and dark in winter

Student top tips

- Join MedSoc before you arrive as its one less expense to keep track of once you're there.
- Join the gym early as it is very popular.
- Don't miss out on the Freshers' Fling as it is a great way to meet people and is an unforgettable evening.
- Purchase a bus pass as it makes travel around the city much easier.
- Make use of rural GP attachment and be proactive in clinical years.

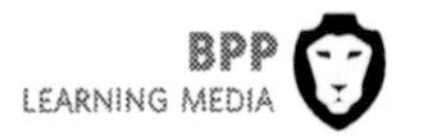

Summary Table

Positives	Negatives
Excellent new facilities (medical and sport)	Cold weather
Medsoc and Gradsoc events	Accommodation not close to campus
Enthusiastic teaching on single campus	Poor exam feedback
Bustling student city	Lack of student union
Remote and rural option and rural GP placement	Lack of ERASMUS programme

Belfast

Queen's University Belfast
University Road
Belfast
BT7 1NN
Northern Ireland

www.qub.ac.uk/mdbs

Queen's University was founded as a college in 1885, becoming a university in 1909 in the vibrant and student-friendly city of Belfast. With a lively nightlife established around the city's ever developing cosmopolitan outlook students are offered a wide variety of multicultural restaurants, café-bars and ground-breaking entertainment centres, which regularly attract some of the world's biggest acts.

Belfast is a very compact city with a dedicated student area giving it a campus-feel, with the added benefits and attributes of city life on your doorstep. In relation to other university cities in the UK, Belfast is a very affordable place to study, with high quality, convenient accommodation available within walking distance of the medical school.

The medical school itself is part of the largest faculty within the university. The course is designed around lecture-based, student-centred learning as opposed to problem-solving.

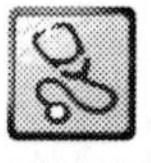

The medical course

Key facts

Course Type	Traditional	Degree Awarded	MB BCh BAO
Basic Entry Requirements	AAA	Entrance Exams	UKCAT
Year Size	270	Open Days	April
Admissions Website	www.qub.ac.uk/schools/mdbs/medicine/Prospectivestudents/		

Getting in – student tips

No interview process takes place for school leavers, however all graduate entry applicants and school leavers who have had to re-sit individual A level modules or whole subjects in an institute outside their school are subject to interview. Questions asked include your reasons for choosing Queen's University to study Medicine, as well as ethical dilemmas demonstrating the applicant's competency in decision-making skills and judgment. School leavers are encouraged to put great emphasis on their intent to study Medicine at university in their personal statement and provide examples of their communication skills and initiative.

Course details

Foundation / Pre-Med	N/A	**Graduate**	N/A
Student Population	Male: female ratio: 40:60	**Term Length**	Pre-clinical: 12 weeks Clinical: 12-18 weeks
Erasmus / Foreign Exchange	Yes – Final year. Desination is student's choice	**Elective Period**	End of year 4 – 6 weeks

Intercalation

Stage	After year 2, 3 or 4	**Degree Awarded**	BScMedSci (Hons)
Requirements	Good standing within the university	**Subjects**	Anatomy, Physiology, Biochemistry, Microbiology, Pharmacology, Cardiovascular Science, Neuroscience, Pathology

Anatomy teaching

Four hours of anatomy teaching each week in the first and second year with groups of five to six students having their own cadaver to dissect (under the guidance of various anatomy demonstrators) along with teaching with pre-prepared prosections in the dissection rooms. This is further complemented with anatomy lectures given by the heads of the Anatomy and Physiology department. An additional Student Selected Component can be undertaken in the

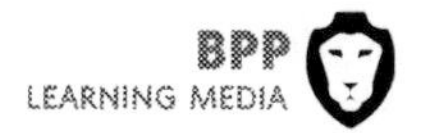

second year for those with a keen interest to dissect the muscles and structures of the back. Also intercalated degrees, BSc (Hons), can be taken in Anatomy after the second year.

Pre-clinical/Years 1–2	
Topics	***Year 1:*** Genes Molecules & Processes, Cells Tissues & Organs, People & Populations, Anatomy, Therapeutics & Pharmacology, Clinical Skills, Personal & Professional Development, Physiology – Cardiovascular, Respiratory, Renal. ***Year 2:*** Anatomy, Epidemiology and Public Health, Individual in Society, Microanatomy, Medical Statistics, Microbiology, Pharmacology, Mechanisms of Disease, Immunology, Microbiology, Clinical Skills, Physiology – Neurology, Gastrointestinal, Endocrinology, Musculoskeletal, Reproductive System.
Teaching	Lectures, practical demonstrations, self-directed learning.
SSC Periods	One is taken in the second semester of the first year and then one in each semester of the second year. Topics vary from year to year and students can apply to have their own SSCs created, if they are deemed viable and there is support from the appropriate staff.
Exams	Format varies from examinations to essays or practical demonstrations. Mark awarded in SSC doesn't contribute to your final mark in Medicine, only a pass mark is required.

Clinical/Years 3–5	
Topics	***Year 3:*** General Medicine, General Surgery, Dermatology, ENT, Endocrinology, Haematology, Musculoskeletal, Nephrology, Neuroscience, Ophthalmology, Pathology. ***Year 4:*** Obstetrics & Gynaecology, Preoperative & Emergency Medicine, Paediatrics, Cancer Studies, General Practice, Geriatrics, Radiology, Fractures, Psychiatry. ***Year 5:*** General Medicine, General Surgery, other topics are chosen dependent on the students interests.
SSC Periods	Three weeks are devoted to SSC at the start of each semester in the third year, so not to get in the way of clinical teaching.
Exams	Clinical Examinations (OSCES and written). Exams consist of MCQs (not negatively marked), EMQs, OSCE, written papers. 50% pass mark. Students who fail exams must re-sit them at the end of the year, if re-sit is failed, then the student must repeat the year.

Hospital placements/academies

Accommodation is provided by the university in halls of residence in peripheral hospitals. In hospitals within the greater Belfast area it is expected that you are able to obtain long-term accommodation in Belfast itself. The accommodation provided is similar to that in university halls of residence with individual, well furnished rooms with sinks, kitchens and common rooms for students to relax in. Placements can vary depending on which speciality you are currently doing eg one week for dermatology, or 12 weeks doing General Medicine/Surgery. Most hospitals have libraries and computer suites for students to use. The Medical Biological Centre (MBC) in Belfast has a Clinical Skills Education Centre where students are taught how to perform clinical skills, as well as being able to book out rooms to practise and use equipment, that would otherwise be unavailable. Student numbers can vary from small groups of five to six in peripheral hospitals to up to 20 in central Belfast hospitals, which are regional centres for excellence eg Endocrinology and Neuroscience. The Royal Victoria Hospital in Belfast is the biggest hospital in Northern Ireland and contains many regional centres of excellence, which provide good opportunities for students to learn.

Hospitals and Travel Time from University	
Royal Victoria Hospital	5 minutes
City Hospital	2 minutes
Mater Infirmorum Hospital	10 minutes
Musgrave Park Hospital	10 minutes
Ulster Hospital	20 minutes
Antrim Area Hospital	20 minutes
Craigavon Area Hospital	30 minutes
Altnagelvin Hospital	1 hour 15 minutes
Causeway Hospital	1 hour 30 minutes
Erne Hospital	1 hour 30 minutes
Tyrone County	2 hours

The medical school

Work	✚	✚	✚			Intense but manageable
Facilities	☕	☕	☕	☕		Medical Biological Centre and Medical libraries, as well as Clinical Skills Centre
Support	👥	👥	👥	👥		All tutors and lecturers are very helpful and will respond to all of your question in person or will email you answers very promptly
Feedback	📋	📋	📋			Feedback is usually not in great detail

Facilities

Facilities at QUB are very modern with the state of the art CS Lewis Library on the main campus. There is also a library in the Medical Biology Centre (MBC) itself where the majority of pre-clinical teaching takes place and most of the medical textbooks are housed. The MBC also has the Clinical Skills Centre, anatomy rooms, microbiology suite, computer suite and practical physiology rooms.

All hospitals have some form of library and computer suite available, and the Royal Victoria Hospital houses a large selection of books, wireless internet suite, computer room and common room.

Student support

A special building has recently been built beside the Queen's University bookshop, which houses the Student Guidance Centre. This Centre houses the Admissions and Access Service, Careers, Employability and Skills, Counselling Service, Disability Service, Income and Student Finance Centre, Learning and Development Service, Student Finance Centre, Welcome and Orientation and the Widening and Participation Centre.

The University Health Centre at Queen's is a General Practice that provides both student-focused and general National Health services.

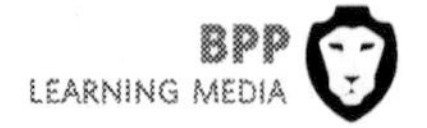

The Health Centre also provides university-funded, non-NHS services, for students of Queen's. For the medical students, a special society has recently been created by third year medical students in which a buddy system for new first year students had been put in place to help them with problems such as course material and revision for exams, with two third year students assigned to help look after groups of first years. Tutor mentors from university staff are also assigned to groups of students and are readily available for advice and support. There are 13 different chaplaincies in the university, which cater to every religious denomination, all within walking distance of the main university buildings.

Medical societies

The biggest and most popular medical society in Queen's is the Belfast Medical Students Association (BMSA). This is a very popular society which organises various themed nights out that involve all five years of the medical faculty, as well as the main event of the year, the BMSA Mystery Tour during which 500+ students travel to various different clubs and pubs in Northern Ireland and the Republic, a definite must to go on! Other societies include Belfast Marrow (a society run by medical students, which tries to recruit students to join the bone marrow register to help fight leukaemia), also Scrubs, our surgical society, which organises many extra-curricular workshops in practical procedures and emergency medicine. Another big society is the Student Working Overseas Trust (SWOT), which is an organisation run by fourth year medical students which raises money in order to purchase medical supplies to send to hospitals in the developing world when students visit them to take their electives. The highlight of their year is the SWOT Fashion show which uses the fourth year students as models for some of the trendiest shops in Belfast to model clothes and raises in excess of £40,000 a year. There is also a medical rugby team that meets regularly at the Queen's Physical Education Centre.

Finance

There is hardship funding, the amount eligible is related to individual circumstances. There are various different scholarships that can be obtained throughout the course of Medicine, and are usually given out for outstanding academic achievement.

Student opinion

'Queen's is fun, interesting and exciting. There is never a dull moment with the new friends you make or all of the different society nights out.'

The university

Accommodation	Non-campus halls of residence
Further Info	Queen's accommodation website - www.stayatqueens.com

Accommodation

Most first year students live in the Queen's halls of residence – Elm's Village. It's a great way to meet new people on your course as everyone is always nearby. It's a 20-minute walk to the MBC in the morning which is the best way to spot fellow med students as they'll be the only ones up at 9.00 in the morning!

Study facilities

The main libraries used by medical students are the MBC library, the library at the Royal Victoria hospital site, and the Seamus Heaney Library (which is open 24 hours a day in the run up to the exam period). The multi-million pound CS Lewis Library will take over as the main library, replacing the architectural anomaly that is the current tower block. Each library has an extensive IT suite with wireless facilities throughout the building as well as offering some of the best views in Belfast.

University sports & students' union

Queen's student union is opposite the main university building on University road, and has recently had a £9 million facelift. In the union, there are three bars, which serve food, an SU shop, snooker rooms, Clements Café, bookshops, chemist, IT suites, various different canteens and a refurbished area called The Space which is full of sofas and chairs and is used regularly for club and

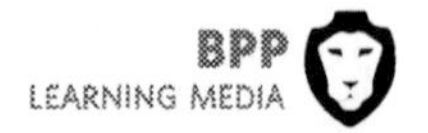

society meetings as well as relaxing. Downstairs in the union is the Mandela Hall which is used regularly for concerts.

An all inclusive membership at the Queen's Physical Education Centre (PEC) is available. In the last few years £10 million has been invested in PEC to provide it with state of the art facilities which include: a swimming pool, free weights area, strength and conditioning suite, climbing walls, indoor basketball, badminton, table tennis, a 120-station fitness suite, outdoor training facilities, air conditioned cycling and dance studios.

Freshers' Week usually lasts for up to two weeks, just before the start of term in September. Events include: freshers' festival: sign up for clubs and societies, freshers' party: the key social event, speed dating: get to meet new friends... (quickly!), Vice Chancellor's welcome, BBQ and entertainment at the Elms student village centre, sport tester sessions to try out a new sport and international food fair. There are also freshers' workshops on dealing with transition and change; getting organised and action planning; managing and spending money and job shop opportunities. There are a variety of different functions at various sites throughout the university, which change from year to year. There is also a freshers' bazaar in which students can sign up and join a variety of different clubs and societies, as well as the medical student-run ones.

Student opinion

'It is a friendly and welcoming place to study, with everything a student would ever need very close by.'

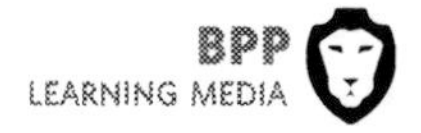

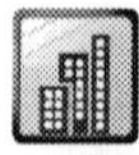

The city

Safety						Belfast is generally safe for students
Nightlife						Most of the best bars and clubs are within walking distance of the university
Transport						There is lots of parking available in nearby residential areas. But while studying in Belfast, transport isn't needed, unless placements are in peripheral hospitals
Cost of Living						Rent is usually around £200/month depending on which area you live in. A taxi to anywhere in Belfast should never cost more than £5. Pints are usually around £3 and entry into clubs is usually £3–5

Things to do

Belfast has a wealth of visitor attractions, which provide the ideal opportunity for an enjoyable day out and a chance to soak up the local culture and heritage. The city is compact and intimate, with a rich legacy of Georgian, Victorian and Edwardian architecture, which includes Belfast City Hall, the Grand Opera House, Queen's University and Belfast Castle. There are local museums and places of interest including the Titanic's Dock and Pumphouse and the Ulster Folk Transport Museum which offer an insight into industrial heritage and times gone by; while award winning attractions including Belfast Zoo and W5 Interactive Science Centre provide great days out. Students tend to go to the city centre, Queen's campus and the nearby Botanic Gardens to chill out and relax.

The main student nights out vary from club to club with each establishment offering something different on each night. The biggest student nights' out are usually at the student union on a Monday or a Thursday. All the best student pubs and clubs are within walking distance of the university. Belfast also has great shopping spots within easy walking distance of each other. From the prestigious Victoria Square Shopping Centre development, numerous high street stores, family businesses, luxurious designer boutiques and specialty shops. Whether it is high street or budget shopping, designer or couture, the city offers a wealth of choice for every taste and pocket. This is a pleasant and easy city to live in with everything a student could want within easy access.

Places to Go		
Place	**Brief Description**	**Entry Fee/ Opening Time**
Students' union	Best Monday night out	£5, 9.00pm–1.30am
The Botanic Inn	Club upstairs, with live music downstairs on Wednesdays	£5, 9.00pm–1.00am
M Club	Cheap entry £1 a drink on Tuesday nights	£3, 9.00pm-1.00am
The Box	Giant club at the Odyssey arena with three different DJs and great drink offers on a Thursday	£5, 8.00pm–1.00am

Student opinion

'Belfast is a constantly changing city with new and exciting things happening all of the time, which makes it very enjoyable to live in and be part of student life there.'

Student's view

Pre-clinical

'My first two years at Queen's were easily my favourite and the best advice I can give is to enjoy the free time while you can! The pure lecture format of these years is the only chance you'll get to experience true student life before you're forced into your shirt and tie and embrace the alcohol free joys of responsibility. Take every opportunity you can. I joined about six clubs in my first month! It's a brilliant way to meet people from other courses as well as

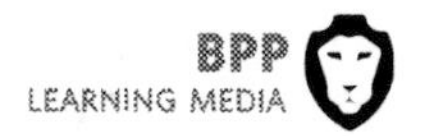

giving you a wide and varied university experience plus a little extra to write on the dreaded MTAS form!

As for the teaching itself, I can promise you now the first semester is as dull as dishwater, but don't despair, the interesting stuff will start from Christmas onwards! That's when you have your first daunting trip into the Dissection Room, as well as the beginning of your physiology, pharmacology and the not so fun epidemiology... Personally I found the physiology/anatomy surprisingly interesting but I've always been a bit of a closet nerd about how things work and how the body is the ultimate machine.

A typical day is 9.00am–5.00pm apart from Wednesday afternoon, which is set aside for sports...cough...sleeping! Two afternoons a week are usually dedicated for SSCs although this varies, as does the workload for each so think about your choice...especially before coming up to exams, nobody wants a 10,000 word essay on the ethics of the NHS the night before an anatomy exam!

Exams can be tough, especially at the end of the first semester, not because they're particularly hard but the step up from A level to university can be tricky for many students. The best way is to try to keep good notes right the way through and stay on top of things, a little bit every day will stop you turning into a caffeine fuelled wreck around exam time!

Highlights for me from QUB are endless; I had a healthy balance between working during the year and enjoying every single second of university life, then getting my head down around exam time...I believe it's called cramming? The mystery tour is one of the highlights of the year and a great way to get to know your fellow students–maybe some a little closer than others!

Good luck or as they say in Irish... Go n-éirí an t-ádh leat! Ádh mór ort!'

Clinical

'A normal day usually begins with getting up early and heading for the hospital that you're placed in for about 9 o'clock (sometimes earlier if you're trying to catch the early morning ward round or going to watch surgery). In the morning you are usually taught by various different consultants and registrars on topics that they

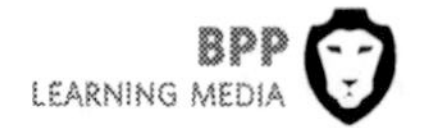

specialise in, followed by seeing a patient that may or may not exhibit this condition, as well as taking a good group history and examining them. The rest of the morning is usually spent by trying to find patients for yourself to write up and present to consultants the following day. After lunch there is usually additional teaching to be had, as well as presentations by each individual student to the group to further the group's and your own understanding of a topic selected by the consultant that you are assigned to. Any time left in the day is again spent by speaking to more patients or looking through notes, going to assigned clinics or surgery, or watching various different procedures occurring. The days usually finish around 4.00 or 5.00pm.

Depending on what placement you are on, attachments can last from one week, to up to 12 weeks, depending on what speciality you are doing and what hospital you are based in. The majority of the course is taught via specific set teaching given by the consultants, a learning and teaching DVD that you are expected to work through, throughout the year, as well as your own private study. Personally I found that in the majority of hospitals that I have been placed in the teaching has been exemplary and all the staff very helpful and friendly, however there are always exceptions to this depending on what you are studying and where that is. Examinations are generally ok provided that you have been working steadily throughout the year in each different placement that you have been in. I always find that if you leave everything to the last minute, then you rush to cram everything in, as a result can miss out key learning points and information, and Medicine isn't just about passing the next exam (although it may seem like that!) but constantly adding to your knowledge base to make you a good doctor. Aspects that I particularly enjoyed included my General Medicine and Surgical placement as I felt that I was being included and being made part of the whole team, and not just getting in the way.'

Once you get in...

Once you get in, you are sent a time and date to turn up for initial registration, in which you are given your welcome pack, timetable, and general initial information as well as student card. You are also given information on how to sign up to the various different medical defence unions and student organisations. As well as this, the various student run medical societies organise nights out in which all first year students get to meet each other eg pyjama parties and three legged pub crawls! During your first week you are exposed to a variety of different classes that you have never had before eg anatomy, microbiology, clinical skills, as well as getting taught in lecture theatres for the first time. You also get to meet your tutorial group that you will be with for the next two years and very quickly strike up brand new friendships. The best tip is to enjoy your first couple of weeks and make as many new friends as possible!

The Best Thing	Meeting new people and going out on lots of nights out with friends
The Worst Thing	Exam time stress!

Student top tips

- Join a sport club or society to make lots of new friends
- Go on every medical society night out to get a sample of Belfast, especially the BMSA nights out.
- Never be afraid to ask a lecturer a question at the end of a lecture, or email them afterwards.
- Enjoy yourself!

Interesting facts

- Biggest faculty in the whole of Queen's.
- One of the only UK medical facilities that give you a BAO (Bachelor of Obstetrics) as well as your normal medical degree.
- If everyone in the final year passes their examinations on the first go, the names are read out while wearing white gloves.

Summary Table

Positives	Negatives
Very good teaching	Exam time stress
Very good social and night life	Occasional lack of guidance for exams
Friends are easy to make	Price of gym membership
Belfast is an easy and nice city to get to know	
Good atmosphere in the summer	

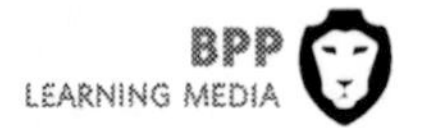

Birmingham

College of Medical and Dental Sciences
University of Birmingham
Edgbaston
Birmingham
B15 2TT

www.medicine.bham.ac.uk/index.shtml

Some may know Birmingham as the heart of the Midlands, the home of chocolate enthusiasts' Cadbury World and for the infamous '*brummy*' accent. But those better informed know it as a prospering, exciting city with a bright future. There truly is something for everyone in Birmingham: the Bullring provides a huge range of modern accessible shops and cafés; sports fans will know that the city is surrounded by famous football, cricket and golf grounds – including the stadiums of Aston Villa and Birmingham City, with Edgbaston Cricket Ground and Edgbaston Golf Club within walking distance of university accommodation. If you're seeking culture then the well acclaimed Symphony Hall hosts not just the Symphony Orchestra but also jazz, rock, pop, folk music and even stand-up comedians. Equally Birmingham's museums and art galleries host highly renowned work.

The university itself boasts a beautiful campus with a peaceful atmosphere promoted by its greenery and aesthetically pleasing architecture.

The medical course

Key facts

Course Type	Traditional	Degree Awarded	MBChB
Basic Entry Requirements	AAA	Entrance Exams	None
Year Size	Approx 300	Open Days	September and June
Admissions Website	www.medicine.bham.ac.uk/		

Getting in – student tips

Birmingham will interview any applicant that has a personal statement demonstrating an academically able candidate with an affinity for science; proof that the candidate has the determination to study medicine and knows (eg from work experience) what the medical profession entails; that the applicant is concerned about human affairs and the welfare of others and that the applicant has a range of others skills and interests, for instance a flair for communication.

The interview panel consists of two or three interviewers made up from academic staff from the medical school, consultant staff from teaching hospitals / practices and medical students. Make sure you know your personal statement well enough to effectively answer probing questions about anything in it.

Course details

Foundation/ Pre-Med	N/A	**Graduate**	Yes
Student Population	Male: female ratio: 40:60	**Term Length**	Pre-clinical: 12 weeks Clinical: 15 weeks
Erasmus/ Foreign Exchange	N/A	**Elective Period**	5 weeks after Year 4 exams

Intercalation

Stage	After year 2, 3 or 4	**Degree Awarded**	BScMedSci (Hons)
Requirements	Places are awarded on academic achievement	**Subjects**	Clinical Sciences, Cell and Molecular Pathology, Physiology, Cardiovascular Science, Neuroscience, Pharmacology, Biochemistry, Healthcare Ethics and Law, History Of Medicine, Behavioural Science, International Health, Public Health and Epidemiology, Psychological Medicine

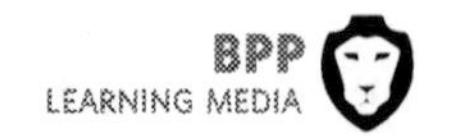

Anatomy teaching

In the first and second year: two to five hours of anatomy small group tutorials per week with two to three anatomy lectures per module. This is supplemented by three prosection sessions per term. The sessions are one to two hours long; groups of three to five students spend time with a tutor being led round a variety of differently dissected cadavers, the tutor leading and testing the students through the necessary anatomy. You are expected to have prepared a pre-designed question/answer booklet on anatomy for each session. These can vary in length from five to 20 pages and can be very time consuming. While Birmingham has been criticised for its anatomy teaching, the teaching staff at the medical school are aware of this and are constantly striving to improve it.

Pre-clinical / Years 1–2	
Topics	***Year 1:*** First term: MTM (Molecules to Man); CEP (Cell communication – Endocrinology – Pharmacology); NAS (Neurones and Synapses) and PPP (People, Patients & Populations). Second term: MJM (Muscles, Joints & Movement); IRM (Introduction to Respiratory Medicine); DIS (Digestive System) and DPS (Doctors, Patients and Society). ***Year 2:*** First term: BAB (Brain and Behaviour); CAN (Cancer: Causes to Cures); CVS (Cardiovascular System) and DEM (Decision Making). Second term: IIH (Infection, Immunology and Haematology); RED (Reproduction – Endocrinology – Development); REN (Renal System) and HES (Health Services, Chronic Illness and Disability). Community Based Medicine and Integrated Problems are also taught during the course of the two years.
Teaching	Lectures, small group tutorials, online material eg assessments, one day per two weeks spent at a General Practice.
SSC Periods	***Year 1:*** One week in November to study a topic of your choosing and write a brief account; one week in February to pick a topic from a range of about 20 staff led projects that involve basic teaching and direction of research by a leader – normally a tutor within the medical school; finally two weeks at the end of the third term, one week is again staff led and the other again up to you.

	Year 2: Students must produce an interactive presentation and a 3,000 word written project on subjects of their choice. Topic selection opens in September and students have until April to produce their work.
Exams	During the term ICAs (in-course assessments) are used to test recently acquired physiology knowledge and account for 20% of each of the six Basic Science modules. MCQs and EMQs take place in January for the majority of modules covered in the first term and make up 30% of those modules. In May/June there are SAQs, MCQs and EMQs to examine everything covered during the year. Students need to obtain a score of 50% to pass; if they don't obtain this mark then they re-sit the module/s they failed in August.

Clinical/Years 3–5	
Topics	***Year 3:*** Integrated Medicine and Surgery Hospital Placements. Neurology. Opthalmology. A&E on calls. General Practice. Clinical Sciences (Pathology, Immunology, Haematology, Clinical Chemistry, Infection) Epidemiological Methods. ***Year 4:*** Cardiovascular, Renal, and Urology. Trauma, Orthopaedics and Rheumatology. Opthalmology, Metabolic disease, Geriatrics. Oncology. Anaesthetics, Respiratory and Intensive Care Medicine. Psychiatry. General Practice. ***Year 5:*** Medicine and Surgery. Accident and Emergency. Dermatology. ENT. Genito-urinary medicine. Neurology. General Practice. Obs and Gynae. Paediatrics.
SSC Periods	***Year 3**:* Take seven half days over the course of each of the two Medicine and Surgery placements to explore an area of interest and prepare a presentation for your lead consultant. In addition, one two-week special study module chosen from a list after third year exams. There is an ongoing group public health project over the course of the third year in which to prepare a research study, an audit or a service evaluation, which is an excellent opportunity to get a publication to your name if you work hard. ***Year 4**:* Four-week clinical SSA placement in a specialty you are interested in. Additionally, time given to complete a clinical audit and prepare a poster presentation on your audit, which is a fantastic opportunity to get a publication.

	Year 5: Six-week post rotation period is available for a student study project. It could take the form of in depth studies of particular conditions, shadowing work, research projects, service evaluations or audits. Again another good opportunity to achieve a publication.
Exams	***Year 3:*** OSCE, EMQs, MCQs. ***Year 4:*** MCQs, EMQs. ***Year 5:*** SAQs, MCQs, EMQs, OSCEs. Pass mark is 50%. MCQs and EMQs are not negatively marked, but they are made harder because of this! If students fail once, they are given one more chance at re-sits. It is uncommon for students to fail re-sits in the clinical years as extra support is given prior to re-sits if you fail an exam. Prizes and distinctions are awarded for exceptional performance.

Hospital placements/academies

Basic accommodation is provided for students undertaking evening on calls, and basic accommodation is provided at Hereford, the most distant placement. Medicine and Surgery placements in the third year last for 15 and 11 weeks. In the fourth year, you go through a rotation of seven five-week blocks in different specialties. In the fifth year placements are generally five-week blocks, with a long 10-week block for specialties experience. You are normally placed into firms of between two and six students for each block. UHB Queen Elizabeth Hospital is world renowned for research, cancer, burns and plastics. And Selly Oak hospital is famous for its trauma centre, where many UK servicemen and women are treated for major trauma injuries. Most hospitals are reasonably easy to get to, but it is useful to have a car once you get into clinical years, as public transport to some placements can be quite complicated and time consuming.

Hospitals and Travel Time from University	
UHB Queen Elizabeth	2 minutes
Womens Hospital	2 minutes
Barberry	3 minutes
UHB Selly Oak	5 minutes
Royal Orthopaedic Hospital	5 minutes

Birmingham City Hospital	15 minutes
Birmingham Children's Hospital	15 minutes
Whittall Street Clinic	15 minutes
Heartland's Hospital	20 minutes
Alexandra Hospital	25 minutes
Russell's Hall Hospital	25 minutes
Sandwell General	25 minutes
Good Hope Hospital	30 minutes
Walsall Manor Hospital	30 minutes
Worcester Acute	30 minutes
New Cross Wolverhampton	35 minutes
Hereford County	75 minutes
Royal Shrewsbury	75 minutes

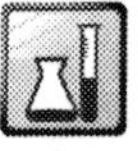

The medical school

Work						Can be difficult to find the right work/ life balance with so much to do
Facilities						Medical school library and computer cluster
Support						Varies depending on the people allocated to support you. But good online support via med school website and email
Feedback						Formative assessments throughout the year and emails to/from tutors good. OK feedback after exams but could give more overall feedback for everything

Facilities

The medical school itself has a deceptively antique looking exterior. Inside it boasts a newly refurbished and comfortable common room with vending machines; on the floor below this is a modern canteen which offers breakfast and lunch or sandwiches, drinks

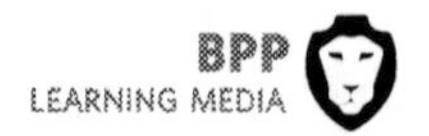

and snacks for during the day. Perhaps more importantly, it has a spacious library where silence is always respected and a large computer cluster with free printing. Furthermore there are a number of large lecture theatres with first class acoustics and many more small teaching rooms.

Student support

Great support can be found online at Birmingham with people ready to email back almost immediately and give helpful advice or organise a time and place to meet and chat. However, the support given to you in the form of people greatly varies depending on the person. In the first year you are assigned to a PM group. In this group you have a medical school 'mum and dad' and a personal tutor (who is changed in consecutive years), the idea being that a medical school 'mum and dad' are there to text and meet you if you're struggling with something or just need advice. As with real-life mums and dads some may smother you, bombarding you with unnecessary advice and forever texting you wanting to meet up; while others may be completely negligent and barely reply to your texts. This is also true of personal tutors, who you organise meetings with via email.

Medical societies

Medsoc is the well renowned medical society for medical, biomedical science, physiotherapy and nursing students at Birmingham. Well structured and avidly run by a range of students, it has a number of sports teams from 'medpong' (table tennis) to Medsoc football. All of the teams have their own social events and are a great way to meet new friends. Medsoc also has a range of societies for students wishing to further their future careers, such as 'Surgsoc', the surgical society which allows its members to attend a range of lectures given by surgeons and take part in surgical courses. Medsoc regularly sends out emails advertising any events and also allows its societies and sports teams to send messages. Perhaps Medsoc's most advertised event is 'Medbar' which takes place most Fridays and gives medics a chance to socialise at a reasonable price.

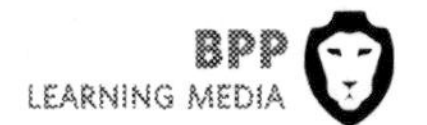

Finance

There is a Birmingham Grant and a Birmingham Scholarship available to UK students from low income backgrounds, which can be as much as £1,300. There are also prizes and scholarships provided each year for excellence in examinations.

Further info: www.undergraduate.bham.ac.uk/finance/

Student opinion

'The modern medical school coupled with the fantastic clubs and societies available make your time at Birmingham Medical School very enjoyable.'

The university

Accommodation	Non-campus halls of residence
Further Info	www.guildofstudents.com

Accommodation

Birmingham offers a huge range of accommodation, greatly varying in price, location and layout. The majority of the accommodation is located in a luscious part of Edgbaston known as the Vale. At the centre of the Vale is a picturesque lake and many of the halls loosely surround this, meanwhile life on the Vale centres around the Hub – a small complex containing the reception for the halls of residence, laundrette, canteen and bar. The most expensive of these halls is the most recently constructed Mason Hall and at around £5,000 for the year it could be mistaken for a 3 or 4 star hotel with every room containing an en-suite bathroom with walk-in shower. However, Mason does lack the communal spirit of Tennis Court, a large set of halls across the road. There is still more accommodation dotted around Edgbaston and Selly Oak and the majority of the halls are within, at the most, 10–15 minutes' walk of the medical school and university. Birmingham's comfortable accommodation is one of its greatest lures as a university.

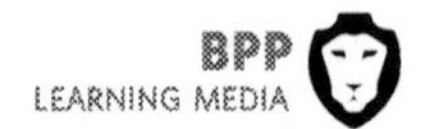

Study facilities

The University of Birmingham library has an impressive range of resources and offers a perfect place to study, although it can be difficult to find a seat during the exam period. However medical students will generally keep to the medical school, which has its own library and computer cluster for work.

University sports & students' union

The university has a well equipped gym in the sports hall with two rooms of machines – a number of running machines, bikes and resistance machines, and a large separate weights room. Excellent services don't come cheap, for a pass for the gym and swimming at the university pool will cost around £200. As you would expect the gym does get busy around peak times, but early morning and evening does see the gym empty a little. Birmingham prides itself on sporting excellence, and most university teams are within at least the top 10 in the country.

Freshers' packs can be bought online with tickets for all available events; alternatively packs with slightly fewer events may be bought from reps when arriving at halls. There will be a freshers' fair running over several days of the week with information on a range of societies students can join and support facilities along with a number of helpful free items, such as a frisbee. Separate to this, there is a sports fair. Every sport on offer at Birmingham, from football to American football to ultimate frisbee, will have a stall set up at the sports hall with a chance to sign up and give any sport you fancy a go. Remember to take your wallet.

As with the university freshers' and sports fairs, there is a Medsoc fair where medics can sign up to Medsoc sports and societies, along with organisations such as the MDU, MPS and BMA. Again remember to bring a chequebook. A number of popular Medsoc events are organised, so it's important to sign up for the tickets as soon as you can. If anything, this week is better organised than that of the halls, while there are fewer events, more memorable times are assured on trips such as the 'River Boat Shuffle', and a 'Meet & Greet' ensures you recognise at least one or two medics in the lecture theatre. For medics, lectures begin in the second week and are often on mornings after freshers' nights out, but it doesn't spoil the fun or make the lectures harder – it just means a rather busy, tiring week.

Student opinion

'The newly built Mason Hall is a fantastic place to live and Edgbaston campus is a great place to make friends and to relax after lectures.'

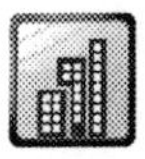

The city

Safety	🛡	🛡	🛡			Birmingham is a generally safe, student-friendly city
Nightlife	☾	☾	☾	☾		Super-clubs, smaller clubs, several bars and pubs
Transport	🚌	🚌	🚌	🚌		Train station right outside the uni (University Station), quick and cheap taxis, fairly regular buses, good parking spaces at halls and in houses in Selly Oak (second year onwards) but let down by very bad traffic
Cost of Living	🐖	🐖	🐖	🐖		Expect to pay about £275 a month for rent, £6–8 (but only about £1–2 if sharing) for a taxi, £5–6 to get into big clubs and expensive drinks puts the cost of a good night at about £20–30

Things to do

Edgbaston where the university and halls are situated is a 5–10 minute £5 taxi ride away from Broad Street. Here, and its adjacent streets and complexes, contain the majority of the city's attractions. Broad Street in particularly is where the popular bars and clubs are. Aside from clubbing, Birmingham is also outstanding for shopping with its famous Bullring. The Bullring is a massive shopping complex accessed via Broad Street and has a whole range of shops. For a slightly more upmarket atmosphere, for those who can afford it, there is the Mailbox just around the corner from Broad Street. The Mailbox is tucked away from busy traffic and offers designer shops, and a number of highly rated hotels and restaurants. Museums and art galleries are also not far from Broad Street but take a little more research to find.

As the city is centred on a number of busy main roads, its atmosphere isn't quite as calm and picturesque as other university's cities. However, because the clubs and bars are mostly located along one stretch, they are very well policed and this makes Birmingham a very safe place to go out of a night.

Places to go		
Place	**Brief Description**	**Entry Fee/Opening Time**
Bristol Pear	Medbar host on a Friday evening. Make sure you try a Heidi!	£Free, Mon–Sun 11.00am–11.00pm
The Soak	Friendly, relaxed pub/bar in Selly Oak with pool tables and big screens for sports events	£Free, Mon–Sun 11.00am–11.00pm
Oceana	Popular Superclub, with differently themed bars and 2 big dance floors	£4 Student Night. Mon and Wed 9.00pm–3.00am
Gatecrasher	Newly refurbished Superclub	£4 Student Night. Wed and Fri 10.00pm–3.00am.
SportsCafe	Sports Oriented bar on Broad Street with massive screens for all major (and minor) sporting events	£Free Mon–Sun 12.00pm–2.00am

Student opinion

'A busy, bustling urban city with fantastic modern shopping facilities. There is always something to do.'

Student's view

Pre-clinical

'The first year is a true test of stamina on a course that requires a lot of energy. It is also a test of your commitment to Medicine. It's difficult to ignore the allure of organised nights out in Birmingham and spending time with new friends, while also setting aside enough time to keep up with studying and enjoy all the sports and societies the university has to offer.

Furthermore, you'll find yourself spending a lot more time during the week in lecture theatres and small group teachings than flatmates with less demanding timetables. Teaching on Wednesday finishes by 1.00pm to allow the afternoon free for sport but you'll be in the medical school from 9.00/10.00am to 5.00/6.00pm on numerous other days. As a result, it's important to use the spare hours between lectures in the medical school to go over lectures or prepare for small group sessions (or have a power nap if you've been out the night before). Providing you work steadily throughout the year, making sure you understand the lectures and making notes, passing exams won't be a problem.

If I could master time and space itself and throw myself back to the start of my first year I would change a few things. First, I'd get involved in more societies and sports teams – they offer the perfect way to expand your friendship group and have some great nights out and fun times. On a similar level I'd attend more events organised by and for medics and join more 'Medsoc' societies. Finally, I'd make sure that I worked steadily throughout the year building up my notes and filling in my anatomy folder – trust me when I say 'it'll make the future a lot earlier'. Birmingham medical school understands that the first year is a busy and exciting time for you and provides a challenging yet accessible course that requires steady work but allows time to enjoy a host of extra-curricular activities.'

Clinical

'A normal day starts at 9.00am. You may go to a clinic, where you may be allowed to clerk new patients and present them to the Consultant or Registrar in charge. Or you may observe the clinic, examine patients as necessary, and be quizzed and taught by the doctor in charge. Alternatively, you may spend the morning on the wards, taking histories off patients and performing examinations as practice, taking bloods, inserting cannulas and practising other clinical skills. You may then have an hour of organised bed-side teaching with a Consultant which is always very interesting and useful. Lunch is taken as and when you have the time, on some days you may get more time than others! In the afternoon, you could be doing much the same, or alternatively you could be going to observe surgery in theatres and, if you are lucky enough, be allowed to scrub in! The average day finishes at about 4.00pm usually, but can go on till 5.30pm if you are in a clinic.

In the third year, you have quite a lot of bedside clinical teaching, which I found was the most useful part of my learning. You normally get one lecture a day on an important disease while on placement in addition to the opportunities to attend clinics, ward rounds and theatres. It is also important to practise your examinations and histories as much as possible to make your third year OSCE easy! In the fourth year, there tends to be a lot more clinics, and sometimes this can become quite boring, especially if you are not being allowed much responsibility or given much teaching during the clinic. In the fifth year there tends to be more ward work, which is useful as it is the staple of what you will be doing in a year's time as an FY1. Staff in theatres are normally keen to explain what they are doing, quiz you on anatomy and even let you scrub in. A couple of real highlights for me were scrubbing in on an open Laparatomy for a four-hour lower GI operation, and being the cameraman for a laparoscopic Cholecystectomy in the third year.

Another really useful part of the clinical years is the on-calls. You are expected to spend a number of days where you stay until at least 10.00pm in either A&E or EAU and clerk new patients and perform clinical skills. There is no better place to learn Medicine than at the front door when you can see the signs and symptoms and early management of a patient for yourself.

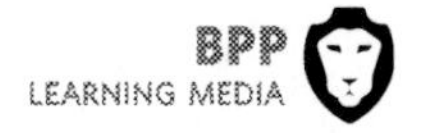

The advice I would give to a student in clinical years is take all the opportunities you get to go on call. And don't be scared of giving a new clinical skill a go, the more you try the better you'll be!'

Once you get in...

Birmingham will send you a pack welcoming you to the university. The pack contains a number small leaflets, many of which will be about the sort of support you can access through the university eg financial support, support for your own wellbeing etc. There will also be information about the gym and other facilities in the university. You should already have received and sent off some forms regarding housing and student finance and you may receive more information. Finally, you will receive a welcome pack from 'Medsoc' with a booklet containing information about 'Medsoc' sports and societies; information about your timetable for the first week (eg meet and greet events and a tour of the medical school – NOT about lectures, you will receive information about lectures when you attend the tour of the medical school and introductory lecture) and purchasable tickets for 'Medsoc' freshers' week events. It is important to be proactive once you get in and search the university website and 'Medsoc' website for more information and tickets for freshers' week. Be sure to join as many facebook groups as possible as these are an invaluable source of information for where to get tickets and what to expect during your first week at the university.

The Best Thing	Very enthusiastic lecturers and doctors in hospitals are always keen to teach
The Worst Thing	With such a large number of people in the year, it is easy to get lost in the system

Student top tips

- Don't miss out on the Medsoc freshers' package, the HOP is unbelievably good fun, and the riverboat shuffle is also an awesome experience.
- Join up with the University Medical Practice early on, it's free!

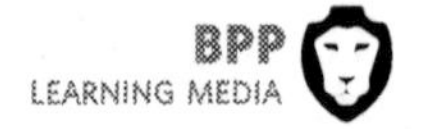

- Join a Medsoc team or society, it's a fantastic way of getting to know other medics as well as keeping your extra-curricular activities and fitness up.
- Join a university club or society in addition to a Medsoc club. Medics can be quite cliquey and it's good for getting to know a wide variety of different people in the university. I can highly recommend the skydiving club!
- Don't miss out on MedBall. It may be expensive at over £50 per ticket, but it is more than worth it! They have top DJs, inflatable toys, photos, casinos, free champagne and lots more!

Summary Table

Positives	Negatives
Beautiful campus area with lots of greenery	Anatomy teaching is poor
Excellent facilities within the medical school	Easy to get lost in the system in such a large year
Enthusiastic teaching	Poor feedback on exams
Comprehensive MedSoc society with lots of activities to get involved with	Reimbursement for petrol costs is poor
Lots of opportunities to enhance your CV with publications	Poor public transport system
MedBall!	Getting out of the city in rush hour
Big city and campus with lots to do	Big city and campus which can be overwhelming

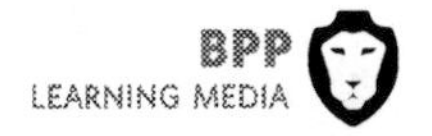

Brighton and Sussex

Brighton and Sussex Medical School (BSMS)
BSMS Teaching Building
University of Sussex
Brighton
East Sussex
BN1 9PX

www.bsms.ac.uk/

Vibrant, dynamic, inclusive, fun, and always challenging the usual status quo; Brighton is certainly a fantastic place to spend your student life. The same words also capture the spirit of BSMS, the new medical school that began taking in students here in 2003. This course is not constrained by tradition, and is continually refined to improve academic standards while meeting the needs of individual students.

With access to facilities from both Brighton and Sussex Universities, opportunities for developing other interests (in sport, arts, activism, or elsewhere) are almost boundless. Brighton itself is also a hotpot for creativity, with a music and arts scene unrivalled in a town this size. Gigs, clubnights and theatre shows happen every night of the week, and the year is dotted with events such as the Brighton Festival, Pride, and the Great Escape Festival. Everything is easy to access (within walking or cycling distance), the beach is never far from view, and the usual high-street shops exist in addition to the unique boutiques and cafés in the famous Lanes. For anything else, London is less than an hour away.

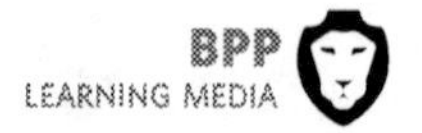

The medical course

Key facts

Course Type	Integrated	Degree Awarded	Bachelor of Medicine Bachelor of Surgery (BMBS)
Basic Entry Requirements	AAA or A*AB	Entrance Exams	UKCAT
Year Size	140	Open Days	July to mid-August
Website	www.bsms.ac.uk/index.php		

Getting in – student tips

BSMS looks for personal statements that demonstrate a realistic attitude to studying Medicine and possession of qualities that will enable you to become a competent, caring and compassionate physician. Evidence of academic achievement and potential are important, but if you have particular achievements or interests outside of academia use them to make yourself stand out and to demonstrate a commitment to caring for others, the ability to work effectively within a team, to appreciate other people's point of view, and a willingness to accept responsibility. Gap years are favoured as long as useful and beneficial activities are undertaken.

The interview panel consists of two interviewers from clinical and educational departments within the university, local hospitals and GP practices. A trained medical student is often also present. Think about why you want to be a doctor (with an emphasis on *you*), what you could contribute to the medical school, and why you are considering Brighton. Interviewers are not trying to catch you out, and questions generally refer to your personal statement – however, some knowledge and opinions on current scientific, medical and ethical issues are necessary too. Demonstrate self-confidence, enthusiasm for Medicine, and good communication skills and you will be halfway there!

Course details

Foundation / Pre-Med	No	Graduate	No
Student Population	Male: female ratio: roughly 40:60	Term Length	Pre-clinical: 10 weeks Clinical: 16 weeks
Erasmus / Foreign Exchange	N/A	Elective Period	Year 4 - 8 weeks (Sept)

Intercalation

Stage	Most commonly between year 3 and year 4	Degree Awarded	BSC or MSc
Requirements	All students with good academic standing are permitted to apply. About 40% intercalate	Subjects	Biochemistry, Biomedical Sciences, Experimental Psychology, Medical Neuroscience, Molecular Genetics, Molecular Medicine and Pharmacological Sciences. There are also Masters degrees available in Leadership and Management in Healthcare, Child Health and Public Health

Anatomy teaching

A highlight of the course is the regular opportunity for dissection that begins almost from day one. As a new medical school, BSMS can boast state of the art facilities, and about three hours' dissection a week (undertaken in small groups of eight) which focus on the systems studied in the rest of the module take place through years 1 and 2. Computer-assisted teaching and use of X-ray/CT/MRI imagery complement the dissection in addition to regular 'living anatomy' sessions in groups of 12. Taught within its clinical context and examined by viva each term, anatomy is certainly a strong point of the BSMS course.

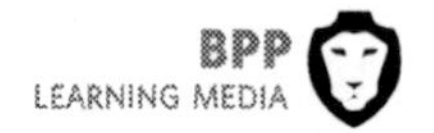

Pre-clinical/Years 1–2	
Topics	***Year 1:*** Foundation of health and disease; Heart, lungs and blood; Nutrition, metabolism and excretion; core Clinical Practice module. ***Year 2:*** Neuroscience and behaviour; Reproduction and endocrine systems; Musculoskeletal and immune systems; core Clinical Practice module.
Teaching	Teaching is systems-based and integrated, including anatomical, physiological, biomedical, and pychosocial aspects. 25% of learning is clinically based at this stage, including hospital and GP visits, and an individual patient study each year.
SSC Periods	A large range of choice, three SSCs a year with one SSC each term/module. SSCs relate to what is being studied that module, with a large variation from lab work to clinical.
Exams	Exams are modular (every 10 weeks) and include Multiple Choice Questions (not negatively marked), Extended Matching Questions, Short Answer Questions and anatomy vivas. Pass Mark ~ 50% (depending on difficulty of paper). The clinical aspect of the course is assessed via a clinical OSCE and an in-depth patient report. SSCs usually require an essay or presentation to be passed but are not graded.

Clinical/Years 3–5	
Topics	***Year 3:*** Scientific Basis of Medicine module (includes: Research methodology, Infectious diseases, Pharmacology and Therapeutics, Immunology, Metabolic medicine, Cancer biology and treatment, Stem cell biology, Imaging, Neurobiology, Genetics, Cellular pathology). Clinical rotations in a Clinical Foundation Course, Medicine, Surgery, Obstetrics and Gynaecology, Paediatrics, Elderly Medicine, and Mental Health. ***Year 4:*** Clinical Elective, Individual Research Project, General Practice, Population Medicine and Palliative Care.

	Clinical rotations in Neurology and Neurosurgery, Dermatology, ENT, Rheumatology and Orthopaedics, Infectious Diseases and HIV/GUM, Oncology and Haematology. ***Year 5**:* Clinical rotations in Medicine, Elderly Medicine, Surgery, Obstetrics and Gynaecology, Paediatrics, General Practice, and Mental Health.
SSC Periods	***Year 3:*** Four blocks of eight weeks. Students rank their choices from a selection of approximately 60 options on a huge range of topics, including: philosophical thinking, the role of imaging, molecular neuroscience, literature and medicine, and bioterrorism. ***Year 4:*** Individual Research Project – one day per week for the entire year. Students can conduct research in almost any area of their choice, provided a supervisor is available and ethical approval is granted. These can range from lab-based research, to clinical audits, to literature reviews. Can be self-designed or can join existing research being conducted. Opportunities for publications. ***Year 5:*** One-month option after finals where students can work in a clinical or research department of their choice. Opportunities for audits, research and publications.
Exams	Exams at the end of the year on all rotations include Multiple Choice Questions (not negatively marked), Extended Matching Questions, Short Answer Questions. Pass mark ~ 50%. Also an exam on subjects studied in Scientific Basis of Medicine module. Clinical modules are also assessed at the end of rotations with a Case-Based Discussion, lasting 10 minutes presented to two consultants.

Hospital placements/academies

In the fifth year there are three placements lasting two months each, based in the hospitals listed below in and around Brighton. Rotations in hospitals one hour away from Brighton have accommodation provided – these are next to the hospital and are of adequate standard, normally with students sharing kitchen and bathrooms between four to six people and having their own room.

Each placement has about 16 BSMS students at a time, but there are also students from other medical schools (such as King's), so there are opportunities to meet and work with new people. You can choose between two to four people in the year with whom you would like to be placed so people can stay with their friends and share lifts etc. Teaching in all hospitals is generally of a good standard, though like anywhere it is dependent on the particular consultant or firm that you are attached to.

Hospitals and Travel Time from University	
Brighton General Hospital	20 minutes
Royal Sussex County Hospital	25 minutes
Haywards Heath Princess Royal Hospital	30 minutes
Worthing Hospital	30 minutes
Eastbourne General Hospital	45 minutes
Redhill Hospital	1 hour
Chichester Hospital	1 hour
Hastings Conquest Hospital	1 hour

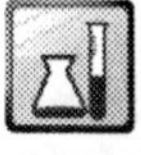

The medical school

Work						Good work life balance
Facilities						Many computer clusters, libraries on Sussex and Brighton campuses
Support						Small, personal environment. Personal tutor, clinical academic tutor, and student parent scheme provide great support
Feedback						Limited feedback on exams/projects, but usually available if requested

Facilities

The medical school on campus has a very large computer cluster for medical students, and shares clinical labs with Sussex Biomedical departments. There is no shortage of computer clusters available on either Brighton or Sussex campuses. The lecture theatres and seminar rooms on both campuses are less than seven years old, with state of the art AV systems.

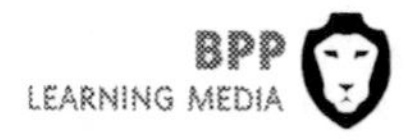

Student support

Being small and new, the environment at BSMS is friendly, personal and supportive. Each student has a personal Academic Tutor in years 1 and 2, and a Clinical Academic Tutor for years 3 to 5. As well as that, it is easy to build up good supportive relationships with many of the tutors and consultants involved with teaching, and most are more than happy to offer help, guidance, support, and advocacy if necessary. While the traditional hierarchical relationships in Medicine are still important at BSMS, consultants and tutors seem to make a point of being more approachable than perhaps at other universities. Both Sussex and Brighton universities have chaplaincies, and UNISEX provides a drop-in sexual health service.

Finance

BSMS students are included in the University of Brighton's bursary scheme, worth from £540 to £1,080 per year to those whose family income is £40,330 or less. All third and fourth year students will receive from £200 to £650, depending on means, to assist with the longer terms in those years. The University of Sussex's bursary scheme is inapplicable, but you may apply for a University of Sussex Chancellor's scholarship.

Student opinion

'BSMS is special in a number of ways. Its size makes it more personal, between fellow students and also the faculty. Its young age means that the course reflects the aims of the GMC's Tomorrow's Doctors publication, and it is constantly being refined and adapted. The fact that it belongs to two universities means that extra-curricular opportunities are doubled, though sometimes more disjointed. Brighton itself has been voted the best place to be a student in recent years, for very good reason. You won't be bored here.'

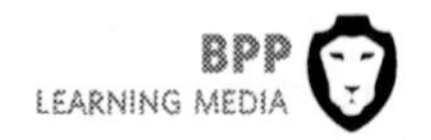

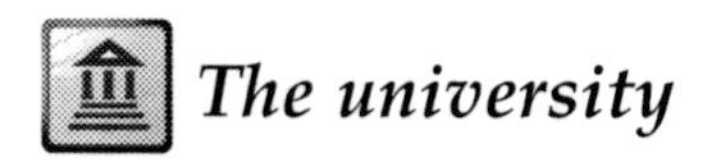

Accommodation	Campus halls of residence
Further Info	www.ussu.info/

Accommodation

Halls of residence are located on the Falmer campus of Brighton or Sussex Universities. Both are about 5-10 minutes' walk across campus to the medical school. Brighton halls are mostly only a few years old and of very good standard, consisting of approximately six students in each complex with shared living space, kitchen, bathrooms – some are en-suite.

Sussex has a wide range of accommodation, differing in type, price and quality. Lewes Court are the nicest halls but are furthest from the medical school and most expensive. Lancaster House, York House and Kent House consist of corridors with basic shared kitchens / bathrooms. Park Village and East Slope are the cheapest. There are also brand new blocks of accommodation. The Sussex campus has better bars and shops, and more green space.

Study facilities

Sussex University library is the biggest library in South East England. The medics use the university libraries for reference and studying, and can find many of the books on the reading lists at them. Sussex library is open 24 hours a day, which is handy for late night revising as exams approach!

Students' union

If there is an area Brighton and Sussex Universities were lacking when we were there, it was a huge student union area. The problem is that with Brighton so close and student friendly, if students want to go out anywhere they can just go into Brighton and they are spoilt for choice. Brighton university students' union offers a number of exciting student nights (www.ubsu.net). Sussex University has several bars and a club called The Cube.

Student opinion

'Our first two years at BSMS followed the age old 'work hard play hard' mentality often taken by medical students. BSMS has an exceedingly well thought out curriculum and enthusiastic teaching staff, making the work easier to do and more enjoyable. As BSMS is a small medical school, you soon get to know everyone so often large groups of medics hit Brighton at the same time. Brighton is one of the most accepting and diverse places you could go for university, with exciting experiences waiting around every corner.'

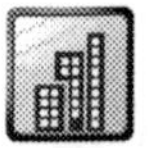

The city

Safety	🛡	🛡	🛡	🛡		Brighton is safe and people are friendly, though there is crime like in any city
Nightlife	☽	☽	☽	☽	☽	Brighton has some of the best nightlife in the UK, catering for all tastes
Transport	🚌	🚌				Cycling is the best option, but car maybe useful in the fifth year
Cost of Living	🐖	🐖	🐖	🐖	🐖	Living is expensive, rent = £65–100/week

Things to do

With two universities in the city, the student nightlife is huge and after five years you can still find new places to go and bands and DJs to see. There are a number of clubs along the seafront, and pubs and bars line almost every street even in most of the residential areas. Safety is not usually an issue to be worried about. There are three cinemas (including an arthouse one with homemade carrot cake!), and shoppers are well catered for: North Laine and South Lanes offering something different from the usual high street options. Life can be expensive in Brighton, so you have to budget well.

Famous attractions include Brighton Pier, the Sealife Centre, and of course, the beach! These are great from one point of view, but

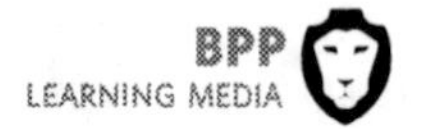

it does mean that the city is crowded with tourists as soon as the summer season starts, which can be tiring (but mean it's not hard to find a job for some extra cash!). For those who like to get out of the city, the surrounding countryside (including the Downs) is easily accessible by car or train for days out to clear your head.

Places to go		
Place	**Brief Description**	**Entry Fee/Opening Time**
Concorde 2	Big club away from the centre, hosts big names	£6-12, Mon-Thur 10.00pm-1.00am, Fri-Sat 10.00pm-5.00am
Honey Club	Famous seafront dance club	£3-6, Mon-Sat 10.00pm-2.00am
Rikitiks	Bar in the centre, good Thai food too	£Free, Mon-Sun 11.00am-1.00am
Audio	Basement club with cocktail bar upstairs	£Free-£8, Mon-Sat 10.00pm-2.00am

Student opinion

'Brighton is a great place to be a student – trying to balance all the nights out and days on the beach or in town with such a challenging course certainly improved my time-management skills! I wouldn't have it any other way though as there's never a dull moment.'

Student's view

Pre-clinical

'The BSMS timetable is based around lectures, and I spent much of my first two years trying to frantically remember as much as I could in lectures to minimise the amount of work that needed to be done in my own time. I had always had a lot of extra-curricular activities (as do most med students) before uni and I wanted to keep these up, along with being able to go out and have a good time and make new friends.

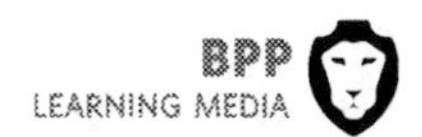

Fortunately, with basic time management skills it is easy to do this. Doing a little bit of work when you have the time to slot it in saves you from having to do massive amounts when deadlines come in and your mate's birthday is tonight and you really need to get out and have a good time etc. Birthdays are fantastic, with about 140 people on the course you can be expecting a birthday every few days, and as this is quite a small number of people to be spending these years with, you know most people pretty well so expect many good times!

Our first two years at BSMS followed the age old 'work hard play hard' mentality often taken by medical students. BSMS has an exceedingly well thought out curriculum and enthusiastic teaching staff, making the work easier go do and more enjoyable. As BSMS is a small medical school, you soon get to know everyone and often large groups of medics it Brighton at the same time. Brighton is one of the most accepting and diverse places you could go for university, with exciting experiences waiting around every corner.'

Clinical

'The third and fourth years remain a balanced mix of lectures and clinical experience. Clinical lectures are normally in groups of around 20, while scientific and General Practice lectures happen once a week with the whole year group. It can be crowded on ward rounds and free clinics are sometimes hard to come by, but the minimum requirements are always timetabled.

The third year rotations are pretty full on and the exams are hard, but the clinical experience gained during the year is a highlight, and you can look forward to your elective at the end of it. Prepare yourself for earlier starts, a full five-day week, and some on-call sessions. This was a tiring year, but in many ways it was also the best part of the course as we could really get stuck in to the practical side of Medicine and start interacting with patients on a daily basis. By the end of the year your confidence in talking to patients, taking structured histories, and considering differential diagnoses will have improved dramatically. You also get many opportunities to gain experience in practical procedures such as taking blood, examining patients, and assisting in theatre.

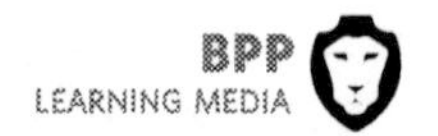

The fourth year allows more time for self study, particularly on your research project, but clinical exposure is reduced as you are only on rotation for three days a week. At this point you have to learn to manage your own time and motivate yourself well, or you can fly through without gaining as much as you should. General Practice is a key focus of this year (with lectures, a placement, an essay assignment, and an exam) and this encourages a different approach to the hospital-based model.

The final year is perhaps the most enjoyable clinically, as your experience increases 100-fold and the teaching over the last few years finally starts to fall into place! The chance to practise medicine in different hospitals, to meet students from other medical schools, and to take on a bit more responsibility while also revising for finals allows you to prepare yourself for life as a Foundation doctor.'

Once you get in...

Make sure you sign up to the Medsoc as they organise all of your events and belonging to Medsoc gives you discounts on all these events, saving you money fast! Then again, we may be a little biased, as we were the social secretaries for Medsoc in our second year, planning all the events.

Use the freshers' guides you get in the post to think about what you may enjoy. There are non-alcoholic alternatives to major events and contacting flatmates by facebook is always a good way to start to get to know what you are expecting and help you feel a little less nervous!

The first week seems a bit daunting as you have to go to lectures at the same time as having a freshers' week, but they are nothing too difficult and this is nothing to worry about, many med schools seem to do it, unfortunately.

The Best Thing	Enthusiastic teaching
The Worst Thing	Expense

Student top tip

BSMS is the first medical school in the UK to integrate personal digital assistants (PDAs) into undergraduate teaching.

Summary Table

Positives	Negatives
Supportive environment	Fairly high living costs
Modern course, appropriate to tomorrow's doctors	Crowded hospital
Individual research project	Lack of parking
Brighton city – all the bars, restaurants, etc	Lots of one-way streets!

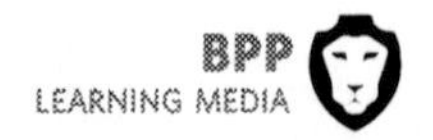

Bristol

University of Bristol
Centre for Medical Education
39-41 St Michael's Hill
Bristol
BS2 8DZ

www.medici.bris.ac.uk/

Once the home of pirate ships and Wills' Tobacco, Bristol is famous for Banksy's street art and its stunning architecture such as the Clifton Suspension Bridge. Bristol University celebrated its centenary year in 2009 and both the city and medical school have seen money invested in new buildings and facilities. Bristol is one of the oldest medical schools in the country and prides itself on both its modern facilities and academic excellence. The medical school offers a traditional course with a strong history and excellent anatomy teaching. The city and surrounding areas make Bristol a brilliant place to be a student with lots of things to see and do in the green Southwest. The city itself is compact with most attractions within walking distance of the university precinct and this helps to build a strong student community. The numerous hills and large open spaces are ideal for those who are keen on keeping fit and Bristol features numerous sports clubs and societies.

Bristol boasts modern appeal against a background of rich history and the medical school offers a traditional course in a friendly and relaxed setting.

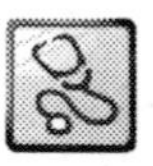

The medical course

Key facts

Course Type	Traditional	Degree Awarded	MBChB
Basic Entry Requirements	AAB	Entrance Exams	None

Year Size	216	**Open Days**	End of June and end of September
Admissions Website	www.bristol.ac.uk/study/		

Getting in – student tips

Bristol looks for a personal statement demonstrating a realistic interest in Medicine, a commitment to helping others, a wide range of interests, a contribution to school / college / community activities and a range of personal achievements (excluding exams).

Bristol has particular focus on social medicine with one of the country's leading epidemiological departments.

All students will be interviewed for a place at Bristol. The interview panel consists of two interviewers from clinical and medical science departments within the university, local hospitals and GP practices.

Bristol interviewers often ask typical questions, for example, why do you want to be a doctor? Why do you want to study Medicine? Why do you want to come to Bristol? Together with ethical scenarios and interesting points from your personal statement, interviewers are looking for your reasons for wanting to study Medicine, awareness of current developments, an ability to communicate, self-confidence, enthusiasm, determination to study and an ability to cope with stress. Gap year students are favoured provided they can show that it has been beneficial.

Course details

Foundation / Pre-Med	Yes	**Graduate**	Yes
Student Population	Male: female ratio: 40:60	**Term Length**	Pre-clinical: 10 weeks Clinical: 15 weeks
Erasmus / Foreign Exchange	Erasmus European exchange possible in Year 3	**Elective Period**	End of year 5 (March) 8 weeks

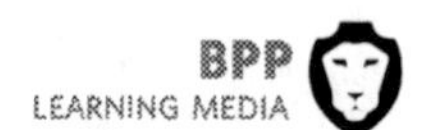

Intercalation

Stage	Usually after year 2 but possible after years 3 and 4	**Degree Awarded**	BSc or BA
Requirements	Usually need to be in the top 40% of the year group, but exceptions can be made	**Subjects**	Anatomical Science, Biochemistry, Bioethics, Cellular & Molecular Medicine, Pharmacology, Physiology, International Health, Medical Humanities and Neuroscience

Anatomy teaching

Three hours of anatomy teaching each week in the first and second year with cadaveric prosections in the dissection rooms. Trainee surgeons prepare the prosections. There is 1.5 hours of small group (six to ten people) teaching around cadavers or isolated organs. The teaching is interactive, enthusiastic and covers all you need to know. The remaining 1.5 hours of teaching is done in the anatomy suite. Here one can look at further prosections, use computer assisted learning and learn more independently. Bristol medical students do not feel they miss out by not doing dissection. Well prosected cadavers allow more time for learning and there is an anatomy dissection Student Selected Component in the second year for those with a keen interest in dissection.

Pre-clinical/Years 1–2	
Topics	***Year 1:*** Molecular and cellular basis of medicine and Human basis of medicine. ***Year 2:*** Systems of the body.
Teaching	Lectures, small group tutorials, online tutorials, GP Visits.
SSC Periods	***Year 1:*** No SSC. ***Year 2:*** A written library project and a choice of options from learning a foreign language to a dissection project.
Exams	Multiple Choice Questions (Negatively Marked), Extended Matching Questions, Short Answer Questions and anatomy spot tests in January and June. 50% pass mark.

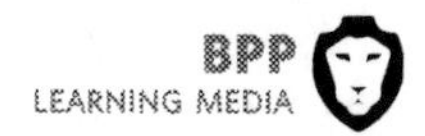

Clinical/Years 3–5	
Topics	***Year 3:*** Hospital Medicine & Surgery Attachments, Orthopaedics, ENT, Emergency Medicine, Ophthalmology, Psychiatry, and Ethics. ***Year 4:*** Obstetrics & Gynaecology, Pathology, Anaesthetics, Paediatrics, General Practice, Care of the Elderly, Dermatology.
Elective	Offered at the end of year 5 after finals.
SSC Periods	There is a four-week SSC period at the end of the third year. This is a fantastic opportunity to complete an audit, research project or get published.
Exams	MCQs (Negatively Marked), EMQs , OSCE, OSLER. 50% pass mark. There are no re-sits for Finals, students failing any component (written, long case, OSCE/DOSCE) are required to re-sit the entire year.

Hospital placements/academies

Placements last eight weeks and consist of around ten students attached to a specialty with time divided up between ward work, theatres, clinics and doctor-led teaching sessions. Accommodation is provided for students on site where necessary and ranges from modern en-suite bedrooms, at Swindon, Taunton and Gloucester to basic hospital digs at Bath and Yeovil.

All hospitals feature undergraduate academies where undergraduate co-ordinators organise teaching and help students with any problems. All academies have a library, IT, common rooms and clinical skills rooms with Bath, Taunton and Bristol having particularly excellent facilities for students.

Bristol Royal Infirmary and Bristol Children's Hospital are keen to get students involved in audits and research and Frenchay has a large plastic surgery department where consultants are keen to take students interested in plastics for SSC periods.

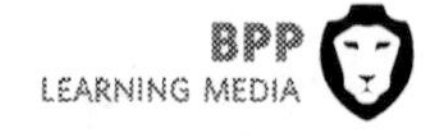

Hospitals and Travel Time from University	
Bristol Royal Infirmary	3 minutes
Southmead Hospital	10 minutes
Frenchay Hospital	15 minutes
Weston Hospital	45 minutes
RUH Bath	50 minutes
Gloucester Hospital	1 hour
Cheltenham General	1 hour
Musgrove Park Taunton	1 hour
Swindon Hospital	1 hour
Yeovil Hospital	1 hour 15 minutes

The medical school

Work	●	●	●	●		Work life balance good until exam periods
Facilities	●	●	●	●	●	Medical library
Support	●	●				Parent system for first year but support during exam periods can be poor
Feedback	●	●				Poor feedback on examinations

Facilities

The medical school features a medical library, complete with coffee shops and IT facilities. There is a student common room with fantastic views overlooking the city. There are two main lecture theatres: E29 located in the medical school and St. Michael's Hill 1.4, which also contains small tutorial rooms. There is also a simulation suite, clinical skills lab and histology lab for teaching practical skills.

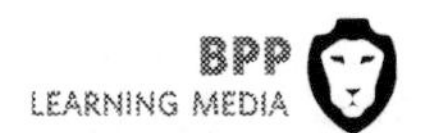

Student support

Galenicals, the Bristol Medical School society, named after the famous Greek physician Galen, organises regular social events and careers evenings for students. Scrubs, Bristol's surgical society, is ideal for those with a keen interest in surgery and offers suturing workshops and surgical careers evenings. There is a range of medical sports teams including football, rugby, cricket, netball, hockey and cheerleading. Galenicals has a fantastic relationship with Nantes University, France and every two years there is a tour to Nantes for all the medical sports teams. Every other year Bristol hosts Nantes. Most of the sports teams also participate in NAMS, which is the national medical sports tournament. Furthermore Bristol has links with numerous other university medical sports teams. There is also a strong musical theme with a medics' choir and string orchestra.

There is a pre-clinical and clinical review each year put on by the medical students. This is a play which satirises the lecturers, and is a must see for all medical students.

Famous across the whole university is the medic strip-show Clicendales that annually raises around £10,000 for the Clic Sergeant charity.

Finance

The university offers bursary packages of up to £1,135 a year. Top-up bursaries of £1,025 a year are available to local students and a variety of scholarships are also offered.

> **Student opinion**
>
> *'The new facilities, enthusiastic lecturers and social events make the pre-clinical years absolutely amazing.'*

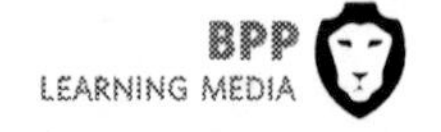

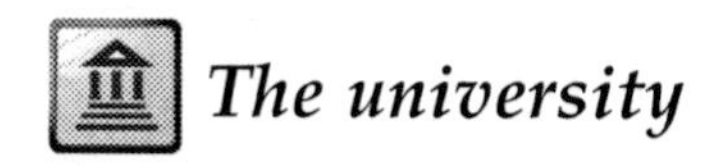

The university

Accommodation	First years: non-campus halls of residence
Further Info	www.bristol.ac.uk/study/ www.bristol.ac.uk/accommodation/ www.ubu.org.uk/

Accommodation

Most first years live in halls of residence in either Stoke Bishop or Clifton. Stoke Bishop is a good 30 to 40-minute walk to the medical school across the Downs', whereas Clifton is around a 20-minute walk to the medical school. There is also less popular accommodation just a few minutes' walk from the medical school. Student areas of the city include Redland and Clifton where the majority of students rent properties.

Study facilities

The two main university libraries are the Arts and Social Sciences Library and the Law Library, housed in the incredible Wills' Memorial building. Bristol also has a 24-hour computer lab for when the libraries close. As previously mentioned the medics have their own refurbished library.

University sports & students' union

Despite being housed in an unattractive, concrete building the union features regular live music and the re-launched Bar 100. The union is not the centre of Bristol students' socialising, (although it is one of the stops on the annual medical school pub crawl!) however it is a large building and completes its function providing rooms for all the university societies. There are plans to build a new union in the future. A university sports pass grants access to the Pulse fitness suite and swimming pool. The gym is relatively small and can get very busy at peak times.

Wednesday afternoons are kept free for sport and most teams train at the Coombe Dingle sports complex. The university has strong rugby, waterpolo and rowing teams.

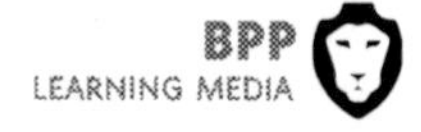

Student opinion

'I was in Wills' Hall, the place was amazing with beautiful buildings and grounds. Wills' and Churchill were the most popular though all the halls are fun and run brilliant social events.'

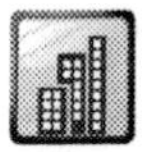 *The city*

Safety	🛡	🛡	🛡	🛡		Bristol is a generally safe city for students
Nightlife	☾	☾	☾	☾		The majority of clubs and bars are located in the Triangle area and Park Street
Transport	🚌	🚌	🚌			Parking can be a nightmare but a car is very useful for clinical years
Cost of Living	🐖	🐖				Expect to pay around £350 pm for rent

Things to do

Bristol has a rich history and features many beautiful buildings. The city itself is compact with most shops, bars and areas of interest located in close proximity. This makes for a small, community atmosphere in what is in fact a major city. For shopping the recently constructed Cabot Circus in the city centre houses boutique shops, restaurants and a cinema complex. Bristol Hippodrome features theatrical performances and the Bristol O2 Academy regularly hosts famous bands.

During the summer months students are known to relax and socialise in one of the many parks and grass expanses in Bristol and the surrounding areas of the South West offer days out. Bristol Zoo and waterfront make for great trips as does Bath Spa.

For those who enjoy a night out Bristol has a vibrant collection of bars, clubs and pubs. The standard is Lizard Lounge located on the Triangle and frequented by most of the university. There are numerous small pubs and bars throughout the city with the

White Lion at the Avon Gorge Hotel offering spectacular views of Clifton Suspension Bridge.

Places to Go		
Place	**Brief Description**	**Entry Fee/Opening Time**
Lizard Lounge	Popular club on The Triangle	£3; Mon-Thur 10.00pm-3.00am
Syndicate	Superclub located in Broadmead	£5; Wed & Fri 10.00pm-3.00am
Thekla	Club located on a boat	£3; Mon, Thur, Fri 10.00pm-3.00am
Mr Wolf's	Cool bar with live music	£Free; Wed-Sat 6.00pm-4.00am

Student opinion

'Bristol is incredibly beautiful and is a huge contrast to most city universities. There is loads to do and the new shops at Cabot Circus are fantastic.'

Student's view

Pre-clinical

'The first year focuses on the Human and Molecular Basis of Medicine with lectures given by enthusiastic, knowledgeable lecturers. Bristol has a strong anatomy department and we are fortunate enough to have Dr Alice Roberts (of Time Team, Coast and Dr Alice Roberts: Don't Die Young) teaching.

Work-life balance is excellent with Wednesday afternoons kept free for sport and most days lasting from 9.00am to 5.00pm. A typical day begins with the 40-minute walk from halls alongside numerous other students discussing the events of the night before. Lectures begin at 9.00am in the medical school and usually last 50 minutes to one hour with an hour break for lunch. Lunch can be bought in the medical school or from one of the cafes on St Michael's Hill or if you are really organised you can bring your own. Afternoons are either more lectures or small group teaching with tutors.

In the second year most afternoons are free for Student Selected Components. Examinations can be tough with negatively marked multiple-choice questions and feedback from exams is fairly poor. If you learn the lectures as you go along and work through the online tutorials you will encounter little difficulty.

I found that Bristol Medical School appreciated that getting a medical degree is not just about learning Medicine. It also makes sure you enjoy life 'as a normal student' as much as possible with so many societies covering all areas of interests and lots of well attended social events. My highlights of pre-clinical years include winning BUSA with Bristol University Rowing Club, Clicendales, the most incredible medics Christmas party and the sports tour to Nantes.'

Clinical

'The clinical years comprise eight-week hospital placements in various specialties at hospitals around the South West. It is particularly enjoyable working in areas such as Bath and Taunton, however, being placed in Yeovil for eight weeks can be pretty lonely. Holidays are reduced with terms now lasting 15 weeks leaving two weeks for Christmas, one week for Easter and four weeks for summer vacation.

A normal day consists of attending an 8.00am or 9.00am ward round followed by morning ward work with the F1 doctor till lunch. Ward work consists of taking blood, putting in cannulas, taking patient histories and chasing up request forms. Lunch is usually taken in the Doctors' Mess or canteen and then the afternoon may be spent in clinics, back on the wards or in a teaching session with the other students.

The majority of the surrounding hospitals are keen to involve students and most F1s are friendly and helpful.

Personal highlights from the clinical years include enjoying morning coffee with Mo the academy co-ordinator in Bath, spending time in

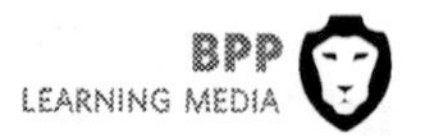

theatres with eager consultants and being taught by the enigmatic Professor Andy Levy at Bristol Royal Infirmary.'

Postgraduate

'I was 34 years old, working in the armed forces and enjoying the experience. At the same time, I was involved with Medicine through voluntary work in the Ambulance Service. I read a magazine talking about being a mature doctor and that set me thinking. I took a deep breath and went for the plunge and, before I knew it, I was sitting in the lecture theatre surrounded by lots of young students.

You hit the ground running on the Bristol 2in1 course, with lectures from both the first and second years crammed in to the first year, reducing the five-year course to just four years. The modular systems-based learning suited me and I got on well with the lectures that, on the whole, were good. It was 'big boys' rules' as you were left to yourself to sort out timetable clashes and catch up on missed learning. The days were full, but well laid out in the first year. However in the final term, when lectures started to clash, I remember running downstairs to set up a sound recording in a lecture theatre and then running upstairs to attend another lecture; catching up on the recording in the evening. As a group, our 2in1 group worked well in supporting each other and that made a huge difference. We were told from the outset that we had to work out a lot on our own and it was certainly the case. Teamwork was essential. Once in the clinical years, you followed the course the same as the other students.

I really enjoyed the learning experience and would recommend the Bristol graduate scheme.'

Once you get in...

Expect to be sent a packet containing a lot of documents. The first piece of information will be about choosing halls of residence. You will get information on what all the halls are like and you will be required to make a first and second choice on where you would like to live.

You will also get information on the sports facilities. If you are going to join the university gym it is best to sort this out now saving you time when you arrive at the university. Another tip is to try to book your induction to the gym as soon as possible, as these get booked up very quickly. You can book an induction by going to the reception at the gym.

The union will send you a booklet on the societies and clubs that you may wish to join. This is worth reading so you know if there are any particular stalls you want to visit at the freshers' fair. It also has a lot of helpful tips on what to bring to university, and how to make freshers' week less hectic.

Galenicals will send you a helpful booklet about the medical school and how to join the society before you get to university.

Finally you will receive a Fresher's' Week timetable from the medical school. This will help you to know what you will be doing, and what lectures you will need to attend and where you are meant to be.

The Best Thing	Relaxed atmosphere and enthusiastic teaching
The Worst Thing	Lack of feedback and support during exam period

Student top tips

- Take your autograph book as Justin Lee-Collins and the cast of Skins can often be seen wandering the streets.
- Get your Freshers' Ball ticket, gym membership and Galenicals membership before you get to Bristol to save time and effort.
- Get your gym induction sorted early on to avoid delay.
- Don't join a society straight away at the freshers' fair; sign up and give details but do not hand over a cheque until you are absolutely sure you will go to the society, otherwise you will waste a lot of money!

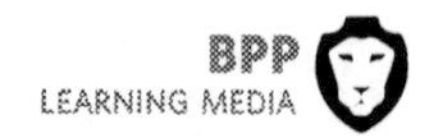

Summary Table

Positives	Negatives
Strong anatomy teaching	Poor feedback on exams
Fun, relaxed atmosphere	Minimal support during exam periods
Galenicals social events	Small university gym
Enthusiastic teaching	Lack of parking
Beautiful city and surrounding areas	Lots of steep hills

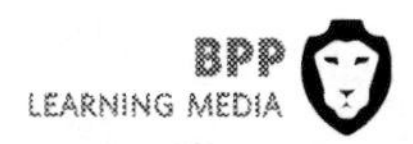

Cambridge

University of Cambridge School of Clinical Medicine
Addenbrooke's Hospital,
Box 111
Hills Road
Cambridge
CB2 0SP

www.medschl.cam.ac.uk

The University of Cambridge can trace its history to 1209 when scholars fled from hostile townsmen in Oxford. 800 years later Cambridge is recognised as one of the top teaching and research institutions in the world. Many great medical discoveries were made here; for instance the structure of DNA by James Watson and Francis Crick. The picture that most people have of Cambridge, of its beautiful Colleges, the beautiful river Cam, and its age old customs, is indeed real. For a student studying in this unique city, Cambridge will also be some of the best years of their lives. The medical course in Cambridge is very traditional, and is separated into pre-clinical and clinical stages. The strength of the Cambridge course is that it places great emphasis on the scientific basis behind clinical medicine. This ensures that not only will well trained doctors graduate from Cambridge, but that they will perhaps contribute to the constant advances in medicine. A defining feature of the Cambridge course is the use of supervisions. Supervisions are personalised teaching sessions given to groups of two to four students by academics who will be experts in their field. They allow students to check that they understand the core material, as well as to discuss any topics of interest in greater depth.

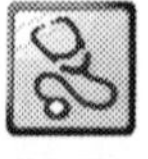

The medical course

Key facts

Course Type	Traditional	Degree Awarded	MB BChir
Basic Entry Requirements	AAA	Entrance Exams	BMAT

Year Size	330	Open Days	Start of July
Admissions Website	www.medschl.cam.ac.uk/education/prospective/		

Getting in – student tips

The official and also generally true assertion is that Cambridge picks you based on your academic ability alone – specifically, in science. Those not offering three science A levels are expected to show the equivalent ability and having just one science is a serious disability, although not technically a bar to success.

This ability is primarily judged by A level predictions, BMAT score, and your performance at interview.

Course details

Foundation / Pre-Med	No	Graduate	Yes, approx 20 places
Student Population	Male: female ratio: 50:50	Term Length	Pre-clinical: 8 weeks Clinical: 15 Weeks
Erasmus / Foreign Exchange	Up to three places for a one year exchange with the Massachusetts Institute of Technology in Year 3	Elective Period	Start of Year 5 7 weeks July-August

Intercalation

Stage	Year 3	Degree Awarded	BA Hons
Requirements	Madatory, graduate students cannot intercalate	Subjects	Biological Anthology, Biochemistry; Genetics; History and Philosophy of Science; Mechanisms of disease; Neuroscience; Pathology; Pharmacology; Psychology; Physiology & Psychology; Physiology, Development, & Neuroscience. A small number of students take other non biological subjects such as Linguistics, Management Studies or Philosophy

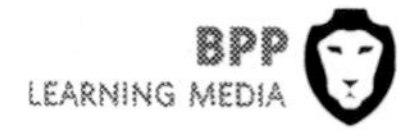

Anatomy teaching

Anatomy teaching is intensive and thorough: students attend four hours of practical classes a week and learn using dissection on cadavers. This allows the whole of human anatomy to be covered in Year 1. Students also learn from models and prosections. Students are supervised by demonstrators, who are usually retired or trainee surgeons. There are usually around only six students on each dissection table. This is supplemented by three anatomy lectures a week. A unique feature of the Cambridge course are the weekly supervisions-students are given small group teaching (two to four students) to facilitate a greater understanding in the theory behind Anatomy. At the end of every term there are mock practical exams called 'steeplechases'. In additions students attend a two hour seminar every two weeks which covers clinical procedures that link in with the lectures and dissection. This system of teaching ensures that all students will be prepared for the challenging end of year Anatomy exams as well as for their clinical studies.

Pre-clinical/Years 1–2	
Topics	***Year 1:*** Functional Architechure of the Body – or Anatomy – Biochemistry and physiology are also studied, though similarly under a different name. Small exams cover statistics/epidemiology and social medicine. ***Year 2:*** Diseases, drugs, reproduction, and neuroscience are covered, again under their own unique headings. ***Throughout*:** Preparing for patients gives various patient contact and discussion opportunities, and PBL sessions fit into the main subjects. As a traditional course, neither are substantial.
Teaching	The teaching is in part supervision (generally very small groups in one-hour sessions with the relevant fellow at your college) – which is very variable and not necessarily on topic, but a valuable opportunity, with the rest made up of lectures and practical sessions in all the subjects.
SSC Periods	There are no SSCs in the pre-clinical years, other than the intercalated BA which is free choice.
Exams	Examinations are an arcane process leading to what is called 'Exemption from 2nd MB' and with funny marks distributions all part of the 'Tripos', (what Cambridge calls the degree course). The larger exams are at the end of the year with pass-marks (and so numbers failing) set by each department.

Clinical/Years 3–5	
Topics	***Year 4:*** Clinical Introductory Course, Hospital General Medicine and General Surgery, SSC, General Practice, Law and Ethics, Public Health. ***Year 5:*** Paediatrics, Obstetrics and Gynaecology, Neurology, Rheumatology, Orthopaedics, Psychiatry, Oncology, Infectious Diseases, Cardio-thoracic medicine, General Practice, Law and Ethics, Public Health. ***Year 6:*** Elective, SSC, Acute Care, ENT, Dermatology, Ophthalmology, Care of the Elderly, Radiology, Palliative Care.
Elective	Students are free to choose any medical institution in the world, provided it is safe. Up to three destinations are permitted. Thus students may go to developing countries and then head off to one of the prestigious American medical schools. Electives are usually clinical but they can be research-based. A 1,000 word report must be submitted. Prizes and limited funding are available from the medical school. Funding may be available from some colleges.
SSC Periods	There is a five-week SSC in Year 4 and a four-week SSC takes place in Year 6. A wide range of SSCs from many specialties are on offer, which may be clinical or lab-based in nature. SSCs are usually restricted to the East Anglia region. Topics are highly varied ranging from Cardiothoracic surgery to Spanish. Some students undertake audits and research projects. However non medical related SSCs such as languages are equally popular and students are also encouraged to organise their own. An example of a popular SSC is Medical Law. Last year some students had the chance to attend GMC disciplinary meetings.
Exams	Objective Structured Clinical Examinations, Multiple Choice Questions, Extended Matching Questions, essay questions and data interpretation. Exams take place after at the end of Year 4, 5 and 6 and after some specialty attachments. The Pathology exams in Year 5 are notoriously difficult. Several students resit these exams. For Finals, students must repeat the year if they fail a clinical exam or more than one written paper, otherwise resits are possible.

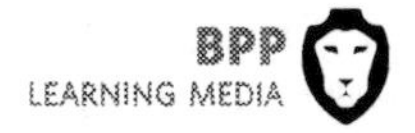

Hospital placements/academies

Depending on the clinical year, placements last from five to nine weeks. Accommodation is situated close to the hospitals and varies a lot between placements. In general it is basic but satisfactory. Ipswich and West Suffolk boast four bedroom flats with Wi-Fi, a kitchen stocked with utensils and a shower, while Hinchingbrooke and Bedford are more basic with no internet. However the Clinical School is constantly reviewing the quality of accommodation. Addenbrooke's Hospital is part of the Cambridge Bio-Medical Campus, one of the largest medical research centres in Europe, making it a popular choice for students when it comes to SSCs. Ipswich is always a favourite due to a combination of lot of organised teaching and a great Doctor's Mess that boasts its own bar!

Hospitals and Travel Time from University	
Addenbrooke's Hospital	15 minutes
Papworth Hospital	25 minutes
Hinchingbrooke Hospital	40 minutes
West Suffolk Hospital	40 minutes
Peterborough District Hospital	55 minutes
Bedford Hospital	55 minutes
Luton & Dunstable Hospital	1 hour 15 minutes
The Queen Elizabeth Hospital King's Lynn	1 hour 15 minutes
Cross University Hospital	1 hour 15 minutes
Ipswich Hospital Whipps	1 hour 30 minutes

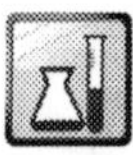

The medical school

Work						Work load is often full on
Facilities						The medical school is extensively equipped to maximise learning
Support						College supervisors and tutors ensure there is constant support
Feedback						Brief regular feedback is provided

Facilities

At the pre-clinical stage students are taught by individual subject departments, and as such there is no pre-clinical department of Medicine. Facilities are therefore provided by these departments and the Colleges. At the clinical stage there is the Clinical School which is located next to Addenbrooke's Hospital. The heart of the Clinical School is the Sherwood Room, where the clinical students relax. It boasts a pool table, table tennis, table football, computers, a widescreen TV and plenty of sofas. Next door there's a very small café, seminar rooms and lecture theatres. The Medical School library is located upstairs. The library is very large and meets all learning and postgraduate research needs. There are several modern IT suites of which two are dedicated for medical students. The Clinical Skills Centre is located over in the hospital and is accessible 24 hours a day.

Student support

At the pre-clinical stage, students will meet up twice a term with their College Tutor (a non-medical academic) and their College director of studies (a medical academic) to discuss their progress. They are the first point of call if students have a problem and students are also free to 'drop in' at regular times. On a more informal level most Colleges have a College family system. Freshers are given parents whom provide academic advice but are usually more proactive in organising socials! At the clinical stage students are adopted by a new Clinical School family. Clinical School supervisors provide weekly bedside teaching to small groups of students and often they are invaluable when it comes to academic problems. Otherwise most Colleges have a chaplaincy and a health centre and there is also a University Counselling Service.

Finance

Cambridge offers some of the most generous financial support schemes of any university. The Cambridge Bursary Scheme offers bursaries for UK students of up to £3,250 per year. The amount depends on parental income and there is no limit to the number of these bursaries. There are also bursaries for graduates and international students and there are additional hardship funds and scholarships offered by the Colleges.

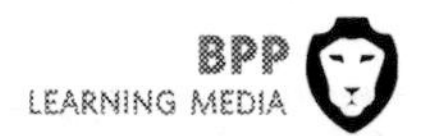

Student opinion

'My first few years here were intense, in terms of balancing the truly world class course with an equally intensive schedule of socialising in College and playing sports.'

The university

Accommodation	First years all in college
Further Info	www.cam.ac.uk

Accommodation

Accommodation is one of those things that varies hugely by College. On the plus side they all will rent you a place to stay for every year at Cambridge, no rent payable on holidays and a reasonably wide choice in the later years. First years are generally in College, so a matter of metres away, but the College itself might be nearer or further from the medical teaching.

Study facilities

There are too many libraries to visit at Cambridge, with normally at least one per major subject, one per College, one often in any large teaching facility, plus the University Library and more. They are all normally accessible but the nearest will mostly have what you want. IT is well integrated and while a lot of people use their own computers, some don't use them at all and some make great use of the facilities available at each college, which are normally fine.

University sports & students' union

The Cambridge University student union does exist and runs club nights, deals with some admissions/welfare issues, and has a significant role in university government. However College student unions are more important to the day-to-day student life and these tend to run the College bars, events, and so forth. As the people running them changes yearly, the good ones that have a lot on aren't always the same – but in most cases all students make good use of other College's provisions. There is no main sports centre for Cambridge and this is a bit of a bugbear; however there are sports clubs for most things and they use public facilities or get their own from somewhere. The athletics club does have a good track and of course rowing is a big thing here with most Colleges having a sizable boathouse and fielding a few teams of considerably variable ability.

Student opinion

'Cambridge is a great place to study – with world-leading academics, research, and teaching facilities, it more than deserves its good reputation, and a heavy academic focus – while sometimes tiring – can really push you to achieve. However it's also a great place to be apart from all that. The atmosphere, the buildings, the fact that there are countless bars and/or churches within about five minutes from anywhere and countless students in between mean that you are surrounded but the separation into Colleges means you can also feel at home and manage to get to know all of your year!'

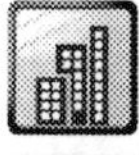

The city

Safety	🛡	🛡	🛡	🛡		The city has a reputation of being safe
Nightlife	☾	☾				There are only a handful of clubs in Cambridge
Transport	🚌	🚌	🚌	🚌		Departments are within walking or cycling distance from the centre. Bus services are very good, although owning a car will be very convenient for clinical attachments
Cost of Living	🐖	🐖				Rent varies from £89 to £130 per week

Things to do

Cambridge is a beautiful city intertwined with a rich history, and as a result it is a magnet for tourists from around the world. The city is unique in that the university and its Colleges are the main tourist attraction. King's College Chapel is world famous and seen as the symbol of Cambridge. Punting is popular among students who want to enjoy a relaxing trip down the River Cam, enabling them to appreciate the beauty of the Cambridge Colleges and various historical bridges, each with their own story. Cambridge has recently opened the 'Grand Arcade' a much needed shopping mall in the city centre. This complements nicely the range of existing restaurants and coffee shops located conveniently in the small city centre. Since Cambridge is a very compact city, students will find that nowhere is further than a 25-minute walk away on foot in the city! Students frequently visit the Corn Exchange, ADC theatre, or the Cambridge Arts Centre to take advantage of the diverse performances on offer. At night students generally socialise in their own College bars. Colleges host regular student nights known as ents which are a fantastic way for medics to meet other students. The city nightlife is lively but limited. Perhaps the most popular club is Ballare which students go to on Tuesday and Wednesday nights. There are student nights on most days of the week but oddly, there are not any student club nights on Friday or Saturdays. Otherwise students can attend formal hall on most nights at a College. By and large Cambridge is a safe city, but it is not without its alcohol related violence at night.

Places to go		
Place	**Brief Description**	**Entry Fee/Opening Time**
Ballare	Popular club, also known as 'Cindies'	£4.50: Mon-Sun 10.00pm-3.00am
Revolution	Club and bar, popular with medics	£4; Mon-Sun 12.00pm-2.00am

Student opinion

'Everything about Cambridge is unique. Whether it is punting in the summer, playing frisbee on the College backs, my time in Cambridge will certainly be memorable'.

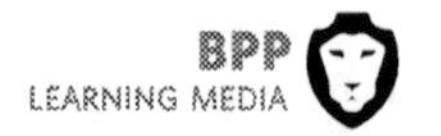

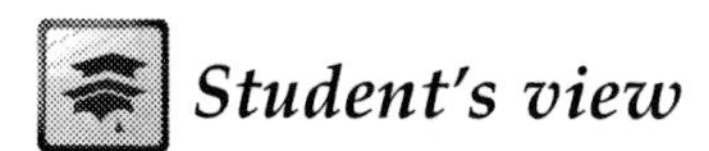

Student's view

Pre-clinical

'The pre-clinical study at Cambridge is traditional and a non-integrated course. And when they say that, they mean it – science is top of the agenda and you will see a couple of hours worth of patients all year. I was a little non-plussed with the degree to which essays held sway as the supreme test of learning, science sometimes seemed more important than useful Medicine, and I couldn't lift my textbooks with both hands. But really you can almost always see the practical application of what you're learning and most people here liked academic science – and were good at it – before they came. The course isn't really all that scary, and though you need to apply yourself, there is seriously plenty of time for fun as well, and I have found that compared to other universities there is actually as much if not more going on, all the time – plus it is so varied that no matter your tastes, you will enjoy something.'

Clinical

'The clinical stage at Cambridge is intensive, and split into three stages. The biggest shock for many are the short holidays. Students get two weeks off at Christmas and Easter, and three weeks in the summer. Each stage consists of attachments lasting five to nine weeks. In Stage 1 the priority is to get to grips with the main clinical examinations and how to take to take a history based on Cambridge's own system, the Calgary Method. Stage 2's attachments focuses on the different specialities, while Stage 3 focuses mainly on preparing students for the transition to an F1 doctor and allows them to as far as possible be involved with patient care. Typically a day in Addenbrooke's hospital in Stage 1 starts off with a ward round at about 8.30am, and this is a fantastic way to learn on the job and to find out which patients have got good signs. After the ward round students assist the junior doctor with ward work, such as cannulations, taking blood and inserting catheters. Much of what one does on the wards is self-directed, which may not suit those who are used to being spoon-fed. A priority for the day is to practise clinical examinations on one patient, preferably with good signs, and to take a full medical history from a consenting patient.

After this is written up and checked with the notes, students usually head off for a much needed lunch break back in the Sherwood Room in the Clinical School. After catching up with friends on different firms, students join up for a series of afternoon lectures consisting of Pathology, Radiology and teaching based on a clinical case study. Other afternoons in the week may be replaced by a Clinical Skills session on how, for instance, to suture a wound. In Stage 2 and 3 more time is spent on the wards, but formal teaching is still provided either at the bedside or in the form of small group teaching seminars. Students tend to enjoy regional placements as doctors usually have more time to teach students on the wards. It is especially fun at the large regional attachments like Ipswich. Firm sizes at placements are small with two to seven students.

There are never more than two students in the Stage 3 making teaching extremely effective. Throughout the Stages, students regardless of their rotation come back to Cambridge for ten Review and Integration weeks, when a comprehensive series of lectures are delivered to students. The clinical course is challenging and students can be very competitive but there are several highlights in the year to let off steam; the Addenbrooke's pantomime and the medic's ski trip in the Christmas holidays. The best tip for students is to read up on conditions as and when they see it on the wards. That way they can hang the theory onto a real person, and this will make revision a lot easier.'

Once you get in...

All the normal things apply – vaccinations and CRB check – but yet again what you get as an applicant, how you have to prepare and so on really does depend on the College, so as with the rest of the information here, it is best to ring or better go in person and ask, see the place, talk to current students. That applies very strongly before and after the application.

The Best Thing	Supervisions and teaching given by some of the best experts in their field
The Worst Thing	An intense and competitive environment that can take it toll on some students

Student top tips

- Choose your College carefully by going on open days; Colleges differ on many aspects such accommodation, grants, location and size. However they are more similar than dissimilar.
- If you are lucky enough you may get to see Steven Hawkins outside his College.
- Make sure you make friends with medics from the bigger Colleges so that they can get you tickets for the decadent Mayballs that their Colleges host.
- Research your intercalated year carefully as you can choose from many of the subjects Cambridge has to offer.
- Try to demonstrate to the admissions tutors what appeals to you specifically about the Cambridge course.

Summary Table

Positives	**Negatives**
Extremely thorough anatomy teaching	Demanding course and competitive peers
The long holidays in the pre-clinical stage	Students have to reapply to Clinical School
Emphasis on the scientific basis of medicine	Limited nightlife, especially on weekends
College supervision system	The eight-week terms can seem to be too short
London is only 45 minutes away	Real clinical contact only begins in Year 4

Cardiff

Cardiff University School of Medicine
UHM main Building
Heath Park
Cardiff
CF14 4XN

http: / / medicine.cf.ac.uk / en

Founded by Royal Charter in 1883, Cardiff University has an excellent international reputation for high standards of teaching and research. Situated in the beautiful city of Cardiff, with its modern city centre, the Portland stone buildings of the civic centre, and beautiful parks, it attracts students and staff from all over the world.

The School of Medicine is world renowned for its high standards of teaching, research and training. The medical course offers a modern integrated approach with an excellent reputation and outstanding teaching in anatomy. Cardiff is a wonderful place to live for a student, as almost everything is within walking distance.

The medical course encourages a drive for excellence in a friendly and relaxed environment.

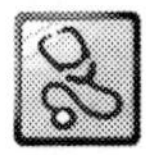

The medical course

Key facts

Course Type	Traditional	**Degree Awarded**	MBChB
Basic Entry Requirements	AAA	**Entrance Exams**	UKCAT
Year Size	Approx 300	**Open Days**	University: April-September Medical School: July
Admissions Website	http://medicine.cf.ac.uk/		

Getting in – student tips

Your personal statement needs to demonstrate your motivation for a medical career, a caring ethos, a sense of responsibility and non-academic interests. You will also be marked on your academic potential, based on results already obtained. For UK applicants, this is from your GCSE grades and your A level results, if they have been completed.

The interview panel usually consists of three people including a senior medical student and at least one medically qualified person. The interview is mainly based around your personal statement and they are usually very friendly. Above all else, the interviewers are looking for your communication skills and enthusiasm for a career in Medicine. However, you need to show you have a realistic approach to what medical training will entail and that you have other interests outside of medicine and academia.

Offers are usually made in December and in February / March.

Course details

Foundation / Pre-Med	Yes	**Graduate**	N/A
Student Population	Male: female ratio: 40:60	**Term Length**	Pre-clinical: 10 weeks Clinical: 15 weeks
Erasmus / Foreign Exchange	Erasmus European exchange possible in Year 4 in association with selected universities in France, Italy and Portugal	**Elective Period**	End of year 4, beginning of year 5. 8/9 weeks long. September-October

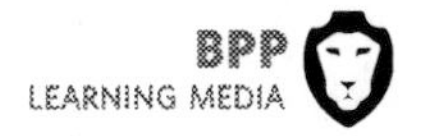

Intercalation

Stage	After year 3 or year 4	Degree Awarded	BSc
Requirements	65 students are allowed to intercalate each year. If more than 65 people apply, selection is based on prior exam results	Subjects	Anatomy, Physiology, Neuroscience, Pharmacology, Medical Genetics, Public Health, Psychology and Medicine, Cellular and Molecular Pathology, Neuropsychology & Neuropsychiatry (at Bangor), Exercise physiology (at Bangor). Further subject choices are being developed

Anatomy teaching

Cardiff is well known for its excellent anatomy teaching. Students spend two full days a week studying anatomy in the first year and one day a week in the second year in the dissection room. In groups of 12, students carry out dissection on a full body cadaver, while instructed and taught by surgeons and demonstrators. Three people per table dissect at a time while other students can attend interactive teaching sessions, either by watching videos of surgeons carrying out dissection or by attending teachings by demonstrators, who may use prosections to teach or students may fill in dissection manuals. Overall, anatomy teaching is carried out in an excellent social and friendly environment. Students may also choose to intercalate in anatomy at the end of the third year.

Pre-clinical/Years 1–2	
Topics	***Year 1**:* Anatomy, Foundation Studies, homeostasis, cardiovascular respiratory, alimentary, musculoskeletal, health in society, Student Selected Component and clinical integrative and academic skills (coursework panel). Clinical skills are introduced from year 1 through direct patient contact. ***Year 2:*** Anatomy, neuroscience, homeostasis, mechanisms of disease and therapeutic approaches, alimentary, cardiovascular respiratory, infection and immunity, health in society, development growth and reproduction, student selected component and musculoskeletal, as well as academic skills (coursework panel). Practical teaching includes Lab Based Clinical Skills as well as clinical skills through direct patient contact.
Teaching	Lectures, tutorials, e-learning, interactive sessions. The quality of teaching is of a very high standard and there is something to suite everyone.
SSC Periods	One panel per year is a Student Selected Component forming 25% of the curriculum. In year 1 this includes a presentation and an essay on a topic of choice. In year 2 this includes a language (French, Spanish, German or Welsh), clinical experience (including choices in Medicine, Surgery and primary care) or essay/presentation topics. This takes place during two days a week throughout the first and second semesters. The family case study comprises of two students being allocated a family whom they meet on a number of occasions, on which an essay of the student's choice is written.
Exams	Anatomy exam includes a spot test as well as a radiology test. Pass mark 50%. End of year exams are integrated to allow a theme of clinically relevant topics to be examined. Pass mark is an average of 50% overall. Questions include multiple choice questions as well as simple answer questions. Coursework includes two small exams taken during the year as well as essays. Almost all the coursework provides an element of choice in topic area.

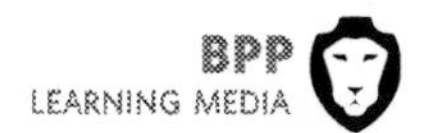

Clinical/Years 3–5	
Topics	***Year 3:*** Rheumatology and Orthopaedics, General medicine and General surgery, General Practice, Cardiology, Respiratory. ***Year 4:*** Paediatrics, Psychiatry, Obstetrics and Gynaecology, ENT, Dermatology, Infectious Diseases, Ophthalmology, Haematology, Care of the Elderly, Neurology ***Year 5:*** General Practice, Secondary Referral, General medicine and General surgery.
SSC Periods	During the third year, everyone does an oncology project where you follow a patient suffering from cancer for six months. At the end of the year, there is a nine-week SSC, where most people self-organise their own project in an area which interests them. The fourth year SSC is an audit in a group of six carried out over the course of the year. The SSC of the final year is eight weeks long which again most people organise themselves in an area of medicine which interests them.
Exams	Most exams take place at the end of the academic year. The written papers are mainly EMQ/MCQs with some SAQs. We also have OSCEs and a long case in Obstetrics.

Hospital placements / academies

Third year placements are eight weeks long and all within south east Wales. The university provides buses to and from the hospitals for this year.

In the final two years, you can be sent anywhere in Wales. You can usually expect four placements within commuting distance from Cardiff, and three placements further away. For hospitals within commuting distance, it is definitely useful to have a car, although you can usually get a lift from a friend, or get on the third year buses.

Accommodation is provided free of charge for all hospitals more than a 45-minute commute away. The quality is generally good, but varied. The best is in Haverfordwest, where you stay in holiday cottages with a swimming pool!

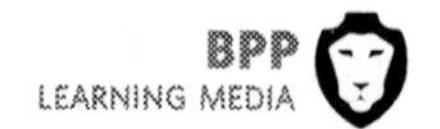

Hospitals and Travel Time from University	
University Hospital of Wales	3 minutes
Llandough Hospital	20 minutes
Royal Gwent, Newport	20 minutes
Royal Glamorgan Hospital, Llantrisant	25 minutes
Princess of Wales, Bridgend	25 minutes
Prince Charles, Merthyr Tydfil	40 minutes
Neath Port Talbot Hospital, Port Talbot	50 minutes
Neville Hall Hospital, Abergavenny	55 minutes
Singleton Hospital, Swansea	1 hour
Morriston Hospital, Swansea	1 hour
West Wales General Hospital, Camarthen	1 hour 15 minutes
Withybush General Hospital, Haverfordwest	1 hour 45 minutes
Brongalis General Hospital, Aberystwyth	2 hours 30 minutes
Wrexham Maelor Hospital, Wrexham	3 hours
Glan Clwyd Hospital, Rhyl	3 hours 45 minutes
Ysbyty Gwynedd, Bangor	4 hours 15 minutes

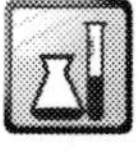

The medical school

Work						Lots of time for fun
Facilities						New undergraduate centre, lecture theatre and teaching rooms
Support						'Buddy' system for first years, plus a personal tutor system for all year groups
Feedback						Formal feedback from exams is bad but this is being improved

Facilities

The first two years are spent at 'Biosciences' in the main university campus in Park Place. Facilities here are good, with a refurbished

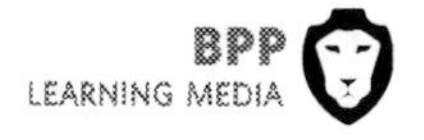

library, lecture theatre and computer room for pre-clinical medical students.

The medical school is within the University Hospital of Wales where there is a large library and computer room. Access to books is only a problem around exam time, when there can be long waits for books so it pays to be organised.

The undergraduate centre at the medical school with a common room and locker room, for use when on placement at the hospital. Every aspect of the medical school (aside from biosciences) will be on the Heath Campus, and will have state of the art technology.

Student support

In the first year, there is a buddy scheme where you are paired with a second year student to help you find your feet.

There is a personal tutor system, but its success largely depends on who you get as your tutor. However, staff in the pre-clinical years are very approachable and supportive if you do have any problems. In the clinical phase, support mainly is in the form of the team who you are placed with at the time. The medical school is usually sympathetic to personal problems, as long as you keep them informed of what is going on.

In addition to the support from the medical school, the university has systems in place, both for financial, emotional and other problems.

Medical Societies

Cardiff Medical Society has an academic, social and welfare committee and they organise some absolutely amazing socials throughout the year, as well as really useful academic resources to help you through the course. As Cardiff medical school only recently merged with Cardiff University, the medical school still has a large number of its own societies.

There are several medics' sports teams, including rugby, football, hockey netball and basketball. The rugby team is particularly successful having won the National Medical Schools Cup in 07/08

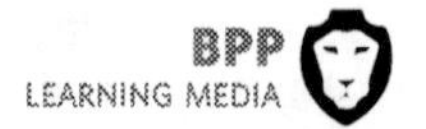

and 08/09. Other societies include a medics' orchestra, religious societies and charities with summer projects working in orphanages in Kenya and Belarus.

The third year students also organise a satirical play called 'Anaphylaxis' about medical school every year. However, if the medical school doesn't offer what you want, or you want a break from the medics' clique, there is a very good chance that the university itself will have what you are looking for with student body of over 25,000.

Finance

Households with an income of up to £39,100 receive a bursary of between £500 and £1,050. The university operates a hardship fund, based on individual circumstances. There are many prizes given out throughout the course, many with substantial monetary reward.

> **Student opinion**
>
> *'Cardiff Medical School is a fun and busy environment. There is so much to get involved with, plus the support is there, should you need it, if times are difficult.'*

The university

Accommodation	Non-campus halls of residence with plenty of variety
Further Info	www.cardiffstudents.com www.cardiffmedsoc.com www.cardiff.ac.uk/for/prospective/residences

Accommodation

There are a number of accommodation sites. Talybont is the main site, about 20 minutes from the university site and 20 minutes from Tesco. University Hall is situated further from the university, however, has a bus that operates on an hourly basis travelling back and forth to the union. All the accommodation in Cardiff is cheaper in price in comparison with other universities, costing on average under £3,000 for the whole year including all bills. Most are self-catered.

After the first year students usually rent a house with housemates of their choice in an area called Cathays aka Student-Ville. 10 minutes from town and five minutes' walk from university, most students choose to live in Cathays with an average monthly rent of £230–250 excluding bills.

Study facilities

There are a number of libraries in Cardiff, as almost every subject has its own, however anyone may use them.

The Biosciences Library is a huge library in a beautiful building with really useful resources. Medics have a habit of taking this over during their exam times! There is also another library on the Heath campus. The resources of both are extremely useful to the extent that while at Cardiff a medical student may only need to buy an anatomy and a physiology book; the rest may be borrowed from the libraries.

University sports & students' union

The student union is directly opposite the Biosciences Building (where most of year 1 and 2 is spent). The facilities include a bar, a restaurant, several shops as well as various sources of help, from the Cardiff Student Letting agency to the Finance Support Centre. Union nights and events are attended by medics regularly as they are quite good and cheap (always a plus in the life of any student!)

Talybont and University Hall (halls of residences) have their own gym and sports facilities. The Talybont sports facilities are what most of the medic/Cardiff Uni Teams use to train. Next to the student union is Cathays Health Centre, containing a gym with good facilities, with various exercise classes and a squash court. The price of these facilities is a one off payment to join the gym followed by a pay as you go payment each time you use the gym.

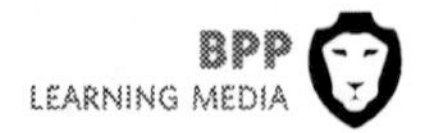

The Heath campus also has its own gym. As well as this Maindy Gym is opposite the main hall of residences, Talybont. Neither of these are affiliated with the union, however, both of these have good facilities and are well priced.

Cardiff Medical Society (Cardiff MedSoc) organises a fortnight of events for medics, not to be missed! Events include the infamous Back to School Party, the Toga Party, Medic Freshers' Ball and much more. Freshers' fortnight provides good opportunity to get to know other medics as well as non-medics, as most of the medic socials are organised to end up in either the union or at the same place as non-medics. This way you'll get to socialise with your flatmates. There is something for everyone.

Upon arrival the medical school and Cardiff MedSoc welcome students separately. MedSoc organises a medic freshers' fayre, which is a great opportunity to sign up to all the charities, societies and sports teams that medics and other healthcare students have to offer. The book and bone sale provides the opportunity to buy second hand books from medics in years above.

Student opinion

'There really is something for everyone, from our International Food Evenings consisting of excellent food and a chilled out evening all the way to Black Tie Dinner Balls with entertainment from our very own Cardiff Jazz Band. Our MedSoc also works with the medical school to provide really useful academic resources and welfare support.'

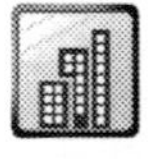 *The city*

Safety	🛡	🛡	🛡	🛡		When taking the usual precautions (eg not walking alone at night), Cardiff is generally safe
Nightlife	☾	☾	☾	☾		Excellent nightlife, with something for everyone

Transport						Parking is difficult in the city centre, but everywhere is walking distance anyway. Very useful to have a car in clinical years when away on placement
Cost of Living						Rent: £240 per month; taxi into town: £5; club entry: £3.50 with NUS; pint: £2.40 in students' union; (all approximate)

Things to do

Cardiff is a great city. It's lively, with all the attractions of a capital city, while remaining friendly and small enough to get around on foot. As nightlife goes, there really is something for everyone, from mainstream clubs to cosy pubs to cool bars and varied music venues. The Millennium Stadium is a great asset, bringing international sporting events and acclaimed music acts to the city. If you haven't spent all of your student loan, shopping in Cardiff is excellent – it has all the usual high street shops plus a number of Edwardian arcades full of individual boutiques, cafés and delis. Cardiff is also home to Europe's largest shopping capital – the St David's Centre, opened in 2009. In summer Cardiff's parks come into their own, with plenty of green space for sunbathing. Upmarket Cardiff Bay is a short train ride away, and boasts the National Assembly for Wales and the Wales Millennium Centre. It's also not far to get out of the city and into beautiful countryside, with the Brecon Beacons National Park only 45 minutes away. Since Cardiff University is not the only university in Cardiff, the city has a huge student population (approximately 30,000) and therefore students are well-catered for, with student nights and discounts aplenty. The downside of Cardiff's impressive nightlife is that the city centre can get a little rowdy on weekends (Cardiff hasn't appeared on 'Drunk and Disorderly' TV programmes for nothing) but if it gets too much then there is always a good night to be had at the students' union.

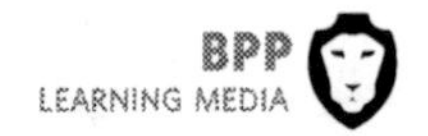

Places to go		
Place	**Brief Description**	**Entry Fee/Opening Time**
Clwb Ifor Bach	Three floors of great (and often live) music	£3–£6, Mon-Sat 7.30pm–3.00am
Buffalo Bar	Chilled-out bar by day, lively club by night	£Free–£4, 7 days a week until 4.00am
Pen and Wig	Cosy pub with board games and great beer garden	£Free, Mon-Fri 10.00am–12.00am, Sat 10.00am–1.00am, Sun 12.00pm–11.30pm
Oceana	Large mainstream club	£Free–£6, Mon, Thur-Sat 9.00pm–3.00am
Woodville	Busy student pub	£Free, 7 days a week until late

Student opinion

'Cardiff feels as if it is made for students. There is something for everyone, with so much to see and do as in every capital city, but without the usual costs.'

Student's view

Pre-clinical

'Upon arrival, you will experience an amazing freshers' fortnight organised by Cardiff MedSoc, who take you under their wing and show you the delights of being a Cardiff medic. Freshers' fortnight gives you the perfect opportunity to meet people in your year, other years as well as non-medics.

In year 1 there are a lot more lectures than in year 2, supported by tutorials. The lectures in both years are based on learning outcomes, which makes putting notes together for exams less time consuming and allowed me to get involved in all the societies Cardiff Union as well as MedSoc had to offer and generally allowed me to enjoy being a student. When an exam or a piece of coursework deadline is completed, MedSoc organised a social to allow students to celebrate. Year 1 is generally spent getting to know your year group and housemates as well as finding your niche. Anatomy is a huge part of it, and something most students come to love as dissection takes place in a social, enthusiastic atmosphere. Early clinical experience through direct patient contact allows students to put some of the anatomy knowledge into practice.

In year 2 you are given a lot more free time as you're expected to do some independent work, which gives students the chance to really enjoy being students as well as providing more freedom with your course. The Student Selected Component module runs throughout the year and allows students to gain more clinical experience in an area of their choice. Again, at the end of any exam/coursework Cardiff MedSoc organises a social to allow students to celebrate. Overall, the pre-clinical years are an excellent way to get involved in student life, be it by getting involved in medic sports, charities and societies or university societies, or indeed by enjoying what delights Cardiff have to offer; from an excellent night life to beautiful parks and historic buildings, not to forget Cardiff Bay! You will find that you have more work than your non-medic friends but that does not mean that you cannot enjoy being a student.

Exam period is always a stressful time but we are lucky in year 2 to finish our exams in April followed by a month of clinical placements in Medicine, Surgery and Nursing in May, followed by two weeks of socials and outings, usually organised by MedSoc to give us a good send off before summer!

Really enjoy these few years, they may be the best couple of years so far!'

Clinical

'The third year is where the hard work begins but is an enjoyable change from the lectures and labs of the first two years. We are attached in groups of three or four students to a team and join the ward rounds and clinics. There is also regular small group teaching by the consultants and registrars. The real aim of this year is to learn how to take good histories and examine patients. At the end of every eight-week placement, there is one week of lectures, which is a good time to recover and have some good nights out (which

are generally a bit more thin on the ground than in the pre-clinical years). Some of the highlights of the year are the halfway ball and it is also the year where you help to produce the satirical play "Anaphylaxis". Even if you don't take part yourself, it's likely that a lot of your friends will have parts so it is definitely worth going along to watch!

However, the exams at the end of the third year are the ones everyone dreads and starts revising for weeks and weeks beforehand. Pass this hurdle though, and you are almost on the homeward run as there are very few people who fail the fourth or fifth year.

In the fourth year we are joined by Swansea students and intercalaters, which helps to spice things up a bit. Because we are all spread around Wales, there is usually just one student to a team, which means you can get more involved and get more individual teaching. It can be a bit annoying being sent for five weeks to Bangor, but it does mean you get to see another part of Wales and it is normally quite fun living with a new group of people. The highlight of the year for me though was delivering a baby!

The final year is a case of actually learning how to be a doctor and you really start to feel like you can be of some help on the wards! The F1s are really friendly and happy to have you around, especially if you help them out with the odd catheter, venflon and drug chart.

Overall they are a great few years, with plenty to get your teeth into but also enough time to have plenty of fun. I have found everyone in Wales really friendly including other students, nurses, patients and even the majority of doctors!'

Once you get in...

The medical school sends you a pack, which includes a memory stick. This contains a welcome from the medical school, a few things about enrolment as well as a book list of what students will require. You will find this useful.

In the memory stick is also the 'Cardiff MedSoc Freshers' Guide' which contains information about Cardiff MedSoc welcoming new students and information about what students may expect all written from a student's point of view. From a contact list and photo of the committee to what students will require in halls all the way to MedSoc's 'No-Nonsense Guide' to year 1, this guide will keep students occupied and will hopefully relieve some anxiety before arrival.

Also in the 'Cardiff MedSoc Freshers' Guide' is information about the freshers' fortnight, what to expect and what to bring. All in all, a good welcome even before you arrive!

The Best Thing	Enjoyable and well thought-out course which is constantly reviewed in response to student feedback
The Worst Thing	Minimal feedback on exams and other assignments, and organisation/administration can sometimes be poor, however this is improving

Student top tips

- Cardiff medics' own bar (formerly MedClub), now called the IV, was relaunched in September 2009 and has gone down a storm! It gives students a place to be during their lunch breaks and is sometimes used in the evenings for socials.
- Be sure to see Wales play rugby at the Millennium Stadium – tickets are cheap against smaller international teams and there is still a great atmosphere.
- Don't buy loads of textbooks before you arrive – try out a few in the library as some may suit you better than others.

Summary Table

Positives	Negatives
Having all Welsh hospitals available for placement means you see a large variety of patients and many beautiful parts of Wales	Having all Welsh hospitals available for placement – sometimes you will be away from Cardiff for several weeks at a time which makes it difficult to keep in touch with friends
Friendly, lively city	Poor feedback on exams and assignments
Well designed course	Difficult and time-consuming to travel to hospitals, unless you have a car

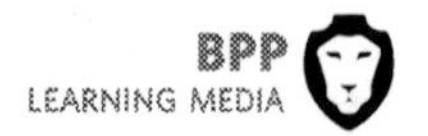

Positives	**Negatives**
Approachable lecturers who are, on the whole, very good	The student/patient ratio is too high at University Hospital Wales (the main hospital in Cardiff)
Excellent selection of SSC (Student Selected Component) projects	Organisation can sometimes be poor, however this is improving

Dundee

Admissions & Student Recruitment
University of Dundee
Nethergate
Dundee
DD1 4HN
Scotland

www.dundee.ac.uk/medschool/

Dundee is renowned for its innovation and research and its medical school is rated as one of the best schools in the UK. The city is well known for being home of the three J's: jute, jam and journalism but is also renowned for its many exciting discoveries both in the medical and geographical field. It homes the RRS Discovery, the ship which was built in Dundee at the turn of the century to take Captain Scott to the Antartic which now proudly sits upon the Tay in the city. More recently, Dundee saw the discovery of the beta blocker Propanolol by Sir James Black and the university continues to lead the way in cancer research. Dundee is a small city that has all the resources. Due to the size, the city is dominated by students and this is obvious in the west end where all the pubs and bars are full of familiar faces which creates an vibrant and friendly atmosphere. Dundee is an excellent place to study and is an ideal central location to access all the sights in Scotland.

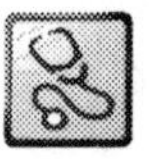

The medical course

Key facts

Course Type	Traditional	Degree Awarded	MBChB
Basic Entry Requirements	AAA	Entrance Exams	UKCAT
Year Size	Approx 160	Open Days	Late June and September
Admissions Website	www.dundee.ac.uk/medschool/		

Getting in – student tips

Dundee is looking for well-rounded individuals who have had at least two weeks of experience in medical situations. Voluntary work in disabled schools and care homes for the elderly are also very creditable. Achievements in other areas such as sports or music are important. The interviewers comprise a number of doctors and academics associated with the medical school. The interviewers ask about outside interests as well as the usual questions about why you want to become a doctor but, in general, students have found that the interviewers weren't too intimidating and it was a fairly relaxed atmosphere. The interview consists of small stations where you rotate around small groups of interviewers who are a mixture of clinical and academic staff. They are also likely to look for an understanding about the type of course taught in Dundee.

Gap years are seen as an advantage as long as they are or have been of significant benefit.

Course details

Foundation / Pre-Med	Yes	Graduate	Yes
Student Population	Male: female ratio: 40:60	Term Length	10 weeks
Erasmus / Foreign Exchange	Five months of year 5 in Malawi is offered	Elective Period	Summer of years 4 and 5. 8 weeks from July/August

Intercalation

Stage	Usually after year 3 but sometimes after year 4	Degree Awarded	BMSc
Requirements	Applications taken on individual basis but generally available to those who have passed Phase One without resits	Subjects	Medical Sciences

Anatomy teaching

The core teaching of anatomy is split into two parts. The first semester of the first year and second semester of the second year. In the first year, all areas are covered except the limbs. There is at least six hours of anatomy teaching a week which compromises at least two hours of lectures and four hours of dissection. Dissection is in groups of three to four per body with one demonstrator for every three bodies. There is also an anatomy library that has a wide range of prosections and X-rays and is available from 9.00am–5.00pm during the week. At the end of semester 1 there is a 50-station spot test.

In the second year, the teaching is during the musculoskeletal block. It is the same format as the first year except the limbs and spine are covered. This is very useful as the anatomy teaching is relevant to the clinical information you are being taught. The anatomy taught during this block makes up a large portion of the end of year exam.

At the beginning of each system, the specific anatomy for that system is reviewed by looking at a number of prosections with the help of a professor and students.

Pre-clinical/Years 1–2	
Topics	***Year 1:*** First semester – Basic sciences – Anatomy, physiology, pathology, biochemistry and public health. Second semester – Dermatology, haematology and cardiovascular. Also weekly primary care teaching and clinical skills relevant to each system. ***Year 2:*** Respiratory, endocrinology, gastroenterology, musculoskeletal, renal and primary care teaching continues. Clinical skills taught per system.
Teaching	Lectures, small group tutorials, online tutorials, teaching boards, primary care teaching and clinical skills. Clinical skills is exceptionally good as there is a centre with a number of GPs who are always willing to help out.
SSC Periods	During the first year the SSC is based on basic sciences and primarily on campus. It runs through the whole year culminating in an essay written by the start of May.

SSC Periods Continued	In the second and third year the SSCs become more clinical and interesting. There are two one-month blocks each year. The university provides a selection of SSCs with a large variety of themes such as learning sign language or a placement in France. As well as these choices the students have the option to self propose an SSC. This can allow an insight into a specialty that you have an interest in and gain experience for your CV. In the third year it is acceptable to go abroad with students going to places such as Ghana and Australia. All of the SSC blocks can potentially have the opportunity to do an audit and/or research with the prospect of a publication.
Exams	From the second semester of the first year till the end of the third year the exam format is the same. There is one online exam consisting of extended matching answers and multiple choice questions covering everything which has been taught in the academic year. As well, there is an OSCE (Objective Structured Clinical Examination) which tests the clinical examinations, history taking and communication skills which you have been taught in each system. The OSCEs progressively have more stations and increase in difficulty. In the third year there is also an oral examination on your Record of Clinical Experience (RoCE). All exams take place at the end of the year, commonly May.

Clinical/Years 3–5	
Topics	***Year 3:*** Neurology, psychiatry, ophthalmology, otolaryngology, paediatrics, aging, obstetrics and gynaecology. Clinical skills and primary care are continued. Two four-week SSC periods. ***Year 4 and 5:*** Task based approach which includes clinical attachments and small lectures. Ten Clinical outblock attachments based around 100 problems. Option for extended GP placements from two to four months in the fifth year and has mandatory Foundation shadowing blocks where you gain invaluable experience for commencing Foundation Year 1.
SSC Periods	The SSCs comprise two four-week attachments in years 2 and 3 and can be carried out in Dundee or in another hospital. The topics can be chosen from a list or can be self-proposed and approved by the medical school.

Exams	The fourth year exams are commonly viewed as the medical finals as they are a written and OSCE format with a portfolio element. In the fifth year there is a portfolio exam that, if passed, acts as an exemption exam from the written examination. In addition to this, there is a progress test, which must be passed, and this is taken every year at medical school with an expected progression in knowledge. The portfolio includes work from the fourth and fifth year and may also include previous work from SSCs.

Hospital placements/academies

The hospital placements vary widely and there is an option to experience rural life in Scotland if you wish during the fourth and fifth year. The placements during the fourth year are generally at district general hospitals and GP practices around Scotland which all offer accommodation that is comfortable and accessible by public transport. Some GP attachments offer home stay accommodation. During the fifth year, there is an option to carry out extended GP placements, which include practices in the outer Hebrides where you are welcomed by the locals and experience a very different aspect of Medicine. Own transport is desirable to access these places but there may be options for two students to be placed together so they can share transport.

The other medical attachments are generally based at District General Hospitals where you spend time in the wards, clinics and theatres and get a very good overall clinical experience. All of the hospitals have guidance on the core clinical problems so that each student covers the essential work required for the exams.

Hospitals and Travel Time from University	
Ninewells Hospital	15 minutes
Perth Royal Infirmary	30 minutes
Kirkcaldy Hospital	45 minutes
Queen Margaret	1 hour
Airdrie	1 hour 30 minutes

The medical school

Work						Lots of challenging work to get through but still plenty of time for everything else
Facilities						Excellent teaching facilities
Support						Good support from senior students with peer tutoring available from an early stage
Feedback						Could improve feedback on exams

Facilities

There is a comprehensive medical library within Ninewells Hospital and an IT suite attached. This is in addition to the campus library that includes medical books and hosts a large IT suite with adjacent café. In addition, there is a clinical skills centre where rooms are available for revision to practise examination skills with other students. These are really popular before exams and are a great way to improve last minute skills. It is also home to Harvey, the virtual mannequin who can have heart murmurs, heart attacks and seizures!

Student support

There is a good support network between students with the common academic family system in place for peer support. There are also a number of counsellors available at the university for help and the staff at the clinical skills centre whom you become acquainted with who often act as an additional support network. Many students also find that the small sports clubs and societies can provide additional support networks.

Medical societies

Medics football has been a huge success with both boys and girls teams competing in the national medic competitions. The sports clubs are constantly growing and rely on enthusiasm from students.

The Dundee University Medical Society hosts a number of events including charity events and encourages students to become involved from first to fifth year so is a great way to interact with the different years and network at medical school. The main social event of the year is the popular DUMS ball, which is held at various hotels within Scotland.

There is an annual sketch show organised by the students at the medical school, which sees students try out their talents on stage. It is attended by most of the school and lecturers and is held at Ninewells Hospital over three nights.

Finance

www.somis.dundee.ac.uk/registry/fees

There are scholarships of up to £2,000 available and these can be applied on an individual basis.

Student opinion

'I had a really positive student experience and found that Dundee was an extremely friendly university and think that it really benefits from being a small campus, which attracts a diverse group of students. Despite its size, there are still the same number of social events at the union and they are always trying new ideas and themed nights. The university tries to provide something for everyone and this is a result of the diverse mix of students from the courses it offers.'

The university

Accommodation	Campus halls of residence
Further Info	www.dundee.ac.uk/studentservices/residences

Accommodation

A large number of halls house the majority of first year students and are on campus so are in the perfect location. For the first semester they are extremely handy as most of the teaching is on campus and

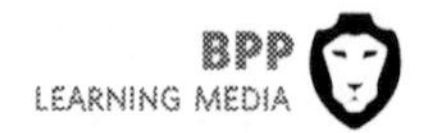

are only 50 metres from the lecture theatre. However, in the second semester all of the teaching moves to Ninewells Hospital. This is about a 5-minute drive or a 20-minute walk. Public transport is good and buses to the hospital are very frequent.

The best halls are the newer ones and they are called Belmont and Heathfield. The other halls are not as new but still have all the important features. Due to the size of Dundee all the halls are a maximum of five minutes from campus. More medics tend to pick West Park Villas as they are advertised as closer to Ninewells, however, they are only about half a kilometre closer and have no other benefit. It is probably best to be on campus as it makes meeting people a lot easier.

Study facilities

The library on campus becomes a second union around exam time especially with medics. Although there is the library in Ninewells Hospital, which holds all the medical textbooks, the campus library is more popular for revision because most students live closer to it. The campus library has recently had a makeover and now has a coffee shop, free wireless internet and a large number of computers available.

University sports & students' union

The students union is at the heart of the university campus. It has three very well stocked bars, a swimming pool, about 25 pool tables and of course, Mono night club. The union is a very busy place with a great atmosphere, especially on a Wednesday and Saturday night when most of the students go there.

With regard to sports facilities there is a new state of the art three-floor gym, which has a great range of machines. Although it can get quite busy there is always enough equipment.

There is no class on Wednesday afternoons and this is when the majority of the university sports teams play. Dundee has some very competitive sports teams including the rugby (men and womens), hockey, netball and rowing teams.

Freshers' week commonly runs in mid-September and runs for one week. Every night has something different with a variety of themes and big name DJs, commonly including Zane Lowe and other Radio 1 favourites. A freshers' pass is available and is worth the money.

The medics have their own society called DUMS. The society holds a number of events throughout the year with the first on the Wednesday of freshers' week. This gives a short introduction to some of the lecturers and people within DUMS and provides an opportunity to sign up to any of the DUMS sports teams or clubs.

There is a freshers' fair on the Friday of the week and this provides the opportunity to sign up to any of the university sports teams or any of the other societies. Although there are all the medic sports teams and clubs, medics have a large influence on the university clubs as well. As you will notice quickly a lot of medics are normally good at more than one thing so you will find large numbers from all years throughout the university clubs.

Student opinion

'Dundee is a university with a great feeling of community. A large amount of money has been put into all the university's facilities and this has only strengthened my experience. You would struggle to find a better atmosphere in any other union in Britain.'

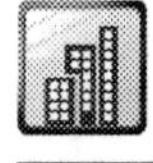

The city

Safety						Safe in the university area
Nightlife						Plenty of small live music venues and friendly pubs
Transport						Difficulty parking at Ninewells, no major airport for trips away. Cheap taxi fares
Cost of Living						Expect to pay around £200–300 per month to rent, £1.50 for a pint and £3–5 for entry to clubs and theatres

Things to do

Dundee is a perfect place for visiting other parts of Scotland due to its central location. It is ideal for many outdoor activities as it is close to skiing centres, mountains and is of course on the Tay so has ideal access for sailing. It is also close to the major cities in Scotland for larger music and dance events. Due to its strong art influences and art school, the city attracts many artists and festivals to the area each year. Dundee is extremely student friendly with most bars and pubs offering student deals.

Places to go		
Place	**Brief Description**	**Entry Fee/Opening Time**
DCA	Dundee contemporary arts centre: bar and restaurant. Food is great and has a small cinema also with some eclectic and foreign films	£Free www.dca.org.uk
Fat Sams	Nightclub: www.fatsams.co.uk	Variable entry fees depending who is playing
Social	Restaurant and bar – great cocktails and fab drinks offers	12.00pm–12.00am every night £Free admission
Underground	Mix of urban beats – fab tunes. Lots of drinks offers	Tues 8.00pm–2.30am Wed-Sun 6.00pm–2.30am £Free before 10.00pm. £6/£3 after

Student opinion

'Dundee is an extremely friendly and safe city and its central location makes trips to the surrounding areas and major Scottish cities a must.'

Student's view

Pre-clinical

'For the first three years you have approximately two hours of lectures every day. Around these are various tutorials, clinical skills, labs and primary care teaching. For the first semester you may feel, "you have done the stuff before" or "it isn't related to medicine", however, as you progress through you realise those first three months are very important. The layout of system teaching is great. While you are getting lectures about a disease, you are also learning how to take a relevant history and examination for that disease.

The work-play balance is great as there is normally at least two afternoons off each week and the occasional late start. Typically the days are 9.00am to 4.00pm. Lectures start at 9.00am, however, due to the closeness of the hospital you can easily leave at 8.45am. They normally last about 50 minutes and the other classes rarely last the full two hours for which they are timetabled. Lunch is a highlight. There is the Ian Lowe centre, which is full of medical students, doctors and other hospital staff. The couches are extremely comfy for a nice hour-long sleep. If you are hungry there are a number of canteens within the hospital and floor 5 is a particular favourite. In the afternoon thankfully there are no lectures, presumably because we all used to fall asleep.

Exams are very different from school. Although none of them are written, they are more challenging due to the far greater volume of information covered. However, I would say just keep on top of it by writing up lectures and you should never have a problem. Also buy 'Clinical Medicine' by Kumar and Clark.

Dundee was always my first choice because of what I had heard about the atmosphere and I knew what Ninewells could offer. There are too many highlights to name from my first three years. The various balls I have been to, the countless number of hangovers, an epic tour to Salou and being given the opportunity to work in a Ghanaian hospital for one of my SSCs. Finally, always make sure you keep a balance between work and play!'

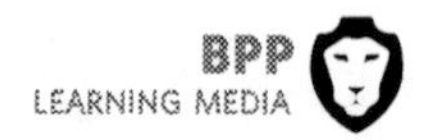

Clinical

'I had only been to Dundee once before I started university and thoroughly enjoyed my whole experience at Dundee and at the medical school. The clinical years were well structured with clear objectives but also gave an opportunity to tailor your course to your interests. There was a good mix of clinical and academic attachments that gave a good basis to entering foundation training.

I felt prepared for work due to the shadowing blocks in the fifth year and found I had a good transition from medical school to becoming a doctor. I would strongly recommend applying to Dundee and found that students seemed to obtain a good work life balance at university and made the most of what was on offer.'

Once you get in...

Once you get in you will receive a number of packages with a lot of scary forms. It is best to organise these and just spend a day filling them all out. You will get a choice of accommodation and this will be the most important form. There are six choices but remember not to get lured in by West Park Villas. Other forms will include information for matriculation. Make sure you have a good photo to send off! There are some very funny pictures on people's badges. There are other forms from the union and DUMS. I would recommend the freshers' pass if you want to be social and it saves a large amount of money.

The first week is a very relaxed affair. Matriculation is normally on the Friday so make sure not to miss it and have your student finances sorted out. Everything else is explained in the vast amounts of paper.

DUMS commonly sends information about book deals. For the first semester you will require books on biochemistry, physiology, pathology and anatomy, all of which are commonly sold by DUMS.

The Best Thing	The familiarity of everyone within the union and the structure of the course
The Worst Thing	Smaller university so clubs are generally smaller

Student top tips

- Bring a large variety of clothing because you will be doing a large amount of dressing up for theme nights in your first few months.
- All the sports teams allow you to play before you pay your membership to encourage people to try new sports.
- Dundee Medical School used to be part of St Andrews University.
- The pioneer of laparoscopic surgery worked at Ninewells Hospital.
- Dundee is called the city of discovery.

Summary Table

Positives	Negatives
Early clinical experience	No foreign exchange
Opportunity to tailor your medical degree	Quieter nightlife than bigger universities
Easy to make friends as smaller university	

Durham

Durham University, Queen's Campus, Stockton
University Boulevard
Thornaby
Stockton-on-Tees
TS17 6BH

www.dur.ac.uk/queens-campus/

Set on the banks of the River Tees, Stockton-on-Tees is the home of the modern University of Durham Queen's Campus. Connected to the main Durham campus via a free bus service, Queen's Campus offers a modern, vibrant and diverse approach to student life. Offering activities ranging from the local 'Tees fringe festival' to white water rafting, students are able to take part in new and exciting experiences.

Providing the pre-clinical years, Queen's campus offers the unique experience of discovering the traditional medical course through innovative teaching methods, led by staff with national achievements in education. This dedication to learning gives students great preparation before their departure to Newcastle to complete their training.

And if anything, explaining the complex issue that you are a Durham student, who lives in Stockton, but will graduate from Newcastle always provides some amusing confused faces!

The medical course

Key facts

Course Type	Traditional	Degree Awarded	MBBS
Basic Entry Requirements	AAA	Entrance Exams	UKCAT
Year Size	Approx 100	Open Days	By arrangement
Admissions Website	www.dur.ac.uk/school.health/phase1.medicine/		

Getting in – student tips

Queen's Campus endeavours to produce the 'Doctors of Tomorrow' and considers that being a well-rounded individual allows this to happen. They emphasise the need for students to give evidence of extra-curricular achievements and enjoyments as they believe that being able to balance this with your studies will set you up in good practice for your future careers. Queen's Campus devotes time to interview all their students due to their keen interest in communication and the social aspect of Medicine. They are held by two interviewers from a range of backgrounds, from GPs to lay members of the community. The informal and friendly nature of the interview doesn't aim to catch students out, but to learn more about the individual from why they want to study Medicine to their clinical reasoning and judgement when faced with ethical or moral clinical scenarios. They enjoy seeing students displaying their personalities and enthusiasm through their answers, and seeing how you are able to build a rapport and deliver information during the period of the interview.

Course details

Foundation / Pre-Med	No	Graduate	No
Student Population	Male: female ratio: 40:60	Term Length	Pre-clinical: 10 weeks Clinical: see Newcastle
Erasmus / Foreign Exchange	N/A	Elective Period	See Newcastle

Intercalation

Stage	See Newcastle	Degree Awarded	See Newcastle
Requirements	See Newcastle	Subjects	See Newcastle

Anatomy teaching

Anatomy is probably the best department in the medical school, as it has very knowledgeable and supportive staff. Learning through prosections and not doing the dissection means that specimens are well presented and you can see all the structures very clearly.

There are two sessions per week, which consist of a lecture on the given topic before going into the anatomy suite. Students are given a work book the week before in preparation for these sessions. The anatomy suite is also open on a Wednesday afternoon for first and second years to allow them to consolidate their knowledge, and staff are always present to help you.

Pre-clinical/Years 1–2	
Topics	The pre-medical years aim to give students a firm understanding of the basic concepts of human anatomy and physiology, and link this with the social aspects of Medicine as well as personal and professional development. A case led approach is used and teaching will revolve around all potential aspects of the patient's care. Topics covered include: Foundation Case, Cardiovascular, renal and respiratory medicine, Nutrition metabolism and endocrinology, Thought sense and movement, Lifecycle, Medicine in the community, Personal and professional development, Student Selected Component, Clinical science and investigatory medicine, Anatomy, Clinical skills.
Teaching	Teaching comprises lectures, seminars, anatomy and clinical skills teaching, laboratory work, patient home and hospital visits and community placements. It is delivered in a structured timetable but also promotes adult learning by encouraging self study. Staff are knowledgeable, but also skilled at delivering information in a way that everyone can understand. With the year group being small, you get to know your lecturers on both a professional and personal level which gives students the confidence to approach staff for extra help should they need it.
SSC Periods	The SSC held in your second year of phase 1 aims to improve key skills such as IT, information retrieval and critical analysis. Students will perform a literature review of a topic of their choice that links in with their community placement or patient study. It gives students the opportunity to explore an area of interest in depth and can range from covering a historical aspect to a current area of hot clinical research.
Exams	Exams consist of written papers and practical exams. There will be OSCEs consisting of three stations, covering some of the basic clinical skills that have been encountered. The written papers will be either MCQs or DIPSEs covering the theoretical knowledge covered in lectures.

Clinical/Years 3–5	
Topics	See Newcastle
SSC Periods	See Newcastle
Exams	See Newcastle

Hospital placements/academies

See the chapter on Newcastle, p. 363.

Hospitals and Travel Time from University	
North Tees University Hospital	5 minutes
James Cook University Hospital	10 minutes
Hartlepool	20 minutes

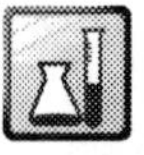

The medical school

Work	●	●	●			Good work life balance
Facilities	●	●	●	●		Newly built campus and accommodation
Support	●	●	●			Peer and education support
Feedback	●	●	●			Verbal group feedback, written individual feedback with appointments on request

Facilities

There are purpose built facilities for medical students. The anatomy suite provides a number of well preserved prosections. There are also clinical skills labs complete with fake arms to practise venesection and an ultrasound machine to get to grips with clinical equipment before Phase II. These rooms are used for structured teaching but also can be used out of hours around exam time to ensure your learning outcomes are met. There is a large lab used for histology teaching which has enough equipment and slides for you and your lab partner.

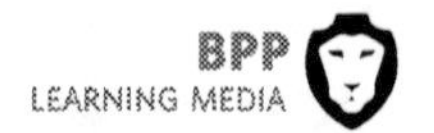

There is a library shared by all students and a fair number of good computers with good internet connection. There are also two cafés on site which are good for relaxing between lectures.

Student support

Queen's Campus is dedicated to making your time at university an enjoyable experience, and understands that there are times when you may need some extra help whether with coursework or just the struggle to adapt to time away from home. There are a number of measures in place to support students. Each student has a tutor who they meet at various times throughout the year to discuss any issues they might have and this involves a free meal! There are also senior residents in the halls of residence that oversee the students, and can be approached for any difficulties you are having with your studies, accommodation or social life. Before arriving students will also be matched with a student with similar interests then assigned a parent in a 'college family' system. More specifically to Medicine, you are assigned a 'peer parent' who is a medical student in the years above you to offer support, and there is also a welfare officer in Medsoc who can fulfil the same role. Finally, all staff at Queen's Campus are friendly and approachable and are available to facilitate additional teaching sessions should you require this.

The main campus at Durham also offers support in the form of chaplaincies, Nightline, a health centre and services for students with disabilities.

Medical societies

MedSoc is at the centre of many students' social life. It is run by students and so is able to cater for all students and liaise with the Newcastle medics by organising joint events to build good relationships in preparation for phase 2.

They organise many a bar crawl and charity events including the 'Medics Full Monty' which allows you to get to know your peers rather too well! As well as this, they are aware that medical students find it difficult to become part of university sporting teams because of clashing timetables, and so they have set up medic sporting teams and organise fixtures with medical schools across the country. They put a lot of time into ensuring all those who want to participate can, as it gives a great opportunity to relax and socialise outside of lectures.

Students can also opt to become part of the Marrow Trust, which is the student sector of the Anthony Nolan Charity, which can involve anything from taking blood from potential donors to representing your university at national meetings.

Finance

www.dur.ac.uk/studying/student-finance/

Student opinion

'Being a student at Queen's is really rewarding. There's quite a family feel, as it's a relatively small campus you have the opportunity to get know lots of people really well and not just people on the course.

The College system also encourages people to get involved in societies, sports and socialising. For a small town, there's surprisingly a lot to do in the local area to keep you more than entertained!'

The university

Accommodation	Both campus and non-campus
Further Info	Union website Accommodation website

Accommodation

Durham is renowned for its college life, and Queen's campus is no different. It offers the choice of two colleges, John Snow and Stephenson, both of which are located in Stockton, and less than ten minutes' walk from university. Both colleges offer a flat sharing system of six to seven people, all rooms being fully furbished complete with en-suite bathrooms and internet access. There is a shared kitchen with all basic equipment provided and enough fridge and cupboard space for each tenant.

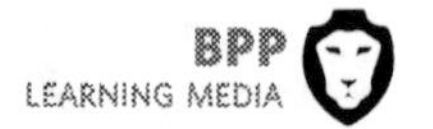

After your first year you find a house to live in. The university holds an accommodation fair around January time when landlords that meet their standards are invited to display the available accommodation. Rent can range from £35-£75/week, but price is no reflection upon standards. Students tend to rent in either Stockton or Thornaby.

Study facilities

There is one library at Queen's campus which is shared by all students. It has a good range of medical text, and books can be requested from the libraries in Durham that are usually transported down that same day. It has group working sections and a quiet room for those who want to study in peace.

There are a number of computers in the library with access to printing and scanning, and wi-fi is available. The internet has a really good connection, and so even when all the students are 'revising' (checking facebook) you are able to view web pages quickly.

Most lecturers tend to print off the lectures notes for you and so you don't have to spend lots of printer credit or be organised enough to remember to do it before the lecture.

University sports & students' union

A gym has opened on campus, and boasts a mixture of cardiovascular and resistance training equipment, as well as plasma TVs to keep you occupied. It is located at the university, and so you can easily go before or after lectures but if not, it is only ten minutes' walk from the furthest college – John Snow. Purchasing a sports card entitles you to a discounted price of £65/ year as well the option to participate in university sport, but you can join for £115 without a sports card.

Students are entitiled to play for either the university sporting teams which would require students to travel up to Durham for training sessions, or to play for their college.

The Waterside is a newly refurbished café/bar on campus that serves as a student union. During the day, it is the perfect place to relax between lectures and serves reasonably priced food and drinks. By the night, students use it as a place to unwind with a beer or for pre-drinks before a night out.

Students tend to take a trip up to Durham on a Friday night for a night out in their students union. They get some big names such as Pendulum. For transport, there is a late night free bus that takes students back to Stockton at 2.00am!

Student opinion

'I loved the small, intimate feel of Stockton, however I know it wouldn't be for everyone.'

The city

Safety	🛡	🛡	🛡			There is rarely any trouble between local residents and students
Nightlife	☽	☽	☽			There are plenty of bars and clubs in Stockton and Middlesbrough, and a free bus to Durham
Transport	🚌	🚌	🚌			There's plenty of parking at uni, although you can manage on foot
Cost of Living	🐷					You can live in nearly new, nice places for as little as £35/week.

Things to do

At the heart of the town is the River Tees which offers great opportunities such as rowing, waterskiing and sailing. There is also a white water rafting course for those looking for the ultimate adrenaline rush.

The town itself is a diverse mixture of history with buildings dating back to 15th century and modern living with the contemporary venue 'The Arc' which shows films and holds a number of courses from salsa dancing to cookery.

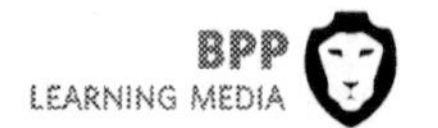

Stockton is also famous for having the widest high street in the UK, which is perfect for holding the market on a Wednesday and Saturday which sells fresh produce at good prices. There are a number of high street shops, cafés, bars and restaurants that keep the students entertained.

Stockton may not seem like other university cities because of its size and smaller student population, but once you have spent a weekend here, you soon realise that it has everything that students need to have a great time and you will create some great memories.

Places to go	
Place	**Brief Description**
Che Bar	The weekly night where everyone knows your name
Joe Riggatoni's	A cool place to eat, right on the waterfront
The Arc	Cinema, gigs, shows, comedy, all under one roof
Weatherspoons	Large pub selling lots of good value alcohol and shows some sports

Student opinion

'Durham is a small, safe city with something for everyone.'

Student's view

Pre-clinical

'Before starting university I was a little sceptical that I would miss out on so much of student life because of the amount of work Medicine would involve and in order to pass I would have to work day and night. While work was tough at times, I was still able to have a great student life.

As the first two years is pre-clinical, we were in lectures from 9.00am to 5.00pm most days but this was split up with lots of practical and interactive sessions. There were lots of concepts to grasp and in hindsight; a lot of the content was in detail which I

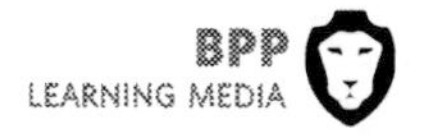

haven't needed in the clinical years. However I feel that it kept us all interested in the topic at hand, and as we are going to spend our whole lives looking at Medicine, it was really interesting to see things from a different perspective. It was really useful to have learning objectives that would stop you learning irrelevant details for the exams, as these had more of a clinical slant to them. We were also given patient contact during these two years which again reinforced the clinical aspects of our lectures.

The amount of teaching and support we were given made it possible for me to be able to balance work and play. Being able to join the rowing team which required 6.00am starts and weekend training didn't get in the way of studies because of the learning and consolidation we would do during lecture times.

From moving to Newcastle, I feel that the main attribute Queen's campus has is its small year group that allows everyone to get to know each other really well – which if anything meant that there was never that panic of who to sit next to in lectures.

Studying at Queen's Campus prepared me really well for the final three years of medical school because it gave me the knowledge to approach clinical practice with excitement rather than dread, and gave the opportunity to make some great friends to support me along this rather scary journey!'

Postgraduate

'Although daunting at first, starting med school as a mature student at Stockton was easy. I anticipated many younger, smarter people all competing like crazy to 'out do' one another and it was soon apparent this wasn't the case at Stockton. Reassured by other mature medics surrounding me, I was glad to see that within a class of 110 people roughly 25% fell into 'mature' category and were keen to share wisdom. Compared to friends starting their medical degrees at various schools across the country I felt lucky knowing that Stockton had a higher proportion of mature students. On a typical day at the Stockton campus you would see a herd of students gathered outside a lecture room sharing stories of drunken antics from the night before and then everyone assembling in their usual seats with their friends surrounding them.

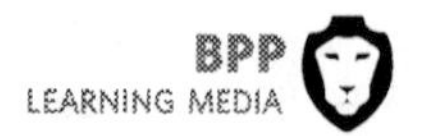

The lecture rooms are flat and there is a more intimate feel compared to your typical lecture theatre. The teaching was good overall with an outstanding anatomy department. They use prosected cadavers and they really made us feel as though they were happy to teach, and that passing exams would be a joint effort. On the other hand, the neurophysiology teaching seemed a little complex, and more importantly, in far greater detail than we needed for exams. Yet support from staff was always at hand and being a smaller cohort we never felt like just a number.

The highlight would have to be the sporting culture I experienced at Stockton/Durham University. The colleges compete with one another and the university plays most sports to a high standard. Often when travelling with the basketball guys to train in Durham, I would feel immersed in a part of England steeped in history that boasts plenty of natural beauty; then we'd arrive at the sports hall with hip hop music bouncing out of the car and my mind firmly back in modern Britain.'

Once you get in...

Once you have been offered a place at Queen's Campus, you will receive a welcome pack. This includes information on both the course and general university living. You will need to fill in accommodation forms including which college you would prefer to be part of, and they try their best to match you and your future housemates according on what you have written. There is also the opportunity to sign up to various freshers' events and buy a sports card etc before you arrive at university. It is recommended to do this as you will have so much admin to do in your first week that it makes life a little easier!

Lectures start during the first week but as these are mainly admin/ introductory lectures, you can still afford to join in on all the freshers' events. It is a good idea to decide which text books you would like from the reading list in advance (a list of recommended texts is usually provided) as you can buy discounted books during freshers' week at the library or from other students.

The main advice is to join any societies that take your fancy and attend all the introductory social events because if for nothing other than the freebies, it's really good to find a hobby that forces you to take time out of studying.

The Best Thing	Small teaching groups meant you weren't intimidated to ask questions or tempted to go to sleep!
The Worst Thing	Some of the societies are held up in Durham and so travelling is required

Student top tips

Stockton is a great place to study, although it may seem different to the stereotypical university town. But you've got to remember that everyone there is set out to have a great time and accepting that Stockton is slightly smaller than most places will allow you to all have just a good a time as anyone at university.

Summary Table

Positives	**Negatives**
Small year groups	Smaller town
Excellent anatomy teaching	Some societies located in Durham
Patient contact from day 1	Fewer bars than most cities
Cheap living	
Free bus to Durham	

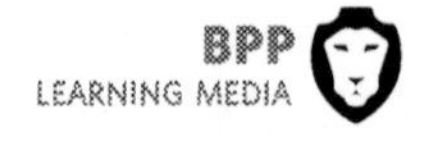

East Anglia

The Undergraduate Admissions Office
Faculty of Health
Edith Cavell Building
University of East Anglia
Norwich NR4 7TJ

www.med.uea.ac.uk

Relics, such as the skyline – the dominating grand cathedral spire and splendid castle, are a reminder of Norwich's medieval heyday as England's second biggest city. Moreover newer constructions have appeared from the horizon, ushering in a more sophisticated future that challenge the city's gauche and archaic stereotype. Examples include the futuristic and contemporary Forum, housing the millennium library and the BBC's Eastern England News Rooms, and the two new sizeable American styled shopping malls. One has even been built under the castle!

The UEA follows along similar lines. Previously attention has been drawn to the 'Ziggurat's', the striking and perhaps best well known pyramidal halls of residence that have personified UEA. However with the nationally renowned Sainsbury centre for arts, and its funky design, and a new, modern, medical school the future looks bright. Furthermore an exciting set of new lecture theatres are being built to add to the medical school's already excellent facilities. Students might even, very possibly, turn up for 9.00am lectures!

The medical course

Key facts

Course Type	Intergrated	Degree Awarded	MBBS
Basic Entry Requirements	AAA	Entrance Exams	UKCAT
Year Size	140	Open Days	October – July
Admissions Website	www.uea.ac.uk/		

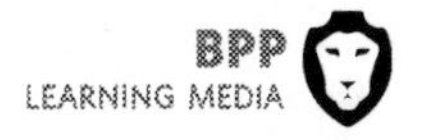

Getting in – student tips

The criteria are capacity for self-directed learning, capacity to work effectively in groups and with colleagues, capacity to take responsibility, motivation, and personal effectiveness.

Candidates are invited to take part in an OSCE style interview. When candidates enter the interview room, they will find a series of booths, known as 'stations'. There will be seven stations to circulate through spending approximately six minutes at each station.

At each station candidates will meet an individual interviewer who will ask one question and mark the response to that question independently. Interview panel members will consist of a mix of academic/lecturing staff from the School of Medicine and clinicians/healthcare professionals from local hospitals and trusts who are involved with many aspects of teaching within the MB/BS course.

Course details

Foundation / Pre-Med	Yes	Graduate	Yes
Student Population	Male: female ratio: 1:3	Term Length	Pre-clinical: 10 weeks Clinical: variable
Erasmus / Foreign Exchange	N/A	Elective Period	End of year 4 – 8 weeks

Intercalation

Stage	Between year 4 and year 5	Degree Awarded	MClinEd, MRes
Requirements	Must be ranked within top two quartiles	Subjects	Clinical Education, Health research

Anatomy teaching

Anatomy is taught in two forms: cohort lectures from the head anatomist and lab-based Student Selected Study Modules (SSSM's, explained later), with the latter an assessment.

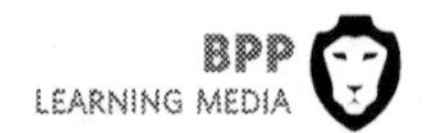

The lab-based anatomy is almost exclusively taught as an SSSM, usually by two members of the problem based learning (PBL) group. The selected group members receive teaching from experienced anatomy tutors through the week, using cadaverous dissection, on specific areas that are to be presented the following week to the PBL group.

During the group presentation, the dissected cadavers are provided to the group for demonstration of the relevant anatomy. This is supervised and appropriately supported by the above tutors. Immediately thereafter, the head anatomist summarises to ensure everyone has a clear understanding of the topic. Neuroanatomy is taught exclusively by the head anatomist.

Every such session is completed with a clinical radiology session taught by an experienced radiologist to integrate the learning, which is particularly useful before hospital placements begin.

Pre-clinical/Years 1–2	
Topics	***Year 1:*** Unit 1: Being a Patient, Being a Doctor (15 weeks) Unit 2: Locomotion (15 weeks) ***Year 2:*** Unit 3: Blood & Skin (12 weeks) Unit 4: Circulation (12 weeks) Unit 5: Respiration (12 weeks)
Teaching	Emphasis in PBL is on learning through group work and self study. Each week topics are covered using a clinically based, integrated teaching approach of the relevant core domains, such as anatomy, physiology, pharmacology, etc relevant to the week. This provides a holistic approach to all the topics.
SSC Periods	At East Anglia these are known as (student selected study) SSS. In years 1 and 2 these consist of analytical review assessments, supported by research methods lectures and ten minute presentations on student selected topics in Biochemistry, Pathology, Physiology, Sociology, Ethics and Philosophy, Epidemiology, Law, Psychology, and Immunity and Infection. Anatomy can also be selected for an SSS topic, although this is assessed through presentations in the anatomy room, integrated into teaching.

Exams	• End of unit and end of year Objectively Structured Clinical Exams (OSCEs). • SSSMs on various core domains, eg physiology, psychology, sociology etc. • Analytical reviews analysing various research papers using the teaching given throughout the year. • End of year written exams in the form of extended matching questions (EMQs) and short answer questions (SAQs), with the latter based around three out of six scenarios provided a week before the exam. • Inter-professional learning (IPL): During years 1 and 2 students are placed into groups with other allied health professionals and work together to produce essays using titles provided by group tutors.

Clinical/Years 3–5	
Topics	***Year 3:*** Endocrinology, Nephrology, Urology, Neurology, ENT, Ophthalmology, Gastroenterology, Hepatology ***Year 4:*** Obstetrics & Gynaecology, Embryology, Neonatology, Paediatrics, Elective Period ***Year 5:*** Psychiatry, Emergency Medicine
Exams	***Year 3 and 4*** A six station OSCE assesses each unit. The integrative period in the summer consists of a large (18-20) station OSCE, an EMQ paper and an advanced notice SAQ paper. ***Year 5***: Six station OSCEs for each unit ***Integrative period:*** A large OSCE only. A written paper may be added soon.
SSC Periods	Years 3 and 4 undertake a compulsory Studies Outside Medicine (SOM) course which runs over two terms. These courses include Philosophy, Archaeology, British Sign Language, French, Spanish and Theology among others. At the end of the second semester, students must either write an essay or take an exam depending on the course in order to pass.
Elective Period	No limitations on location. Eight weeks' duration.

Hospital placements/academies

The medical school organises and funds transportation for all clinical placements not within walking/cycling distance so no student is destined to spend the night in hospital accommodation. Hospital placements last four weeks of every term and of the remaining eight weeks, one day a week is spent in a GP surgery. The NNUH is a new 987-bed hospital which is a five-minute walk from the med school. Although aesthetically pleasing, student numbers are high which can sometimes affect teaching quality, although the school is working on this. The other District General Hospitals (DGHs) are smaller, have a really relaxed atmosphere and generally have a better reputation for teaching quality.

Each PBL group (usually eight to nine students) is allocated to a GP surgery, which may be located anywhere throughout Norfolk, Suffolk or Cambridgeshire. Teaching quality can vary but generally students have great opportunity to sit in with GPs and practice nurses, observe minor operations, go on home visits and perform clinical procedures (taking blood, giving flu vaccinations etc). The GP will also organise for patients with a condition relevant to the topic of the week to talk to students, which is great for developing your own consultation skills and gaining confidence in examining patients.

Hospitals and Travel Time from University	
Norfolk and Norwich University Hospital (NNUH)	2 minutes
James Paget University Hospital (JPUH)	50 minutes
Queen Elizabeth Hospital (QEH)	60 minutes
Ipswich Hospital	90 minutes

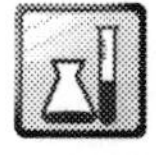

The medical school

Work						Good work life balance
Facilities						Teaching, library and IT facilities are all more than adequate. A new campus building has added more teaching facilities

Support						Each student has a designated personal adviser, with whom they can discuss exam feedback and any personal or course issues
Feedback						Marks may be available if requested

Facilities

The ever-growing medical library is located within the main campus library, which has recently undergone major expansion. The medical libraries and IT facilities at all of the affiliated hospitals are also open to UEA medical students. Purpose built undergraduate clinical skills laboratories are located in both the NNUH and the JPUH, which also have IT labs. The clinical skills laboratories contain simulation wards for students to practise clinical procedures such as venesection, catheterisation, defibrillation, arterial blood sampling and so on. The campus medical school building houses seminar and tutorial rooms, a student common room and an additional IT lab. An anatomy suite and lecture theatres are found nearby on campus.

Student support

First year students have the opportunity to be adopted by a mentor who will act as a student 'parent'. This is great for sharing valuable tips on everything from exam techniques to pub recommendations. Numerous social events take place during freshers' week for both mentor and mentee to get to know each other. As with most universities, a halls of residence tutor is always available to sort out any flat issues in the first year. Each student will be assigned to a personal adviser who may be either a local clinician or an affiliated academic. Students are encouraged to meet with their adviser termly throughout the course to discuss their current academic performance, career ambitions and any pastoral issues they may have. A PBL tutorial tutor and GP tutor will always be on hand to help out with academic issues and to give feedback on your performance and progression. A student counselling service and GP surgery are also located on campus.

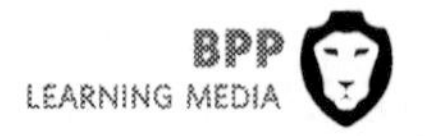

Medical societies

UEA MedSoc is the main society for organising regular social events for medical students. They organise everything from helping you unpack as soon as you arrive to open bus tours of the city to themed nights out to termly formal balls. The medics' rugby and football team (Norwich Medics RFC) are an independent club open to all healthcare related, not just medical students. They are a really enthusiastic bunch of guys and gals open to all abilities.

UEA surgical soc hold regular workshop practicals aimed at developing surgical skills not taught on the curriculum. Regular speciality talks and additional anatomy sessions are also available. Surgical soc has set up a mentor programme with local surgeons from a range of specialities allowing senior students ample opportunity for observing and assisting in theatre. The Ziggurat Challenge is a university sporting competition, which takes place throughout every academic year. Medical students must compete with students from other disciplines in a number of sporting challenges and have consistently come within the top three positions every year.

Finance

Further info: www.uea.ac.uk/services/students/Fin

See scholarships: www.uea.ac.uk/services/students/Fin/grants

There are hardship funds available: www.uea.ac.uk/services/students/Fin/fin_hardship

Student opinion

'Being a relatively small school there is a unique community ethos; you're bound to bump into someone you know whether on campus or wandering about the town. Working in small groups makes the whole learning process much more interactive and regular clinical exposure acts as an incentive to stay motivated and inspired throughout the course.'

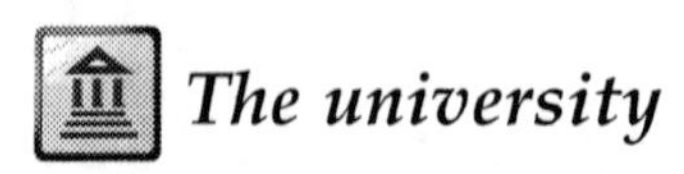

Accommodation	Non-campus
Further info	www.uea.ac.uk/accommodation

Accommodation

Medical students are given a choice from Colman House, University Village, Norfolk or Suffolk terraces or Mary Chapman Court. Most of the university halls of residences are located within a five-minute walk of the medical school, with the exception of the University Village accommodation which is a one-minute walk from UEA campus, and a further ten-minute walk to the medical school. For those who prefer to live in town, Mary Chapman court is a fine choice.

The halls of residence vary in style but all are equally good. Many students agree that whichever hall of residence is chosen, it is guaranteed to be a brilliant start to university life. All of the residences are self-catering, which is an excellent way to bump into your flatmates and also develop your own style of cooking! Usually there are a few fellow medics on your flat, which means that during exam time there is plenty of support close by. There is also a resident tutor who lives in the halls, should any problems occur.

There is not a 'best' hall as such. It depends more on the preference of accommodation. Norfolk and Suffolk terraces have a shared bathroom facility, which is not to everyone's liking but this is balanced out by the unbelievable atmosphere in the halls. Colman House and the University Village accommodations are the newer developments with en–suite facilities.

Study facilities

Generally, medics tend to use the main library and the computer room provided by the medical school.

The library, located opposite the main lecture halls in the middle of campus, comprehensively houses most books for every university course as well as being a public library. The library also has copies of past papers that are freely accessible to students. Stretching over five floors it is simply a massive building and it is easy to find a quiet space to work.

The main IT facilities are located on two floors in the library and feature up to date computers, printers, scanners and photocopiers. It is an excellent environment to work in. Should these floors be busy, every floor has its own set of computers, ensuring that there is never a shortage of computers. There is also an IT helpdesk answering any queries, including personal requests for help fixing personal computers.

For medical student use only, the school has provided a state of the art computer room with an electronic white board. This is located in the medical school itself. Furthermore the Norfolk and Norwich University Hospital, a ten-minute walk from campus, also has an extensive library, which medics have full access to 24 hours a day. Located in the hospital is a student clinical skills area with more IT facilities, again open 24 hours a day.

University sports & students' union

The union is located on the main square above the union pub.

It has a café (The Hive) and ample seating areas, with the freshly baked cakes and smoothies a particular recommendation! There is also a booth to buy tickets to virtually any event occurring in the lower common room (LCR), a helpdesk for any queries, the LCR (the in house club), a graduate only pub, a desk for societies to give or receive funds and an advice and support office run by friendly staff. Around the building is a travel office for train, bus or aeroplane tickets.

The majority of events held at the LCR are student nights. However some major bands and artists have also graced the LCR with their presence, including Calvin Harris, Dizzee Rascal and many more.

Medics use these facilities regularly, especially the bi–weekly student nights! Due to the union's central location and excellent facilities it is also a place visited by medical students after a hard morning of lectures!

As it is East Anglia's largest fitness centre, the sports facilities are vast. There are a wide range of sports available in the Sportspark complex. Some of the highlights include a climbing wall; numerous badminton, squash and tennis courts; a 50 metre swimming pool; dance studios and activity halls; eight multipurpose astroturf pitches; a gym; an athletics track and much more.

Student opinion

'It feels inspiring to be at UEA and it is a fantastic experience to study Medicine here. The motto to "do different" reverberates strongly with different opportunities knocking on the door constantly. As a very welcoming and friendly university, and with something happening every moment, it is a vibrant university.'

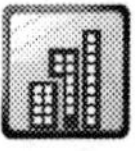

The city

Safety	🛡	🛡	🛡	🛡		Though a city, Norwich is pretty safe
Nightlife	☾	☾	☾	☾		Plenty of clubs and bars to keep freshers happy, and an abundance of cinemas, theatres, specialist restaurants and clubs for the culture vultures
Transport	🚌	🚌	🚌	🚌		Parking in town is expensive, but buses from the campus are frequent. On campus, there is some space for student parking, but not if you live in halls
Cost of Living	🐖	🐖	🐖	🐖		Pretty reasonable. £45-75 per week for a room. Taxi to city centre from campus is £6

Things to do

Norwich has many cultural attractions, with two cathedrals and a castle to visit. The city centre has plenty of clubs and bars, and the Riverside area is particularly popular with students. The UEA and Riverside are also popular venues for gigs. Student discounts are common in the city, especially in restaurants. Popular nights out for students include Brown Sugar, an R&B night at Riverside.

Places to Go		
Place	**Brief Description**	**Entry Fee/Opening Time**
Norwich Castle	A 900 year old Norman keep	10.00am-5.00pm Mon-Sat 1.00pm-5.00pm Sun
The Waffle House	Café/restaurant with great waffles	Open 7 days a week
Brown Sugar @ Riverside /Liquid	R&B and hip hop event	Thursday nights £2
Liquid	Nightclub	Usually free before 10.00pm.

Student opinion

'Both Norwich and the UEA campus manage to hold everything you will ever need, in a compact space. The city has something for everyone, while not being so large it is disorientating.'

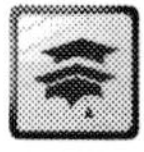

Student's view

Pre-clinical

'The timetable was extremely busy during the first year, especially in the first unit because of the introductory lectures needed to ensure everyone has a similar level of knowledge. There were lots of lectures and clashing seminars, which meant a hectic start to the year reading around the topics beforehand. However we eventually got used to it and found little shortcuts to speed up the process. Moreover there were still generous amounts of independent study and free time given.

In the second year there were fewer seminars and more independent study time, which allowed greater time to read around the PBL topic, understand and summarise it better for the group as well as for personal reading. Obviously the volume and difficulty of material also increased!

Since every day during the week is different, it would be fair to describe a generic week. A regular week includes one day for PBL, lasting for three hours, followed by "wrap-up". The day following this is usually full of seminars to support the PBL outcomes. There is one day near the end of the week for a full day of Primary Care. On the remaining two days there are usually cohort lectures, two-hour lab based anatomy sessions or practical sessions at the hospital.

I was recommended this university by my careers teacher and so I decided to research the university further. I really liked the fact that the course is integrated, the system based teaching approach and the fact that there is early patient contact, which I feel is vital for the development of junior doctors.

My highlights include being a committee and first team member of the UEA squash club and the orthopaedic representative in the surgical society.

The hardest exams were the written exams at the end of the year as it was a completely new format compared to what I had done previously. The first OSCE I did was also a new and daunting experience, as I had not experienced the "station" idea for my interview. However, over the years it has become easier to mentally prepare for them.

My advice is to relax and enjoy the first two to three weeks of the first unit and savour the university atmosphere. Be brave and join new societies to experience as many new things as possible. Keep an open mind with the course, as it is easy to get bogged down early by worrying about learning everything all at once. As a spiral-learning course, some things keep cropping up and so there will be time to cover topics again in other units.'

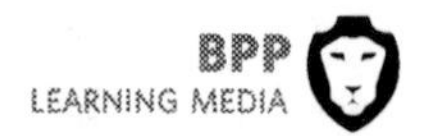

Clinical

'Year 3 is notorious for being one of the hardest years of the entire course as it contains the most of the specialties covered in the curriculum. By the end of year 3, you've covered clinical and academic teaching relating to almost all of the organ systems so clinicians have high expectations of you from a relatively early stage.

The typical week has a similar layout to years 1 and 2 with a termly four-week hospital attachment in years 3 and 4. During year 5, three days of the week are spent in a clinical setting, be it a GP surgery or a hospital attachment and the remaining two days in lectures or PBL tutorials. Clinical placements are generally more hands on in the senior years and students are encouraged to build up a portfolio of clinical procedures they have performed. Towards the end of year 5, students are attached to a particular firm and learn the ins and outs of the common duties of an F1 which really helps smooth the transition from student to doctor.

Studies Outside Medicine (SOM) courses start in year 3 and run parallel to academic teaching. Generally SOM is great for having a break from Medicine and learning something completely different although they can be seen as an unnecessary addition to the workload. The Research Project, although daunting at first, aims to introduce students to the obscure yet sometimes fulfilling world of research. It's all too common for students to be over ambitious with their research ideas and often spend too much time on their research, which can be a major distraction from their normal academic studies.

The end of year written exams really test the breadth of your knowledge as they may include anything from previous years including economics, psychology, law, ethics, sociology and not just basic sciences/clinical medicine. It's physically impossible to cram everything in the weeks running up to the exam and so you really do have to pay attention from day one!'

Once you get in...

Once you get in, you'll receive a letter confirming your place at medical school and a freshers' pack. The latter contains the itinerary of freshers' week, a newsletter about medsoc and forms for medsoc merchandise and to indicate whether you would like a mentor from the upper years.

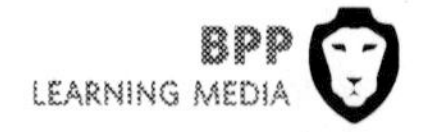

The first week is fairly light in content, which allows you to get your bearings around campus. The first PBL session is slightly intimidating as it is a new experience. There are also a lot of lectures in the first unit, which can result in particularly long days. Finally the first week includes the first Primary Care visit and talking to patients immediately can be a slightly nerve-wracking experience.

A reading list is available online and there is a Waterstone's book store next to the library selling these books. However it is advisable to glance through as many books as you can in the library to get an idea of which you would prefer before buying the relevant books. Contacting your mentor to ask for popular books is also a good way to sort quickly through the reading list.

The Best Thing	The city of Norwich is beautiful, and a wonderful and safe place to study. The course is varied and full of patient contact from the outset, so the first weeks are extremely exciting. The local hospitals are of high quality and within easy reach, making placement teaching well worthwhile
The Worst Thing	The course is still relatively new, so some timetabling issues are still being ironed out

Student top tips

The university is adjacent to the Norwich Research Park which is home to over 1,000 scientists working in several world ranked institutions.

Summary Table

Positives	Negatives
Modern course, mixed curriculum	New school – reputation not yet known
Loads of patient contact from the second week	Course still being refined
Location – Norwich is a great city	Lack of parking on campus
Relatively cheap cost of living	
UEA has vibrant atmosphere, with lots of sport and extra-curricular activities	

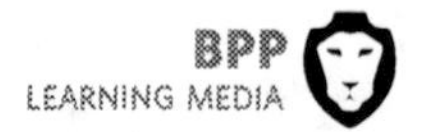

Edinburgh

Undergraduate Admissions
College of Medicine and Veterinary Medicine
The Chancellor's Building, 2nd Floor
49 Little France Crescent
Edinburgh
EH16 4SB

www.mvm.ed.ac.uk/index

Edinburgh, the capital city of Scotland is home to one of the oldest, most established medical schools in the world. In 2002 the New Royal Infirmary together with an adjacent £40 million medical school was completed and houses a new library along with state of the art computer suites and clinical teaching areas. The medical school in Edinburgh boasts a traditional style of teaching with an excellent anatomy department along with a blend of up to date clinical teaching styles. The city of Edinburgh is itself a tremendous area to live in and be a student, it boasts a vibrant city centre, full of 17th century architecture with a modern twist. There are excellent open areas for the keen student to keep fit, for example Arthurs Seat along with the popular Commonwealth Pool. The city is also home to wonderful sights and attractions such as Edinburgh Castle. Edinburgh not only has many areas to socialise in, such as its numerous pubs and clubs, but its residents can be proud of the city's excellent safety record. Overall, Edinburgh University is not only home to a world-class medical school but also a great area for students to live making Edinburgh an excellent place to study Medicine.

The medical course

Key facts

Course Type	Traditional	Degree Awarded	MBChB
Basic Entry Requirements	AAA	Entrance Exams	UKCAT

Year Size	218	Open Days	June and September
Admissions Website	www.ed.ac.uk/schools-departments/medicine-vet-medicine		

Getting in – student tips

Edinburgh has an excellent reputation and so not only asks for outstanding grades at school/university, but also non-academic achievements and interests. They like to see evidence of personal skills (empathy, communications, team working), together with commitment and exploration of career prospects through placements and volunteering. As Edinburgh only interview matures and graduates, it is extremely important to convey your interest and commitment, together with skills and qualities in your personal statement as that is principally what they base their decision on. The interview panel is made up of clinicians and academics. The website states that they will ask you about why you want to do Medicine and what you think it will be like, ethical issues and skills and qualities required. My interview however was more of an informal chat about Elvis Presley, 60's music and how high school is very different to university life, but they all vary!

Course details

Foundation / Pre-Med	N/A	Graduate	N/A
Student Population	Male: female ratio: 35:65	Term Length	Pre-clinical: 10 weeks Clinical: 7 week rotations
Erasmus / Foreign Exchange	Between years 2 & 3 as part of intercalated honours year. Pharmacology in Leiden or Saarland	Elective Period	Between year 4 and 5–8 weeks

Intercalation

Stage	Between years 2 and 3	Degree Awarded	BSc BMedsci
Requirements	Top 90 students in the year wishing to intercalate	Subjects	Medical Sciences

Anatomy teaching

First and second year anatomy is taught primarily in the historic old medical school at Teviot Place. Usually each week there is an introductory anatomy lecture on the areas to be covered in the practical class. The practical classes are 1 and a half hours in length and consist of identifying cadaveric prosections with some embryology and histology. There are professors and senior medical students present to assist the students and there are occasional lectures given by radiographers after the practical sessions. There is an opportunity to visit the Anatomy Teaching Lab out of scheduled teaching hours to bridge any gaps in knowledge. In the second year it is possible to pick Student Selected Components that involve dissections.

Pre-clinical/Years 1–2	
Topics	***Year 1:*** Introduction to life, Health and Society including Medical Ethics, Cardiovascular, Respiratory and Musculoskeletal systems and their related clinical skills. ***Year 2:*** Neuroscience, Nutrition and the Gastrointestinal System, Clinical Genetics, Renal System and the Endocrine System and their related clinical skills.
Teaching	Lectures, problem-based learning (three hours/week in groups of around eight students and a facilitator), small and large group tutorials, online tutorials, clinical skills tutorials. Second year introduces visits to GP practices once a week to begin to put the basic clinical skills and science into practice.
SSC Periods	***Year 1:*** One Student Selected Component in first year covering a broad range of topics from Infection Control after surgery to Communication Skills. The assessment involves creating a poster and presenting it to examiners and other students, there is also and opportunities to present findings to academic groups or publish findings. ***Year 2:*** Two Student Selected Components in the second year. The SSC in first semester has more of an emphasis on reviewing research literature and applying that information in a clinical scenario, tutors and projects are organised by the course organisers. In semester 2 there is a push to get students to produce original research in groups. The projects are organised by students and can be on any topic the students are interested in. These can include anything from research on the latest artificial limbs to a dissection project.

Exams	December and May. Short answer questions, multiple choice questions, extended matching questions and anatomy spot tests. The second year introduces an OSCE. Both years also have occasional in-course assessments consisting of interpreting articles for peer review and resuscitation ability.

Clincal/Years 3–5	
Topics	***Year 3:*** Cardiovascular, Respiratory, Locomotor and GI (medical or surgical). ***Year 4:*** The year is split into three blocks: (1) Obstetrics & Gynaecology, Haematology/Oncology/ Palliative care/ Breast Disease/Renal/Urology, (2) SSC, Senses (Dermatology, Opthalmology, ENT), (3) General Practice, Psychiatry and Neurology. ***Year 5:*** The year is split into five blocks (1) General Medicine, (2) General Surgery with Anaesthetics/ Critical care and A&E, (3) Paediatrics, (4) General Practice and Geriatrics, (5) Elective
SSC Periods	During the third year you have the opportunity to organise three to four sessions shadowing a 'health professional' of your choice, with a presentation and report at the end. In the fourth year there is an eight week block available to complete some research or an audit in any department of your choice. In the fifth year another eight week long elective.
Exams	MCQ (no negative marking) exams at the end of each block. Some rotations also have OSCEs and OSCAs. Pass rate is 60%. If students fail they can re-take, but certain blocks (Obs & Gynae and Psychiatry) are finals and so should you fail, you have to repeat the block (losing your elective).

Hospital placements/academies

On the whole, accommodation is pretty nice, usually a house for four students close to the hospital. They all have a bath/shower but beware internet connection is not provided, and the libraries can close in the early evening and so can be a bit of an issue. There are usually between two and five students on placement for a specific department, although there are also students placed in the hospitals on other rotations. During the fourth and the fifth year, chances are that you will be placed out of Edinburgh for around two-thirds of the year, and so this time can be quite expensive and tricky if you do not have a car. Although it is a bit of a hassle being on peripheral attachments, you get much more experience and teaching as there are fewer of you there. Most of the third year is based in Edinburgh, and throughout the fourth and fifth year certain rotations are always based in Edinburgh, such as neurology, senses and half of paeds. Edinburgh is has a huge amount of research, we have the Regius Professor of Surgery, together with fantastic Cardiology, Neuro and Transplant departments to name but a few. We have the Royal College of Surgeons and Royal College of Physicians in Edinburgh and so you can attend the various courses and educational days that they offer.

Hospitals and Travel Time from University	
Royal Infirmary of Edinburgh	0 minutes
Western General	30 minutes
Royal Hospital for the Sick Children	15 minutes
Borders General Hospital	45 minutes
Queen Margaret Hospital, Dunfermline	50 minutes
Kirkcaldy	60 minutes
Dumfries & Galloway	2 hours
Haddington/Roodlands	45 minutes
Royal Edinburgh (Psychiatric)	20 minutes
Falkirk hospital	60 minutes

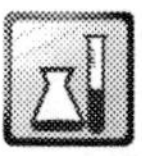

The medical school

Work	✚	✚	✚			Hard work but plenty of socialising
Facilities	☕	☕	☕	☕		New Royal Infirmary of Edinburgh has excellent facilities including library, research labs and clinical skills

Support						Lots of social events, parent scheme in first year if interested, revision sessions and peer-assisted learning sessions gets all years involved
Feedback						Exam feedback is excellent during the first and second year, poor during clinical years

Facilities

At the RIE there is a medical library with 24-hour computing facilities, common room, clinical labs and simulation suites with dedicated, full time staff available to go through any problems.

Student support

Support is excellent; every student has a Director of Studies who can be a clinician or academic. During the first year there are parent schemes if students are interested, and lots of social events throughout the years. Together with specific support for medics, there are the general supports that you would expect for any student, including The Advice Place, Careers Services, Accommodation Services, Night line and a chaplaincy.

Exams are MCQ/OSCE and it is not possible to see past exam papers. Feedback from consultants during attachments is generally excellent, with constructive comments and praise. During attachments you have a consultant as your tutor, and so it is possible to get your references sorted for Foundation applications too!

Medical societies

There is the Royal Medical Society (RMS), Edinburgh Student Surgical Society, Academic Training in Undergraduate Medicine (ATRIUM), Musical Medics...lots basically, not to mention all of the sports ones. The societies tend to have talks and speakers from various specialties, together with courses, revision sessions and conferences, career advice and of course the social events! The RMS also offers bursaries for electives.

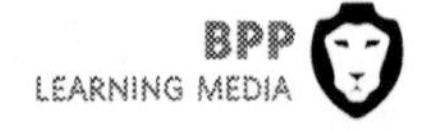

Finance

www.ed.ac.uk/studying/undergraduate/fees-finance

www.ed.ac.uk/studying/undergraduate/fees-finance/bursaries-scholarships

There is a hardship fund that students can apply to multiple times in one academic year. There are also numerous scholarships and bursaries available, together with an accommodation bursary of £1,000. It is best to do some searching early on as many have closing dates many months before you are due to start.

Student opinion

'A fantastic opportunity to experience life in a vibrant city, and make some of the best friends you'll have for the rest of your life!'

The university

Accommodation	Halls of residence: non-campus catered and on-campus non-catered
Further Info	www.accom.ed.ac.uk/

Accommodation

First year accommodation ranges from a 20-minute walk to the medical school from the catered accommodation (Pollock Halls) to a 5-minute walk from the self-catered halls, for example Kincaids Court. Many of the more senior students choose to live in the affluent areas of Marchmont and this makes it easier to travel to the hospitals and clinics dotted around the city.

Study facilities

There is one very large main university library. Spread over five floors, it has many computer suites and there are almost always study areas available up until the middle of exam time. Because of this medical students alone have access to computer suites spread throughout the main university campus along with the libraries in the various hospitals. Royal Medical Society members have access to the RMS library and computing suite.

University sports & students' union

Edinburgh University has four student unions, the oldest purpose built student union in the world (1889) is the late gothic castle styled Teviot Row House (usually called Teviot), by day a coffee shop and bar/restaurant but has large halls where many events throughout the year take place. Across Bristo square lies Potterow, a large open indoor area covered by a clear dome. It houses many student support centres, the RMS and is also home to the Saturday night club event, 'The Big Cheese', popular with medics. Adjacent to the university gym is the Pleasance, home to more bars and restaurants and a popular Tuesday night comedy event. Less popular with medics due to its distance from the medical school and halls is King's Buildings House, again home to bars and restaurants.

A university full peak gym membership costs around £100 per year. The gym is a modest size but is very well equipped. It can get very busy at peak times, especially 4.30pm–6.00pm and Wednesday afternoons. For more information visit www.ed.ac.uk/schools-departments/sport–exercise/home.

The freshers' events are organised both by the university and the Royal Medical Society. Most students move into halls on the weekend around 14 September, usually the Saturday. This gives freshers a good chance to meet their new flatmates and socialise. During freshers' week there are societies fairs where students can join groups with common interests. Many medic freshers join the Royal Medical Society (RMS). There is also a sports fair where students can join sports groups including everything from tennis to skydiving. There are also good opportunities for students new to Edinburgh (or even Scotland) to explore the area and see the historical landmarks. The medical school runs introductory lectures to get students up to date on what it's like to be a medical student with added lectures from senior A&E staff on first aid. The medical school helps the students to get registered with a GP in Edinburgh and helps to get students up to date with their vaccinations. The RMS also organises the annual medics' 'white coat' pub crawl, one of the best opportunities of the year to break the ice and make the friendships you will have for the rest of your life. This all sounds a bit hectic but not to worry as the week is organised very well.

Student opinion

'I was in Kincaids Court, it was a great place and really close to the med school. The uni and RMS always organised fun events to help everyone get to know each other.'

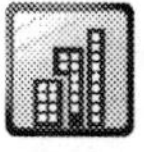

The city

Safety						The city centre of Edinburgh has a very safe feel even in the early hours on weekends
Nightlife						Edinburgh has lots of night clubs. The student union 'Potterrow' puts on 'The Big Cheese' event every Saturday night which is always a lot of fun
Transport						Especially in your pre-clinical years there is no need to use a car, the bus network in Edinburgh is excellent and there is a free NHS shuttle bus students can use during the day to get from hospital to hospital
Cost of Living						Rent can be quite expensive, especially in the city centre, expect to pay >£1,200 pcm for a four bedroom city centre flat. Compared with other cities, the prices of taxis are more expensive. The price of a pint varies from location to location

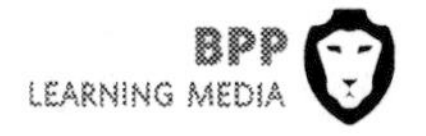

Things to do

The city of Edinburgh boasts many attractions and there are loads of activities for students to do. For sightseers there is the lovely Arthurs' Seat (great for hill walking) and also the amazing Edinburgh Castle for all you historians. Students tend to go to the many cinemas dotted around the city, everything from the massive multiplexes to the indie arthouse cinemas. There are other facilities for leisure – the bowling alleys, pool halls, gyms, swimming pools and so much more. Princes Street Gardens, right beside the castle is an excellent place to just chill, listen to music or have a nap under the sun. Living in the city does mean you tend to pay a little more for everything you do (in relation to other cities in the UK, excluding London) however most clubs have student nights and lots of shops and services offer student discounts.

Places to go		
Place	**Brief Description**	**Entry Fee/Opening Time**
Teviot Row House	The world's oldest (and best) purpose built student union.	Mon-Sun 9.00am–late
Why Not	Why Not is a lively venue with plenty of alternative music nights and vibrant staff.	Mon 10.00pm–3.00am Fri–Sat 10.00pm–3.00am Mon £5 Fri £5 Sat £7.50
Lava Ignite	A fun club with student nights every week.	Wed & Fri–Sun, 10.00pm–3.00am From £2
Brass Monkey	One of the best (small) pubs in Edinburgh. A cool, relaxed bar with a large back room full of cushions and mattresses to laze about on. Shows films every day at 3.00pm.	Mon–Sun 10.00am–late
Black Medicine Coffee	One of the best of the (numerous) places to get a great coffee and a bite to eat in the city.	Mon–Sat 8.00am–6.00pm Sun 10.00am–6.00pm
Doctors	A historic pub situated opposite the medical school, can trace its roots right back to the founding of the medical school.	Mon–Sun 10.00am–1.00am

Student opinion

'I love living and studying in Edinburgh. It's a big city but it feels like a town, there is so much to do and the people are really friendly.'

Student's view

Pre-clinical

'The first year begins with getting the students up to date with the basic medical science side of the course. Each day is filled with mixtures of lectures, practical anatomy sessions and PBL tutorials along with pathology tutorials. Anatomy teaching is very strong at Edinburgh University, especially in semester 1, to get all the students to the same level of basic knowledge. Work-play balance is excellent so long as you plan your time in advance. A typical Tuesday would begin with a 10-minute stroll to the lecture theatre for a 9.00am start. Each lecture lasts around 50 minutes (allowing ten minutes to get to your 10.00am) then a coffee in the RMS while revising the previous lecture before PBL at 11.30am. Lunch would be around 1.00pm and there are many places to get lunch or eat something you prepared yourself. The afternoon would then consist of either learning clinical skills, visiting patients or a practical anatomy class. Other afternoons from semester 2 and beyond would be set aside for working on your Student Selected Component. The second year also introduces visits to a GP practice once a week. The examinations can be tough but they are fair. If you keep up to date with the lectures, the suggested reading material and the online computer assisted learning courses you should perform very well. There is enough time especially in the pre-clinical years to enjoy yourself, whether that be socialising, playing sports, getting involved with societies or having a relationship. The highlights of my pre-clinical years include getting to know some of the most amazing friends anyone could hope to meet, presenting the findings of an SSC to a group of consultants, joining MARROW and attending the medics' nights out. The advice I would give to a first year who is about to start would be to make sure you don't fall behind with the workload but also make sure you have a fantastic time and try not to get too stressed over exams!'

Clinical

'The clinical years are fantastic fun, giving you the opportunity to see what it is like, first hand, to work in different departments. Placements vary between two to eight weeks, with exams at the end. You can get as involved as you like, with the added bonus of knowing that there is someone (usually an F1 or 2) who you can check over anything with before you have the scary responsibility! Days tend to begin with a ward round, followed by some timetabled teaching sessions, either on the ward or in tutorial rooms, followed by 'ward-time'. Out patient clinics are also useful, and it is an excellent opportunity to see progression of disease and a wide variety of patients in a relatively short space of time. The later years give you more freedom, and you can organise your time in the most useful way. Exams are MCQs, OSCEs and OSCAs, which can be difficult and so it is best to get into a group and help and practise with each other.'

Once you get in...

Before you start you will have documents and other official forms posted to you for you to fill in before you begin in September. Some of these will regard accommodation and it's best to apply for accommodation online (as early as possible) as it's much quicker and easier. Expect to get lots of information from lecturers and professors on what medical textbooks to buy. There are booklets provided by the university giving the pros and cons of each but it's best to hold off buying any books until at least after freshers' week. Your freshers' week timetable is provided by the medical school and will help you keep this busy and somewhat hectic week as hassle free as possible.

The Best Thing	Great teaching from some of the highest regarded clinicians and researchers in the world
The Worst Thing	Commuting to and from the various hospitals and GP practices can take up a lot of time

Student top tips

Edinburgh is one of the oldest and most well established medical schools in the UK so read up on the history! Alumni include Charles Darwin who described evolution, Joseph Lister 'the father of modern antiseptics', Sir James Young Simpson who discovered chloroform and its use in sedation and many, many others.

Summary Table

Positives	Negatives
Teaching from some of the leading clinicians and researchers in the world	They have busy schedules and so may change teaching times last minute
Excellent medical library and IT services	Can be busy during exam times
State of the art hospitals with up to date equipment	Commuting to and from hospitals takes up time
Fascinating history involving the medical school and the city itself	Renewal work is ongoing and can be distracting
Beautiful city and surrounding areas	Can be very cold and windy in the winter

Glasgow

Medicine admissions medical school office
University of Glasgow
Glasgow
G12 8QQ

www.gla.ac.uk/medicine

Glasgow Medical School has a worldwide reputation for excellence in both medicine and surgery. Scholars linked with the university include Joseph Lister, who promoted the use of antiseptics to provide a sterile environment for surgery, the influential anatomist and physician William Hunter, Professor Ian Donald, who pioneered the development of diagnostic ultrasound and the current Chief Medical Officer of Scotland, Dr Harry Burns.

The faculty of Medicine is located in the contemporary Wolfson Building and offers a modern approach to educating future doctors. Teaching methods include problem-based learning scenarios and clinical skills training. These are taught in a purpose-built clinical skills suite, which contains its own mock hospital ward and consultation rooms.

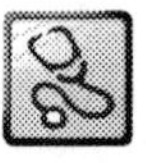

The medical course

Key facts

Course Type	Problem-based learning	**Degree Awarded**	MBChB
Basic Entry Requirements	AAA	**Entrance Exams**	UKCAT
Year Size	Approx 220	**Open Days**	June and September
Admissions Website	www.gla.ac.uk/schools/medicine/		

Getting in – student tips

Glasgow Medical School use the personal statement to judge an applicant's commitment and suitability for a career in Medicine.

Work experience, although useful, is not essential as long as candidates have spoken with their own GP and have researched the realities of a career in Medicine. However, admissions tutors expect potential applicants to display a caring nature, depicted through voluntary or paid work involving care within a community setting.

A selection of applicants are invited to a formal interview. These are normally held between November and March. The interview panel consists of two members of the Admissions Committee, who will be either staff at the medical school or practising doctors. Interviewers expect applicants to display a good knowledge of the Glasgow Medical School course, in particular, problem-based learning. General questions asked in the interview may relate to topical medical issues, the applicant's non-academic achievements and ability to manage stress.

Course details

Foundation / Pre-Med	No	**Graduate**	Yes
Student Population	Male: female ratio: 40:60	**Term Length**	10–15 weeks
Erasmus / Foreign Exchange	Not available	**Elective Period**	There are two elective periods: Junior: end of year 3/ start of year 4 Senior: end of year 4/ start of year 5

Intercalation

Stage	Between year 3 and year 4	**Degree Awarded**	BSc (Med Sci) –1 year (standard) or BSc (Honours) – 2 years.
Requirements	Entry is based on academic performance in years 1 – 3	**Subjects**	Glasgow offers a wide range of intercalated degrees in either Clinical Medicine or Biomedical Science

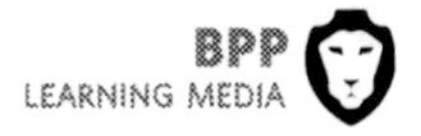

Anatomy teaching

In years 1 to 3 anatomy is generally covered as part of a related problem-based learning scenario. This may then be backed up with a fixed resource session (laboratory class) in the dissecting room or in histology lab.

There is also a dedicated block of anatomy in the first term of the first year which gives a general overview of the subject, covering the upper respiratory tract, the spine and spinal cord, lungs, chest cavity, heart, abdomen, pelvis, upper and lower limbs, the skull and the brain. At the end of the block there is a formative exam to allow students to monitor their progress.

Students are taught gross anatomy using cadavers with groups of no more than eight students per specimen. Several supervisors regularly visit each group so there is plenty of opportunity to ask questions. Prosections may also be used for revision purposes.

There is also the opportunity to take two anatomy based SSCs in the second and third years covering the anatomy of the 'upper and lower limbs' and 'head and neck' respectively. During an SSC you will spend three hours a day for five weeks dissecting cadavers, backed up with a one hour lecture on the same topic everyday.

Pre-clinical/Years 1–2	
Topics	***Year 1:*** Hierarchy of systems, Core values in medicine, Introduction to human anatomy, Determinants of health, Disease patterns, Homeostasis, Risks and responses, Health and illness in communities. ***Year 2:*** Conception, Growth and Development, Musculoskeletal and Neurological Systems, Cardiovascular, Respiratory and Renal Systems, Digestion and Metabolism, Regulation and Responses
Teaching	Primarily Problem-based learning (PBL) backed up with plenaries (lectures), fixed resource sessions (labs/tutorials/dissections/histology/etc), VS (Vocational Skills) and hospital and GP visits.

SSC Periods	There is one SSC period in the pre-clinical years. This occurs in the middle of the second year (between January and February) and lasts for five weeks. There are a wide variety of subjects available for study, from basic sciences such as the anatomy of the upper and lower limbs and skin biology, to more clinical options such as Osteoporosis, Breast Cancer, Sports Medicine and the pathogenesis of malaria. Also, subjects from the faculty of arts, such as languages (Spanish or French) and the history of medicine may be studied.
Exams	Exams take the format of a PBL scenario on which short answer questions are asked. 60% needed to pass. OSCE at the end of the second year.

Clinical/Years 3–5	
Topics	***Year 3:*** Cardiovascular and respiratory systems, Haematology, Musculoskeletal systems, Dermatology, Neurology, Psychiatry, Abdomen and breast. Vocational Skills continues throughout year 3. ***Year 4/Year 5:*** Medicine, Surgery, Psychological medicine, Child health, Obstetrics and gynaecology, General practice.
Elective	During the summer vacations after your third and fourth years, you are required to undertake two, four-week periods of elective study. These are in subjects and locations of your choice.
SSC Periods	There is a wide variety of topics available. Modules are taken in second (one module), third (two) and fourth (two) year. Each module lasts five weeks. Options are vast and encompass titles from Anatomy to Working with children. SSC periods are also a great opportunity to take part in audits, research and publications.
Exams	***Year 3:*** In June you sit an OSCE and two written papers. There is coursework throughout the course of the year which is also part of the summative assessment. ***Year 4:*** No exams. ***Year 5:*** Finals are in February and encompass two written papers and one OSCE.

Hospital placements/academies

Peripheral hospitals offer good accommodation at no extra charge, so it's great to save you having to commute every day to the area and allows you that extra sleep-in which is essential, especially considering the cold Scottish winter days. In the fourth and fifth years, each allocated placement extends over a period of five weeks. I don't think there's a worst/best placement, but peripheral hospitals are known to be cleaner, less chaotic and offer better teaching as the clinician's are not covered head-to-toe with other (more important) things to do, so despite the hassle of getting to the placement, it's not a bad experience after all.

Hospitals and Travel Time from University	
Western Infirmary	2 minutes
Gartnavel General and Gartnavel Royal (Psychiatric Hospital)	10 minutes
Glasgow Royal Infirmary	20 minutes
The Royal Hospital for Sick Children, Yorkhill	15 minutes
Southern General	20 minutes
Wishaw Hospital	45 minutes
Hairmyres Hospital	45 minutes
Crosshouse Hospital	1 hour
Royal Alexandria Hospital, Paisley	40 minutes
Ayr Hospital	1 hour 30 minutes

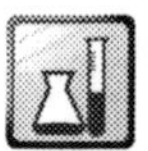

The medical school

Work						Brief summary on volume of work
Facilities						The 'Study Landscape' (medical library) is well equipped and modern, with good access to both textbooks and computers

Support						Students are assigned to an adviser of studies who can help with course or social problems. There is also counselling and health services available on campus
Feedback						Two way feedback very thorough

Facilities

The 'Study Landscape' (Medical Library), located in the medical school, is open 24 hours a day, 365 days a year. There are multiple copies of all the essential textbooks you will use on the course, and as it is not a lending library, the books are always there, so you really don't have to buy any of your own textbooks unless you want to. There are also lots of computers with internet access, as well as plenty of computer programs which supplement the course.

There is also a clinical skills suite housing consultation rooms and a mock ward. These are used for VS (Vocational Skills) classes, and can be booked in the evenings by individuals or groups of students who want to practise their clinical skills outside of class time. During VS sessions, communication skills are brought to life with the use of trained actors who portray a variety of physical and mental illnesses, and may present ethical dilemmas. These sessions can be recorded by video camera and copied onto a DVD so that you can review your performance in your free time as well as gaining feedback from other members of your VS group.

Student support

Each student is assigned an adviser of studies for the duration of the course who they can speak to regarding any personal difficulties they may encounter. There is also an affective Learning Adviser with specific experience of the medicine course who can offer advice on study techniques and exam preparation.

Year co-ordinators and vocational skills tutors can provide support for students when they are facing difficulty with a particular area of the course. Students are also encouraged to visit the counselling

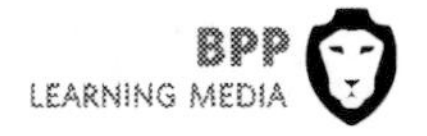

service if they have emotional difficulties which may be affecting their studies.

Finance

For graduate students there is 'Second Degree Fund' which students apply for annually in order to receive additional support.

> **Student opinion**
>
> *'The building is truly an innovative site for the newcomer's eye. A very modern take on architecture indeed, making it the highlight of the university infrastructure really with regard to things that "stand out". For those keen on self-directed learning and who enjoy the challenge of implementing self-discipline, this is the school for you, look nowhere else. The course is highly motivating, inspiring and revolutionary.'*

The university

Accommodation	Non-campus
Further Info	www.gla.ac.uk/studentlife/accommodation/

Accommodation

In the first year, the majority of students tend to stay in Murano Street Student Village that is (self-catering), with between four and ten students sharing a flat. Each flat consists of single bedrooms with a desk / study area, shared living room / kitchen area, bathroom and toilet facilities.

Other student self-catering flats, which are popular with first years, include Queen Margaret Residence, Cairncross House, Winton Drive, and Kelvinhaugh Gate and Kelvinhaugh Street. Wolfson Hall is also popular and is catered.

All halls / student flats are about 15-20 minutes' walk away from both the main campus and the medical school. There is also a free bus service, which runs between 5.30pm and 10.00pm most

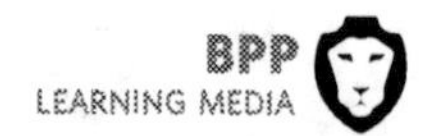

evenings (timetable: www.src.gla.ac.uk/services/minibus/) taking students from the main building on campus, back to each of the main halls. This means you do not have to worry about walking back from the library late in the evenings.

Study facilities

The main library on campus has a lending service – allowing books to be borrowed for up to a month at a time. The Round Reading Room, located opposite the main library, also offers computer and internet access between the hours of 9.00am-5.00pm during term-time.

University sports & students' union

Unlike most universities, which have one students' union, Glasgow has two – each with their own identity. The older of the two, which is also the oldest students' union in Scotland, is Glasgow University Union (GUU), which was founded in 1885. The GUU houses several bars and popular clubs, as well as two libraries, a snooker hall and a convenience shop. This union has a worldwide reputation for debating, having held the world debating title more often than any other university in the world. One of the most popular events in GUU's calendar is 'Daft Friday' – a 12-hour annual ball which is held on the last Friday before the Christmas holidays.

The other, more modern union is the Queen Margaret Union (QMU). This union is famous for great gigs, having played host to bands including Nirvana, the Red Hot Chili Peppers and Franz Ferdinand. The QMU boasts several bars and club nights, which cater to all tastes in music, from Revolution rock night to Cheesy Pop. Cheesy Pop is the longest running student night in Scotland.

Student opinion

'Due to the vast range of leisure activities available at Glasgow, students can easily find time to relax from the pressures of academic life. This also enables them to develop new friendships, meeting both medical students and those from other faculties.'

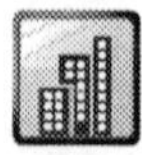

The city

Safety						Glasgow is a safe city, occupied by friendly locals
Nightlife						The city has a great number of affordable bars, pubs and clubs
Transport						Good public transport with regular buses and trains on the subway to and from the city centre
Cost of Living						Rent: £120-300 pcm

Things to do

Glasgow is Scotland's largest city and due to its proximity to the countryside, offers the perfect balance between city life and the dramatic mountains and lochs, which Scotland is famous for.

The city is the second largest shopping capital in the UK, after London. It hosts a vast number of diverse and affordable bars, restaurants and nightclubs.

Glasgow is also renowned for its architecture, ranging from the Victorian gothic grandeur of the university, to the modern Clyde Conference Auditorium (known locally as the 'Armadillo'), and Clyde Arc Bridge (or the 'Squinty Bridge') on the banks of the river Clyde.

Being home to three other universities and several colleges, the city has a large student population meaning that most student activities tend to be reasonably priced.

Places to Go		
Place	**Brief Description**	**Entry Fee/Opening Time**
Curlers	A small pub, a street away from the main university buildings. Serves food throughout the day until 8.00pm. Often hosts MedChir evening events.	£Free, Mon–Thurs: 11.00–11.00pm, Fri–Sat: 11.00 and Sun: 12.30–11.00pm
Viper	Popular student club close to the university.	Mon–Sun: 10.30–02.00 (Closed on Tuesdays)
ABC Glasgow	Popular gig venue which hosts club nights with a mixture of indie, punk, soul and electro music.	£Free entry before 11.30pm and between £3–5 thereafter. Thurs–Sat: 11.00pm–3.00am
The Garage	Offers regular themed nights and plays indie, alternative, rock, R&B, chart, pop music.	Open 7 days a week, 365 days a year. £Free entry before 12.00pm, £3–5 thereafter.

Student opinion

'Glasgow is a modern city with a diverse population and many places to visit, regardless of where your interests may lie.'

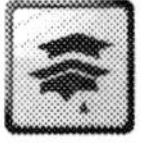

Student's view

Pre-clinical

'The first year follows the format of 'The Hierarchy of Systems', which allows you consider a disease or illness from its molecular foundations through to the cellular and anatomical basis all the way up the hierarchy to the condition's impact on the patient, their family, the community and the wider world.

The weekly timetable at Glasgow for the pre-clinical years is generally less full than lecture based courses (with 9.00am-5.00pm classes) to allow time for independent study.

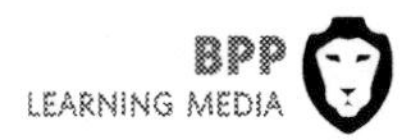

Usually the week begins with a problem-based learning (PBL) session. In first year, PBL sessions tend to take place on Mondays and Thursdays; giving you two to three days to complete each PBL.

During the first session the group (with usually eight to nine students per group) read the scenario and select the main issues that are then used to generate questions. Students in the group research all the objectives to ensure that everyone has a thorough understanding of important concepts.

In the following PBL session, each member of the group feedbacks on the information they have learned from their personal study in order to answer the questions from the first session. The group also begins a new scenario in this session and the whole process begins again.

PBL groups are changed throughout the year, allowing the opportunity meet lots of different people on the course.

The material covered in PBL is backed up with plenaries (lectures) and fixed resource sessions (labs/ dissection/ tutorials). However, as mentioned previously, there is plenty of 'free' time to research PBL objectives and to pursue social and sporting activities.

Before beginning the course students often have reservations about learning via the PBL method, however, the faculty is extremely supportive and several introductory lectures are given during the first week; explaining the process and offering advice on self-directed learning.

Personally, I've found that as well as learning the appropriate objectives PBL has taught me how to approach a clinical problem, to be responsible for my own learning and to gain confidence when presenting my ideas to a group – skills which will be essential when practising as a doctor.

One of my favourite aspects of the medical course at Glasgow is having early patient contact; often taking place within the first few weeks. The majority of patient contact in the preclinical course occurs through Vocational Skills (VS) sessions.

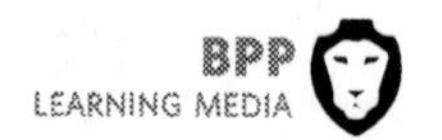

Vocational Skills (VS) sessions, lasting three hours, are timetabled once every week and encompass all the ethical, clinical and communication skills you will require to practise medicine. In addition to this, there are two patient based projects undertaken in the pre-clinical years; the first follows a patient with a chronic health condition, while the second follows the development of a newborn baby to the age of 9 months.'

Clinical

'The final two years of the course, ie the clinical years, are a truly innovative experience to say the least. It's the most exciting aspect of being a medical student. Even though the Glasgow course is unique in that you get hands on experience from day one of the course, it isn't until you reach the fourth and fifth year that you're truly getting the "full throttle" of the clinical world. Both years are divided into a series of blocks, each comprising five-week periods and allocations are made to the following fields: three Medical placements, three surgical, one Paediatrics, one Psychiatry, one Obstetrics & Gynaecology and one General Practice placement. You are allocated to a specific hospital for the duration of the block and assigned to a consultant who serves as your "educational supervisor".

In most cases, it is one student to one consultant, but you may sometimes share an educational supervisor with another colleague. The aims in each block are to get a thorough teaching of examination techniques, recognising and diagnosing the presentation of various clinical conditions and disorders, learning how to analyse imaging reports, test results, etc and building on your patient-history skills and communication skills. Teachings are usually in small groups of four to five students to the bedside to maximise benefit for each member. I loved every aspect of the stratification of the clinical course here at Glasgow University. It truly provided me with extensive opportunity to hone my skills, identify and address weak areas and become increasingly familiar and comfortable with clinical applications, thereby effectively integrating textbook information with the healthcare foundation. A normal days encompasses attending ward round starting at 8.00 or 9.00am, lasting until ~12.00pm, followed by a short lunch break and tutorial or bedside teaching in the early afternoon, or alternatively attending clinics (am or pm).

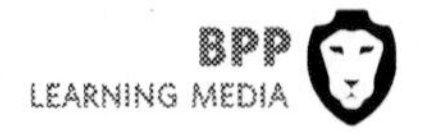

Each of the specialties has specific teaching objectives and schedules to permit students to gain an utmost valuable experience.

All the clinicians are keen to teach and involve students on the wards, and encourage self-confidence. I've never had any problems with this aspect, as everyone is extremely professional, helpful and understanding. They even let you scrub in on surgeries and watch the most experienced of consultant work their magic. I can't imagine a better course for getting the most out of the clinical years which are critical to preparing any medical student for the great challenges and demanding endeavours that lie ahead.'

Postgraduate

'I had never been to Glasgow before applying, but after spending an hour in the city and having my interview, I'd already made up my mind to accept a place if one was offered because I was made to feel as though I belonged here. It's a very friendly medical school, and graduates are really encouraged to apply and there's plenty of support for us once we get here.

Every day is different. I might be in a PBL session in the morning and a lab in the afternoon, I might be spending the day with my vocational studies group in hospital, or I might have just an hour or two of lectures before escaping to the Study Landscape to do independent study for my PBL.

Because I'd already done a science degree that was taught as a very traditional, lecture-based course, I chose Glasgow so that I could come to a medical school where I would be able to learn more independently. It's hard work and you have to be very self-motivated, but it's perfect for me. The highlight for me has been that I've seen patients throughout my first two years – that's what medicine's all about and it's the part I love, and I'm very excited now to start the more clinical years.

It's a busy course with a lot of work, but it's important to get the balance right and there's plenty of time for family, friends, and other activities. I've been able to join a great church community, take up running, and sing all over the west of Scotland with the City of Glasgow Chorus.

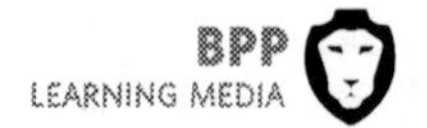

There are plenty of graduates, and we all got here via different routes. I did a Biomedical Sciences degree, but I've got friends who've done degrees in different fields, come through Access courses, had other careers, and had children. As the 'mature students', we all banded together a bit during freshers' week and we all still get on really well, but it doesn't take long at all for the barriers to break down – one of my close friends is in her 30s and another is still a teenager, and it doesn't feel as though there's any distinction anymore.'

Once you get in...

In August, after meeting the conditions of your offer you will receive a 'Welcome Pack' from the University. This contains a letter welcoming you to the faculty of medicine and includes a description of the responsibilities of all Glasgow medical students, a list of recommended textbooks and equipment you will need during your first year (ie a stethoscope, tendon hammer, and white coat), a copy of the medical students magazine SURGO, information on the medical student society MedChir and other administrative forms such as an IT skills booklet.

You will also have to sign up for Vale (the Medical Students Online Learning Environment) and Websurf (online access to other course information) accounts before you begin your studies. The week before freshers' week you will also be required to attend the medical school in order to give a blood sample and to begin the Hepatitis B immunisation programme if you haven't already started this.

The Best Thing	A friendly and supportive environment to learn in with early patient contact within the first few weeks of medical school, allowing you to develop the communication and clinical skills essential to becoming a good doctor
The Worst Thing	A few of the hospitals or general practices can be in peripheral locations therefore it is worth setting a side a bit of extra money for travel expenses

Student top tips

- Don't worry about trying get your Hepatitis B immunisations carried out before coming to Glasgow, as the University Health Service will do this free of charge.
- Don't buy any textbooks before you start (unless you are very, very keen) as there are multiple copies of all the books you will need in the Study Landscape and you can discover which ones you personally find most useful.

Summary Table

Positives	Negatives
Good supportive learning environment	Lack of available parking in university area
Study Landscape open 24 hours a day, 7 days a week – so no need to buy books.	Some hospitals in peripheral areas so you will need to budget for this
Early patient contact	
Anatomy taught using cadavers (which isn't the case in most medical schools)	
Good social environment with plenty of medics' societies and sports clubs	

HYMS Hull York

York:
John Hughlings Jackson Building
University of York
Heslington
York
YO10 5DD

Hull:
Hertford Building
University of Hull
Hull
HU6 7RX

www.hyms.ac.uk

Who said you couldn't have the best of both worlds? One medical school, two very different cities. Over the five-year course you will get to spend time in the picturesque city of York and the fast developing, student city of Hull. York is one of the oldest and most beautiful cities in the UK, with its rambling cobbled streets, ancient walls, the famous Minster and more pubs than days of the year it would be difficult not to enjoy your time here. Then there's Hull, home of the incredible submarium 'the deep', a brand new shopping centre (to add to the two existing ones) and whole area of the city where everything seems aimed at students.

The course combines all the best aspects of the longer running ones with newer elements aimed at equipping tomorrow's doctors with the best education and experience. With clinical placements from year one you can put everything into practice straight away and really feel you're progressing towards your ultimate goal.

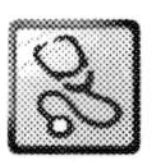

The medical course

Key facts

Course Type	PBL	Degree Awarded	MBBS
Basic Entry Requirements	AAA	Entrance Exams	UKCAT
Year Size	Approx 140 places	Open Days	Five open days a year in March, July and October
Admissions Website	www.hyms.ac.uk		

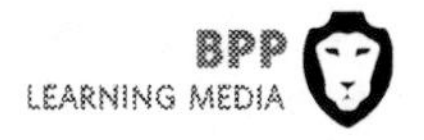

Getting in – student tips

HYMS are looking for evidence of an applicant's motivation to work in healthcare, self-motivation, team working skills, an appropriate level of maturity and confidence and a realistic understanding of healthcare issues and practice. HYMS are also interested in 'unusual qualities and life experience'.

Two people interview candidates; one will be a healthcare professional. Compared to some interviews the HYMS one will seem quite relaxed, you aren't sat across a table from the interviewers so don't feel that they are a judging panel and they are always very friendly to put candidates at ease. In addition to this all of the questions are posted on the medical school website a few weeks before so you can prepare for potential questions. Another element to the interview is that each candidate is given an article to read outside the interview room to then discuss any issues which arise from the article with the interviewers. I was in the first intake where this was done and I actually felt more comfortable when the interview questions started having had a chance to discuss the article first so the initial focus was my thoughts on a separate matter, not me.

Course details

Foundation / Pre-Med	NA	**Graduate**	NA
Student Population	Male: female ratio: 37:63	**Term Length**	Pre-clinical: 12 weeks Commencing: End of Sept Clinical: 16–19 weeks Commencing: Year 3 –1st September, year 4 – second week of August.
Erasmus/ Foreign Exchange	NA	**Elective Period**	First 8 weeks of year 5

Intercalation

Stage	Intercalation is possible between years 2 and 3 or 4 and 5. If you intercalate between years 4 and 5 you have opportunity to do a Masters	**Degree Awarded**	BSc or BA
Requirements	Exam results	**Subjects**	A large variety of subjects are on offer in both Hull and York for example Anatomy, Biology, Medical Ethics and Sports Science. HYMS are also happy for students to intercalate at other medical schools with increasing numbers choosing courses in Leeds, Manchester and London

Anatomy teaching

Anatomy is taught through lectures and the use of models and prosections but if a student would like to try their hand at dissection there are opportunities available in the form of SSCs or just asking the anatomy team nicely. The amount of teaching depends on the topic. For example when studying the musculoskeletal system you have a lot of teaching on anatomy but during weeks where your focus is at a more cellular level you won't have any. As students we don't feel we miss out by not carrying out dissections ourselves as it allows more time for learning and asking questions.

The anatomy departments in Hull and York are state of the art. The staff are the most wonderful thing about anatomy at HYMS and will happily arrange one-to-one sessions with any student who feels they need a bit of extra help.

Pre-clinical/Years 1–2	
Topics	***Year 1:*** foundations of medicine, heart and lungs, Gastrointestinal system, immunology, Brain, Psychology, Endocrinology and Reproduction. ***Year 2:*** Disease Processes, Excretion and homeostasis, Reproductive and child health, Musculoskeletal and nervous systems, Cardiovascular and respiratory systems, Nutrition, metabolism, digestion and excretion.
Teaching	Teaching is done mainly in the form of plenary lectures and PBL sessions. Clinical placement supplements teaching allowing an opportunity to apply knowledge in the real setting of a hospital or general practice. The PBL sessions involve virtual patients who are discussed in groups (which stay consistent throughout the year) and learning outcomes are derived. The students then have a chance to go away and do some learning on their own, answering each learning outcome. In the next PBL session the outcomes are discussed, and questions are answered.
SSC Periods	There are three SSC periods throughout the year. The first two run simultaneously with the regular teaching where classes are attended once a week. The third one however runs for two weeks and classes are attended every day with no other teaching going on.
Exams	There are two formative exams throughout the year. The first one being before the Christmas holidays and the second one being before the Easter holidays. These examinations do not count towards your final mark and the written portion of it is self marked. The marks do go to your PBL tutors however and if they are low you may be called in for a discussion. The HYMS staff do not want anyone to fail and do their best to ensure that students pass. The summative examinations are held once a year and consist of an OSCE and three written papers. Resits are held five weeks later.

Clinical/Years 3–5	
Topics	***Year 3:*** Oncology, cardiorespiratory medicine, dermatology, mental health, gastroenterology and endocrinology. ***Year 4:*** Paediatrics, obstetrics and gynaecology, neurology and musculoskeletal.

Topics continued	***Year 5:*** Begins with the elective period then students spend three blocks of eight weeks working as an intern in medicine, surgery and primary care to ease the transition to becoming a Foundation 1 doctor.
Elective	Students are able to go anywhere in the world. The only times the medical school will object to an elective destination is if there is good reason to be concerned about a student's safety. Students are expected to fund the elective themselves but are given details of where they can apply for grants.
SSC Periods	Students do three SSCs per year each lasting three weeks and typically at the end/beginning of an eight-week topic block. There is a large variety of SSC topics which differ according to which of the sites you are based at, a few examples are 'fraud in the NHS', 'medical hypnotism', 'basic surgical techniques' and 'hill walking'. Students also have the opportunity to propose their own SSC on virtually anything they want as long as they can find a tutor willing to take them on. If students wish to there is opportunity to use the SSC for audits or research.
Exams	Due to years 3 and 4 been viewed collectively as phase II all of the exams for this phase occur at the end of year 4. The exams have both practical and written elements. The exams are difficult especially with two years' worth of work to be examined on but most students do pass.

Hospital placements/academies

During the second year you will choose somebody from your home site to pair up with, the two of you will then be paired with two students from the other site making groups of two Hull and two York students. During years 3 and 4 your teaching will take place in these groups. At the peripheral hospitals there is usually only your group studying a specialty at a time but at the bigger hospitals there may be two or three groups. Having small numbers on each specialty means students have opportunity to gain a lot of experience because there aren't lots of students competing to see the same things.

Other than at the site where you were based in the first and second year NHS accommodation is provided. Over the course of years 3 and 4 students move around four of the five hospital sites (Hull, York, Grimsby, Scunthorpe and Scarborough) spending around six months in each place. Hull and York have the largest hospitals so

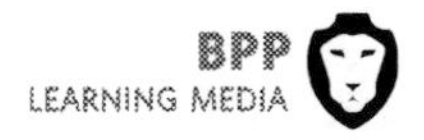

more students are at these sites whereas there may only be 30–40 students placed at the peripheral sites at a time.

The main downside to NHS accommodation is the lack of television and internet access. This doesn't create too much of a problem in Scunthorpe or Grimsby as your accommodation is within a minute's walk of the onsite med school building which has 24-hour access. Some Scarborough students in the past have set up dial up internet and the York accommodation is relatively new so does have broadband.

Other than the York accommodation, which is fit for a king the rest, is pretty basic but you're only there five days a week and you do have everything you need. Having been based in both Scunthorpe and Grimsby I will say that the lack of internet and TV is not quite the end of the world we all expected, everyone gets a lot more work done and the sites are much more sociable because of it.

Hospitals and Travel Time from University	
Hull Royal Infirmary	5–10 minutes
Castle Hill Hospital, Hull	15 minutes
York District Hospital	5 minutes
Scarborough District General Hospital	10 minutes
Goole and District Hospital	35 minutes

The medical school

Work						Can be challenging
Facilities						Each hospital has a recently built/furnished state of the art medical school building with full time staff including a student liaison officer
Support						Small student numbers mean fantastic support
Feedback						Excellent student feedback

Facilities

Each HYMS building at each hospital site has an IT suite, common room (usually with TV), clinical skills lab, tutorial room and simulation rooms. There is no HYMS library but we do have access to the NHS ones.

Student support

HYMS really is brilliant for support. Small student numbers allow you to get to know the staff and other students really well and if you ever have any problems there are numerous people who you'll feel comfortable enough with to ask for help or advice. As a student you do feel valued and the staff will go out of their way to help you.

In the first year there is a buddy system pairing each new student with second and third year buddies who help new students settle into university life, the PBL course and are there to answer any questions and concerns.

All new students are given information on who to contact with problems etc but most tend to speak to their PBL tutors about any worries. Both Hull and York have chaplaincies and counselling services if you don't want to speak to members of the medical school staff.

Finance

HYMS offer bursaries of up to £1,026. Students are also eligible for bursaries from the University of Hull and the University of York.

Student opinion

'With its close knit community, up to the minute course and fantastic facilities it's couldn't be any easier to settle in to life at HYMS. Combine all of that with the never ending social activities and the passionate staff and it's hard to imagine how things could be better!'

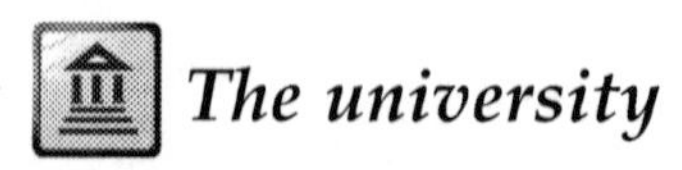

Accommodation	Campus or non-campus
Further Info	www.hyms.ac.uk/undergraduate/

Accommodation

There are various accommodation buildings in York University. Alcuin College is closest to the medical school and the buildings in which lectures are held. However students always end up having an amazing time no matter where they are placed.

Study facilities

The libraries are well equipped both in Hull and York with books relevant to the course. Sometimes however it pays to pick up specific books a little in advance as they can run out although anatomy and physiology is always available. York library does not stay open all night but during exam period they do extend the closing time.

University sports & students' union

HYMS starts its terms earlier than the regular universities and so HYMS students end up getting two freshers' weeks, one that is planned for only HYMS students and one that is planned for the York / Hull students. This is an excellent opportunity for students to get to know not only the medics but the other students as well. Students can sign up for their respective university events online and HYMS sends out specific packages before university starts allowing students to choose events. Although it seems like medics are always buried in work it is extremely easy to find time to join societies like yoga, dance, skiing and many others.

The students' union in Hull has one of the best nightclubs and medics do frequent it often. York also offers a vibrant students' union with regular student nights and even its own iphone app.

York has a well-equipped gym with courts for basketball, badminton, table tennis and others. The gym membership is at an extra cost but it pays off if well used!

Student opinion

'Being a student at York is a wonderful experience. The place is quiet, doesn't have too many people and there are always a variety of activities on hand to partake in. Each residential college has its own café so coffee and lunch are only a minute or two away. It is a truly good experience being an HYMS student in York.'

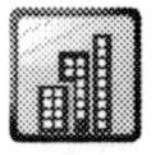

The city

Safety	⛨	⛨	⛨	⛨		Both Hull and York are safe places to be, very few students run into problems
Nightlife	☾	☾	☾	☾		Hull nightlife is cheaper with more going on nightly, York has more expensive venues and pubs with fewer student nights
Transport	🚌	🚌	🚌	🚌		You can manage without a car in years 1 and 2 easily but it would be a struggle in later years without at least one member of your group having a car
Cost of Living	🐖	🐖	🐖			Expect to pay around £50 per week rent

Things to do

Hull is a lively student city with numerous bars, restaurants, pubs and clubs offering student nights and deals. If that wasn't enough Hull University has an impressive students' union (it has been voted best in the country more than once) with its own nightclub, Asylum, and a couple of bars! From comedy nights to fancy dress balls something is guaranteed to be happening every night of the week. For when you aren't busy eating or drinking with friends there's the St Stephens shopping centre, laser quest, ice skating, The Deep, the university gym, a choice of four cinema complexes and several 'learn scuba diving' companies to help you spend what's left of your loan. It's a wonder people still manage to get their work done!

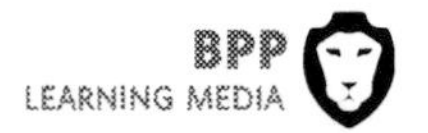

York is a city that is very difficult not to fall in love with. Unlike Hull where things are cheap to attract students York is more expensive because tourists are willing to pay the higher prices although with a bit of local knowledge you'll soon know where to find the student nights! With costs being higher you might only manage a couple of nights out a week but trust me you'll more than make up for any nights in and you'll be spoilt for choice for other things to do! How about a weekend at the races or stepping back in time at the Viking centre or York dungeons, shop till you drop in the city centre then enjoy a cappuccino by the Minster, take a ghost walk around the city at night or dress up for a game of pub golf visiting a few of the more than 300 pubs York is famed for?

The student areas of Hull and York are perfectly safe as long as you don't do anything you wouldn't anywhere else; you wouldn't walk alone down a dark street at night or leave your door unlocked at home. Very few students encounter any problems.

Places to Go		
Place	**Brief Description**	**Entry Fee/Opening Time**
The Deep, Hull	Award winning aquarium.	£7.50, 10.00am–6.00pm daily
Asylum, Hull	The SU night club	£3.50,Mon-Sat 10.00pm-3.30am
Evil Eye, York	Atmospheric bar in York, great for cocktails, mocktails and unusual beers.	£Free, open daily from 12.00pm

Student opinion

'Being a student in Hull is brilliant, the cheap accommodation means having plenty of loan left to make the most of the shops, bars, SU and student events.'

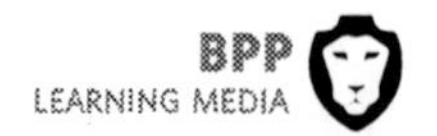

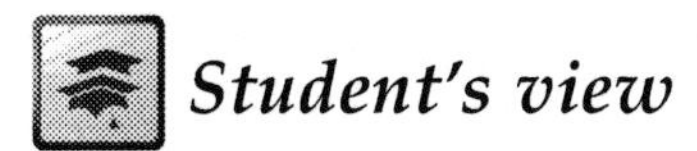

Student's view

Pre-clinical

'I chose the Hull York Medical School for many reasons. Clinical placement opportunity is offered to students from the first year. This is available on a weekly basis and is usually the time of week that students look forward to most. Applying to any medical school is not easy and HYMS is no exception. HYMS looks at well-rounded, knowledgeable students. The way the course was set out, the methods of teaching such as spiral curriculum and PBL set up were all very appealing.

HYMS has a wonderful, dedicated set of staff. I was surprised by the number of times I went to the reception, met different people and was addressed by my name each time. The warmth and care that the staff shows towards all the students is excellent.

The HYMS timetable is very structured although a lot of time is given for other, medical-school unrelated activities if you manage your free time wisely. There is most definitely a balance between work and play but this most definitely rests on your own ability to manage your time well and to create free time for play.'

Clinical

'My favourite thing about the clinical years is that every day is different. Each eight week block is broken down into a topic a week. During the oncology block one of those topics is intra-abdominal cancer. That week we spent time in endoscopy, followed a ward round, observed surgery to remove a bowel tumour, sat in on the colorectal surgeons out patients clinics and met patients at the local hospice with advanced disease.

The only sessions that occur every week are a general practice session where under the guidance of our GP tutor we take most of the patient histories and carry out the appropriate examination. A patient presentation where we each present and discuss a patient with the week's condition and finally on Fridays we have a conference call between all the groups studying the same topic across the sites.

My personal highlight from the clinical years so far has been getting to assist on a caesarean section. I'd only ever been able to scrub in on surgery before, but never actually taken part. I was quite nervous but the scrub nurse and the senior registrar who I was assisting were both very reassuring and talked me through everything. They were both amused by my shock at how much brute force goes into surgery, apparently that takes some getting used to and a fair few medical students get a bit queasy about the tearing that's needed. Having seen c-sections before I knew what to expect but actually being a part of it gave me a whole new perspective. Seeing mum and her new baby boy after felt all the more special knowing I'd helped to bring him into the world.

The only advice I would give to students is to keep notes up to date. Without the threat of exams at the end of the third year a lot of students fall into the trap of not doing enough work which results in a mad panic lasting most of the fourth year as they struggle to get last year's notes up to date for revision as well as keeping on top of the current ones.'

Once you get in...

Once you get in, the HYMS staff and students continue to send you lots of material both on the course and freshers' week. Everything you need to do is well outlined and explained. For York students, you will have to enrol online before a certain date. Other than that, there is nothing else mandatory to do online. You are given a provisional blackboard username and password and this allows you to communicate with the other freshers and the current students.

The Best Thing	The enthusiastic hospital staff that still find students a novelty will go out of their way to help you
The Worst Thing	At some sites you'll struggle to cover a placement's worth of parking with HYMS contribution to travel costs and you do sometimes feel all of your money is being spent on petrol

Student top tips

- Don't buy the Hull Uni freshers' week event pass. With the med school freshers' week at the same time you won't get your money's worth and more often than not you can get tickets on the day.
- Wait for a few weeks to buy any books! There's no rush, the library has plenty of copies of what you'll need to begin with and too many students fall into the trap of buying a £40 book then never using it.
- Make the most of your second year buddies by asking them any questions; it will help you to settle in.
- Don't get in a panic during after your first PBL session. It may seem scary not being told exactly how much work to do but after a few sessions you will find a happy balance and the staff do want you to enjoy the start of term!

Summary Table

Positives	Negatives
Small numbers allow a close staff-student community	HYMS students mainly mix with each other, by the end of term it can be a little claustrophobic
A good excuse to make the most of two very different cities	Hull and York students don't really get to know each other until the third year
Clinical experience from the beginning	Travel in clinical years
PBL gives students confidence in finding things out for themselves, a highly regarded skill in our graduates	The later years 16-19 week terms are a BIG stretch for your loan

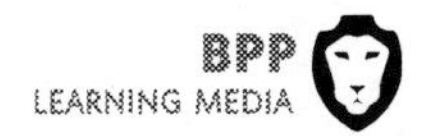

Keele

School of Medicine
Keele University
Keele
Staffordshire
ST5 5BG

www.keele.ac.uk/depts/ms/

Keele Medical School is one of the newest in the UK, having been established in 2003. Keele is situated in the Midlands between Manchester and Birmingham in the city of Stoke-on-Trent. Famous for its pottery production, Stoke is a very friendly city with a diverse cultural background that offers a lot to its visitors. Keele is a campus university and regularly wins awards for student popularity, and years 1 and 2 of medicine are spent on campus. The clinical years are shared between the base hospital in Stoke, University Hospital of North Staffordshire, Stafford District General Hospital and The Royal Shrewsbury Hospital, Shropshire. Community placements are often spread within the counties of Staffordshire and Shropshire so you will have exposure to a wide range of patient cohorts with their differing medical needs, offering you a broad medical knowledge base within a flourishing, enthusiastic medical school in which to start your rewarding career as a doctor.

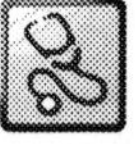 *The medical course*

Key facts

Course Type	PBL	Degree Awarded	MBChB
Basic Entry Requirements	AAB	Entrance Exams	UKCAT GAMAT for graduate entry student
Year Size	120	Open Days	June and August
Admissions Website	www.keele.ac.uk/health/schoolofmedicine/		

Getting in – student tips

The personal statement is your opportunity to tell the admissions team about yourself. It may sound obvious but one of the main things they are looking for are your reasons for choosing Medicine. Keele look for applicants who have work experience in a caring role, this doesn't need to be in a hospital or GP surgery. More important than the specific type of work is that you are able to reflect on what you did and what you have learned from it. Furthermore they are looking for any skills you have developed as a result of the work you did, or if this has changed your views. When assessing the personal statement, academic achievements, hobbies and interests, evidence of team work and communication skills in addition to your determination to study Medicine are considered. If you are planning a gap year you should mention your plans in your personal statement. Having a gap year doesn't increase or decrease your chances of getting in, however if you are applying for deferred entry, the admission panel are interested in reading your reasons for a gap year and what you intend to do during it.

Course details

Foundation / Pre-Med	Yes	**Graduate**	Yes
Student Population	Male: female ratio: 50:50	**Term Length**	Pre-clinical: 10 weeks Clinical: variable
Erasmus / Foreign Exchange	N/A	**Elective Period**	Year 5 – 8 weeks

Intercalation

Stage	Between years 2 and 3 or years 3 and 4 for bachelors and years 4 to 5 for masters.	**Degree Awarded**	BSc, MSc, MPhil, MRes
Requirements	To have passed all prior examinations and be ranked in the top third of the year.	**Subjects**	Medical Sciences/ Humanities

Anatomy teaching

Anatomy is taught in years 1 and 2 with histology and dissection practical sessions weekly. In year 1, the practical sessions are complemented with clinical skills – how to auscultate, examine the ear etc. In year 2 there is more emphasis on human pathology and disease and this is reflected within the teaching sessions.

Pre-clinical/Years 1–2	
Topics	***Year 1:*** Units covered – Emergencies, Infection and Immunity, Cancer, Ageing, Lifestyle and Complex family, each unit is four weeks long. Year 1 is called challenges to health. During year 1 the focus is on understanding how the body works normally. Anatomy and Physiology of all body systems are covered briefly, as are factors affecting health such as lifestyle and psychosocial aspects of health. Year 1 is designed to provide an introduction and overview, as all topics covered will be revisited in more depth throughout the course. ***Year 2:*** Units covered – Inputs and Outputs (eight weeks), Movement (four weeks), Life Support and Defence (eight weeks) and Sensation (four weeks). Year 2 is called integrated clinical pathology. Topics covered in year 1 are revisited, however the focus is on how the process of disease disrupts the normal function.
Teaching	During the first and second year all teaching centres around the theme of that week's PBL case. There are three PBL sessions per week. In the first session the case is read and discussed and the learning outcomes for the week are decided on by the group, and the outcomes are discussed in sessions two and three. All lectures, dissection and practical sessions are related to the PBL case, and the main focus is on the bioscience underpinning Medicine as well as the psychosocial aspects of health. In addition to this there is approximately one experiential learning session. These take place in small groups and can be group discussions, placements or Communication skills sessions. In the first year the aim of Communication skills is to begin practising the techniques used when interviewing a patient and this is done with the help of simulated patients. In the second year the sessions move on to practising taking patient histories and learning how to examine patients.

SSC Periods	There is one SSC period per year. In the first year the SSC period is three weeks, there is a choice of around 100 titles available and if there is any area that interests you it is possible to submit your own title for the project. A wide range of topics are available ranging from Medicine in space to genetics therapies to the history of Medicine. The SSC takes the form of an essay plus a five-minute presentation about your chosen subject. The SSC counts for 10% of the year mark.
Exams	Exam periods are in January and May/June, there are several forms of assessment. The Knowledge papers have both multiple choice and short answer written questions and test material covered in lectures as well as during PBL and lab practicals. In January there is a two-hour paper, which is half multiple choice, half written. In May/June there are two, two-hour papers that assess material covered during the whole of the year; one paper is multiple choice, the other short answer questions.

Clinical/Years 3–5	
Topics	***Year 3:*** General Medicine, General Surgery, Paediatrics, Elderly Care, Mental Health, Clinical Skills ***Year 4:*** Further Surgery, Further Medicine, Child Health, Mental Health, Women's Health ***Year 5:*** Primary care, Acute & Critical Care, Surgical Assistantship, Medicine Assistantship, Distant Elective
SSC Periods	Two SSCs in year 3 which are commonly on a topic of disease studied in the clinical/research setting with completion of a written report. One SSC in year 4 as careers exploration by spending time with doctors from a variety of specialties. Elective in year 5. Publications and audits are possible in any of the clinical SSCs depending on the expected outcomes of the SSC tutor.
Exams	Standard clinical exams include the MCQs, EMQs and OSCE twice yearly, taken towards the end of each semester. MCQs are standardised for the year's performance, therefore approximately 2% of the year must fail – however as long as a pass is achieved in both the OSCE and EMQ the student can still progress. By year 3 and above very few people fail the examinations.

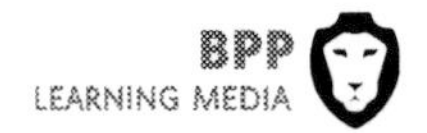

Elective period	The elective period offers maximal flexibility to the student, allowing them to spend 8 – 12 weeks in any subject they are interested in that is related to Medicine. The location of the elective has no limitation, and the majority of students at Keele University decide to experience healthcare overseas. Keele University does provide bursaries for any students at the university to travel abroad during their studies, and many Royal Colleges provide prizes for students attending an elective specific to the College's specialty.

Hospital placements/academies

Keele University is tied to three hospital trusts. Most students attend the large University Hospital of North Staffordshire in Stoke-on-Trent very close to the university, which has excellent facilities, including Cardiothoracic and Neurosurgery, and Paediatric & Neonatal Intensive Care. Onsite is the Clinical Education Centre where the majority of year 3 – 5 teaching is undertaken, with a dedicated health library. Staff are generally helpful and keen to teach. Time on placement varies with module, but tends to be between four and eight weeks, generally with two to four medical students per placement. Students tend to enjoy surgical placements particularly because of the rapid turn around of patients entering and leaving – great for clerking in lots of people – whereas medical wards (especially elderly care) has many long stay patients which can make time on the ward seem a little less exciting. Accommodation is available on Keele campus, but most students choose to rent houses close to the hospital.

Mid-Staffordshire General Hospitals Foundation Trust (based at Stafford General Hospital) is approximately 35 minutes by car away from Keele University, however basic accommodation is sometimes available to students on placement there (depending on demand). This is a medium sized trust and much smaller in comparison to UHNS, however it is relatively new to medical students, and therefore teaching at the hospital is excellent. About eight students study at this trust at any one moment in time.

The Shrewsbury and Telford Hospitals Trust (based at Shrewsbury) is approximately 50 minute's drive from Keele University, however new purpose built accommodation is available to the students attending. Approximately one third of the year is at this trust per semester. Time at Shrewsbury is very popular with medical students as it is also new to teaching students so staff are very keen to help, also it allows the students to experience a new area of the country, and a new nightlife. The student is expected to attend one semester at Shrewsbury between years 3 – 4.

Hospitals and Travel Time from University	
Keele Campus to University Hospital of North Staffordshire	7 minutes
Mid-Staffordshire General Hospitals Foundation Trust	35 minutes
Shrewsbury and Telford Hospitals	50 minutes

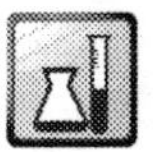

The medical school

Facilities	☕	☕	☕	☕	☕	Great librairies on campus, as well as off site libraries at academies
Support	👥	👥	👥	👥		There are multiple routes available for a student to seek support if they wish
Feedback	📋	📋	📋	📋		Feedback is constantly given from the consultants on the firm or via a print out breaking down student's exam results by module. The student is always aware of subjects on which theyneed to improve

Facilities

Facilities for medical students studying at Keele are very good. Keele University campus library has a dedicated health-orientated section, which is shared between the medics, nurses, physiotherapists and pharmacy students. It is well stocked, however, close to exam time some books may be in demand. Off campus at the hospital site there is a dedicated health library based at the newly built Clinical Education Centre (CEC) at the UHNS, and smaller libraries at Shrewsbury and Stafford Hospitals.

Most clinical skills are taught at the CEC in purpose-designed labs, and this is also the site of the simulated ward environment designed to prepare the fifth year student for entering their Foundation Year. IT facilities are numerous, both on Keele campus and at the hospital sites. There is also a large common room both on campus and at the CEC, and food may be purchased from one of the several shops on the hospital site, or from the large (and cheap) hospital restaurant at UHNS. Stafford and Shrewsbury hospitals also have shops and restaurants for food to be purchased and staff rooms to rest in. Overall, because of the relatively recent nature of Keele University teaching medicine, the medical school's facilities are all newly and purposefully built for medical education, and are highly recommendable.

Student support

Keele School of Medicine provides its own support service for medical students headed by an A&E consultant from the local hospital. It is an easily accessible and friendly service, willing to help on any matters concerning the medical student. The students' PBL tutor, who they will have known for the semester, can address relatively minor problems. Students also see an appraiser yearly who tracks how the student is progressing and also address any problems that may have arisen during the progress of the year.

Outside of the medical school the university also has its own dedicated student support service helping with many problems, including a counselling service and financial support. Keele University students' union also provides its own Independent Advice Unit and Nightline to support students. There is also an on campus health centre that all students living on campus may join. It provides a number of services for students, including sexual health clinics.

Medical societies

There are currently two societies that have originated from the medical school. The main society which most medics join is Keele Medics Society (KMS). KMS organises many nights out for medics throughout the year. The most important night in the medics' social calendar is the pyjama pub-crawl, taking place shortly after the medic-freshers have settled in. This night allows everyone from

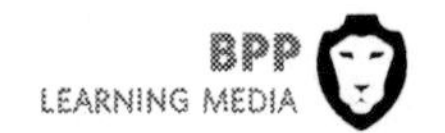

year 1 – 5 to meet and party together. KMS also plans the medic Christmas ball where students get the opportunity to smarten up in their dresses and tuxedos.

Sporting events are also managed by KMS, with frequent football, rugby, netball and hockey matches between medics taking place. A medic versus law student sports day also takes place towards the summer, and the student versus tutor football match is also a highlight of the sporting year. The second society is Keele Surgical Society (KSS), ideal for budding surgeons. KSS runs a number of events such as lectures on careers, interesting cases, etc, suturing sessions, advanced anatomy seminars and day-trips to sites of interest (eg Royal College of Surgeons). KSS also organises the annual summer ball.

Finance

Further info: www.keele.ac.uk/studentfunding/

See scholarships: www.keele.ac.uk/studentfunding/undergraduatebursaries/

Student opinion

'Moving from my family back at home, to Keele Medical School is like saying goodbye to one family and hello to another. As the medical school is so small comparatively, your peers and staff all become friends, resulting in the studying feeling more supported and intimate, with a strong team spirit found throughout all Keele medics. For those who want excellent student support, small class numbers and strong medic camaraderie, then Keele is the place for you!'

The university

Accommodation	Campus
Further Info	www.keele.ac.uk/studyatkeele/accommodation/

Accommodation

There are six halls of residence on campus ranging from 2 to 20 minutes' walk to the medical school. As Keele is a campus university everything is based within walking distance from each hall. All halls are self-catered, there is a catered option, and students are able to purchase a 'meal plan' from the Comus restaurant on campus. The vast majority of medics live on campus for the first year and most choose to stay on campus for the second year too. I lived in halls for two years and really enjoyed my time in halls. I lived in Horwood which is five minutes' walk to the medical school and the main campus and Hawthorns which is a 20-minute walk away, but is slightly out of the 'Keele bubble.' All halls on campus are fairly similar, the newer halls (Holly Cross and the Oaks) are all en- suite, whereas in other halls only a few blocks are en-suite. Halls are made up of several smaller blocks, the number sharing a kitchen and bathrooms is around six to eight, some blocks have slightly less and some slightly more to a kitchen. Each hall is slightly different, but everyone will tell you that the hall or block they live is miles better than all of the others.

Study facilities

The library on campus is used by everyone on campus, it is open from 10.00am - 10.00pm throughout the year and is open 24 hours during exam times. There is also the Health Library in The Clinical Education Centre at the hospital site. This is less busy than the main library and tends to be used mainly by third years and up, first and second years tend to use the campus library, and this reflects where each year is mainly based. Both libraries and the medical school have IT facilities. Both libraries have the recommended books for the course, although everyone seems to want to take out the same book at once, finding copies available for loan is not always possible, but there are plenty of reference copies.

University sports & students' union

The students' union is right in the middle of campus and is used by all students including medics. The union has the university's independent advice unit, print shop and various sales are held there throughout the year. The union campaigns on behalf of the students on many issues and students in charge of the union are always willing to help with any issue. At Keele most people associate the union with nights out, it has several bars and three areas with different music on in each room and, with different events on each night, there is something on for everyone. Live bands such as the Hoosiers and Sugababes have performed at Keele and there are various bands on throughout the year.

The gym has all the usual equipment, with cardio and weights areas, plus Keele is the only university with a kinesis room. Gym membership is around £150 for the academic year or from £3.00 per visit. The leisure centre has a climbing wall, squash courts and many other facilities available for hire as well as classes. Sports clubs and teams are aimed at all levels of ability so anyone can become involved in a sport from complete beginners, who want to keep fit and have a laugh, to those who want to compete at university level.

Student opinion

'When I started medical school at Keele University I felt like I'd joined a family and by now I know the staff well and I am friends with all the people in my year. This is the benefit of attending a medical school where the intake is small. It makes studying easier as there is a wealth of people I can ask when I'm stuck, from my friends and colleagues to the doctors who write my exams. And thanks to the early interaction with patients and the problem-based approach to studying the transition to the clinical years was less overwhelming but just as exciting. I would completely recommend Keele Medical School to anyone looking for a personalised and friendly approach to learning medicine.'

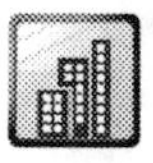

The city

Safety	⛨	⛨	⛨			Keele campus has a good security network and student transport around campus. Take care if out in Stoke and don't go out alone at night

Nightlife						The union is well attended and conveniently on campus. There are clubs in Newcastle-under-Lyme and Stoke itself which are reasonably priced and attract big name DJs – Trevor Nelson played in 2009
Transport						Traffic isn't a big issue in Stoke and public transport is reasonable. A car is pretty much essential as a medical student as community placements are frequently some distance away from your base site
Cost of Living						Stoke is a fairly cheap city to live in, rent is affordable (many properties are owned by med students or their families), taxis are cheap and all facilities are within easy reach. A decent pint will cost around £2.50, but obviously will be much cheaper at the union

Things to do

Stoke is probably better known for Alton Towers, a theme park which offers a great day out. A former area of major industrial production, the city is actively regenerating and has gyms, shopping centres, cinemas, theatres and many fine places to wine and dine at reasonable prices. There are many different cultural groups living in this city and this is reflected in the broad range of restaurants available. As the cost of living isn't very high here it is well within a student budget. Students at Keele tend to go out to the university union or in Newcastle-under-Lyme, the town immediately adjacent to Stoke, where the majority of students in the clinical years live. The junior doctors at UHNS have mess parties most months and students are invited along – a great opportunity to socialise with students past and present. There are clubs and bars in Stoke-on-Trent itself and let's not forget, Stoke is the birthplace of Robbie Williams!

Places to go		
Place	**Brief Description**	**Entry Fee/Opening Time**
Liquid	The main night club in the centre of Hanley	£5, Mon Student Night, 10.00am – late
Trentham Estate and Gardens	Perfect shopping for gifts, good food, or a touch of culture exploring the Trentham stately home estate.	£Free for shops, £6 for students to enter estate/ gardens, 9.00am – 6.00pm
Monkey Forest	Experience monkeys let loose while walking around this nature reserve	£5.50 for Students, Opens seasonally 10.00am – 5.00pm
Lakota	A chic cocktail bar found down the road from Keele in Newcastle-under-Lyme	£Free, All week.
The Club	The main LGBT night club in Staffordshire	£8 Mon (Student night), £10 Fri, inc drinks til 2.00am, open til 4.00am
Fluid	A smaller night club found close to Keele in Newcastle-under-Lyme	£4, Wed Student Night, 10.00am – late

Student opinion

'Stoke-on-Trent, may not strike the reader as a hotspot for things to do, but it actually has an unlimited amount of attractions to keep the student busy – from a bustling night life, an interesting history, plenty of shops, and, of course, Alton Towers. Personally, the highlight of Stoke, for me, is the people who make the city seem so friendly. For people who want to experience city life, but don't want to be overwhelmed by a huge city, and want the safety of campus life then Keele University is ideal.'

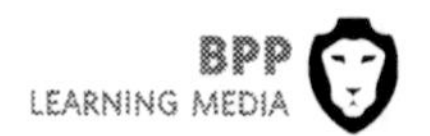

Student's view

Pre-clinical

'I applied to Keele because it is a new medical school with a new course. I also liked the idea of a PBL course as I thought it would be more interesting and interactive than a purely lecture based course.'

The timetable for the first two years is fairly busy, but the timetable changes from week to week, so while some weeks are very busy, this balances out with a quieter week afterwards. As the timetable changes and there are many different sessions it is never boring. A typical day, unfortunately usually starts at 9.00am with lectures and or PBL, the afternoon session may be a lab practical, experiential learning or dissection. As Keele is a PBL course there is a quite a lot of work expected outside of timetabled sessions. However it is easy to balance work and a social life. Personally, I try to get the majority of the work done in the week, leaving the weekends free, however this does change depending what is on during the week. During years 1 and 2, with a bit of organisation, it is possible to manage the workload, be involved in sports teams or societies and find time to go out. A medic's workload is not a reason not to go out, yes it is important to work hard but it is just as important to relax. Sometimes you do find you need a break from Medicine even though studying Medicine is an amazing experience and one I wouldn't change for anything.

For me the highlight of the course has been clinical skills as you get to learn the skills needed on the wards to examine and treat patients, such as venepuncture (taking blood) and patient examinations, I liked this as it provides an opportunity to practise the skills without just being thrown in the deep end on a ward. Outside of the course there are too many highlights to mention, I have had an absolutely fantastic time and met some amazing people, and can't wait to start the third year to see everyone and find out what its like to be in the clinical years.'

Clinical

'There is only one word to describe the clinical years: exhilarating – one day is never the same. My 'standard' Friday on a paediatric placement would typically run like this:

- *8.30am. Wake up (late).*
- *9.00am. Make it just in time to meet the other three medics on this placement with me and get to the ward to meet the doctor.*
- *9.05am. Present histories I took from a patient the previous day to the Consultant Paediatrician, and answer questions.*
- *9.30am. Consultant gives bedside teaching with some of the interesting patients on the ward.*
- *11.00am. Few hours free – I go to the acute paediatric admission ward and clerk in and examine some patients for the junior doctors. They feedback what went well and how I could improve.*
- *1.00pm. Paediatric X-ray meeting – listen to the radiologists interpret the imaging of some of the difficult to diagnose patients on the wards and all the paediatricians give their opinions on what might be the cause. Also gives me time to eat lunch.*
- *2.00pm. Run to the Clinical Education Centre for this week's skills: intraosseous needle insertion, followed by a seminar in developmental dysplasia of the hip and ended with 'Ask The Expert' where a Paediatrician comes in to answer any questions we have on our week's learning.*
- *5.00pm. Home to make tea, watch some TV and do some studying.*
- *10.00pm. Union!*

Because the medical school intake is small, and the UHNS is so large, learning opportunities are ample. The internet sign up system means any time I have free I can fill by choosing from a huge list of clinical experiences (from attending an oncology clinic to assisting a keyhole cholecystectomy in theatre). This gives me the greatest opportunity to extend my clinical knowledge. Clinical placements are well organised and consultant tutors are usually highly enthusiastic to teach. To date my most exciting placement was in cardiothoracic surgery, I felt truly privileged to be able to assist in an operation that consisted of stopping, repairing and re-

starting the beating of a man's heart. Generally, the clinical years are spent with different consultants in an apprenticeship model, putting into practice what is studied over the previous years.

This allows me to learn from the vast experience of the doctors I meet, but the remaining time studying at the medical school protects me from developing any outdated practices from my seniors. To someone about to begin their clinical years the best advice I could give them is... to spend as much time as possible on the wards, even if it means at evenings and weekends. Why? Because while waiting to begin the OSCE or sit the MCQs at least you'll know you've experienced as much as you can in real people – and the examiner will be able to tell that too in your confidence with the patient. Overall, the clinical years really are what studying Medicine is all about, and I'm so glad I've had the opportunity to study such at Keele University.'

Postgraduate

'I graduated as a dentist in 1997 and spent ten years working in Maxillofacial surgery before I applied to Keele Medical School. It was a great shock to come back to full time education but there are many other post graduate students on the course going through the same thing which was a great support. A typical day would involve clinical firms on the ward or outpatient clinic followed by a clinical skills session or macroseminar and during years 3 and 4 one day a week is spent in the community. Every day is different and there are many opportunities to take advantage of to maximise your learning experience – having made the decision to change careers I want to make the most of it and Keele encourages this. I have taken on extra audit projects which I will present at national meetings and have been given the opportunity to contribute a chapter for a book.

The clinical teachers recognise and appreciate a willingness to learn and many go out of their way to help you. The work load is heavy, especially with PBL work on top of firm teaching and I have continued to work as a dentist at evenings and weekends. But it is manageable and there is still time to get back into student life and enjoy a few nights out! The best opportunity Keele has given me was my recent trip to Yale University in the US – I spent nine weeks there on a Bioethics summer school as part of my year 4 and met people from all over the world from many different academic disciplines. Keele has an exchange programme with Yale – medical students come to Keele from Yale and some from Keele go each year on the summer school. In 2010 the first Keele student will be able to carry out their elective period at Yale, and it is planned to send more students in the future.'

Once you get in...

After your offer is confirmed Keele will send out a freshers' pack, containing information about the university, your accommodation, where to find everything on campus and your timetable for freshers' week. The pack also contains some forms, which you need to fill in and hand in when you register at the medical school on your first day, as well as information about how to register for the doctors on campus. During the first week there are a few introductory lectures, and an opportunity to meet your PBL group and get to know each other with a few group activities before the course starts properly on the Thursday. Reading lists and course information are given out on the first day with the year handbook. During freshers' week you probably won't stop all week, between the introductory sessions and the freshers' fair in the day and the events at the unions and various socials in the evenings. The main thing to remember is that the first few weeks may seem a bit overwhelming, but remember everyone else is feeling the same thing but will be too scared to admit it. Later in the term we all admitted to being terrified and thinking that it was just us who felt like that. It takes a few weeks to get used to Medicine and being at university.

The Best Thing	The opportunity to study at Yale
The Worst Thing	Stoke-on-Trent is not the most picturesque of cities although the surrounding countryside is very accessible and well worth visiting

Student top tips

Property prices are comparatively cheap in this area and there would be opportunity for students to purchase here and get on the property ladder early.

Summary Table

Positives	Negatives
Small year group size	Recent curriculum changes to Keele MBChB, problems yet to be identified
Opportunity to study at Yale	The project option has been removed from the new curriculum therefore less chance to have work published or carry out audit projects
Newly established – enthusiastic consultant teachers and teaching fellows	Some GP placements can be as far as away as 40 miles from base so having a car is essential, little chance for reimbursement for travelling expenses
Opportunity to sit finals in January of year 5	
New hospital buildings – updated technology	

Leeds

Room 7.09 Worsley Building
University of Leeds
Leeds
LS2 9JT

www.leeds.ac.uk/medicine

Most medical students would advocate their medical school as being the best and I am no different. Arriving at Leeds I immediately felt at home. The medical school, while not in a particularly inspiring building was full of welcoming and helpful people, and this continued when term started. The school guides you through your first year in a way which makes it easy to settle in and succeed from the outset. The course is well managed and is varied and interesting. The only way to describe Leeds itself is buzzing! The city centre has all the shops you could ever want with everything from Primark to Gieves & Hawkes. There is such an innumerable number of nightclubs that it takes you your entire first couple of years to discover them all! For the sports enthusiast, Headingley boasts Premiership rugby league and union, as well as test match and ODI cricket. For those interested in the arts, there are two large theatres which offer many of various stage productions including the much acclaimed Opera North. I can guarantee you one thing; you will never be bored in Leeds.

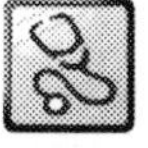

The medical course

Key facts

Course Type	Intergrated	Degree Awarded	MBChB
Basic Entry Requirements	AAA	Entrance Exams	UKCAT
Year Size	220	Open Days	Held regularly throughout the year
Admissions Website	www.leeds.ac.uk/medicine/admissions/		

Getting in – student tips

Leeds are not looking for a load of academics but rather well rounded individuals who are likely to throw themselves into extra-curricular activities as hard as their studies. It is important to remember this when writing your personal statement. At interview there is normally a senior consultant or GP, a member of medical school staff and a medical student. All they have during your 20-minute interview is your personal statement, so it is important to know it inside out and also to include some interesting information in it, so that the panel can allow you to show off your personality to the best. After the interview, the medical school do not leave you hanging around for months, and let you know their decision within two weeks.

Course details

Foundation / Pre-Med	No	Graduate	Yes
Student Population	Male: female ratio: 40:60	Term Length	Pre-clinical: 10 weeks Clinical: 14 weeks
Erasmus / Foreign Exchange	N/A	Elective Period	End of year 4 – 8 weeks

Intercalation

Stage	Year 3 to year 4 and year 4 to year 5.	Degree Awarded	BScMedSci (Hons)
Requirements	Depends on the faculty with which your are intercalating	Subjects	Anatomy, Biochemistry in relation to medicine, Biomedical ethics, Clinical sciences, Genetics in relation to medicine, History of medicine, Human physiology, International health, Medical Education, Medical Imaging, Microbiology in relation to medicine, Neuroscience, Pharmacology, Pharamacology (at Bradford), Primary care, Psychology, Sports science in relation to medicine, Zoology in relation to medicine and veterinary sciences.

Anatomy teaching

In my opinion the anatomy teaching at Leeds is the best part of the undergraduate course. From Christmas in the first year to December in the third year, weekly full body dissection sessions are held, with around four students per half body. These classes are well supported by a full programme of lectures and small seminars. Leeds is one of the few universities offering true full body dissection and it is a brilliant opportunity to learn.

Pre-clinical/Years 1–2	
Topics	***Year 1:*** Basic Biochemistry and Psychology. The anatomy, pharmacology and physiology of the Circulatory, Respiratory, Renal and Gastrointestinal systems. ***Year 2:*** Biochemistry and basic pathology, the anatomy of the upper and lower limbs as well as the spinal cord. Neuro-anatomy and neurophysiology. Examination of diseases of both the central and peripheral nervous systems.
Teaching	The teaching is generally of a high standard and normally takes the form of lectures supported by practical sessions including lab sessions and small group seminar work. On the whole it is varied and interesting.
SSC Periods	Three SSCs are undertaken in the first year and two in the second year. This includes one major literature review. The pre-christmas SSC in the second year is a highlight as it focuses on non-medical issues. Students spend two weeks away from university, doing things as diverse as spending time with West Yorkshire Police, teaching sex education in local schools, or spending time with the inmates at HMP Leeds.
Exams	Exams are normally taken at the end of each term, with a final exam taken at the end of the year, encompassing everything which has been taught that year. In general the exams are demanding but just less than 8% of people fail each exam.

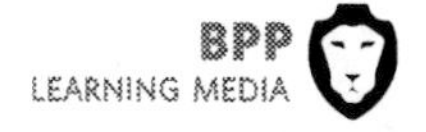

Clinical/Years 3–5	
Topics	***Year 3:*** *This is the final year of Phase I (Preparing for clinical practice). Phase I runs from the beginning of year 1 through to year 3.* During this year there are two Integrated Core Units to be covered. ICUs are modules that cover the basic underlying scientific knowledge in relation to the main medical topics. ***Year 4*** (Phase 2 – Clinical practice in context): During this year the medical and surgical specialties are covered through a combination of lectures and clinical placements. Topics include obstetrics, gynaecology and sexual health, paediatrics and child health, primary care, anaesthetics, accident and emergency, dermatology, rheumatology, infectious diseases, psychiatry, public health, oncology, palliative care and orthopaedics.
SSC Periods	Student selected components (SSCs) give you the fantastic opportunity to explore an area of Medicine outside of the core curriculum. There is always a range of topics to select from and these are really the main opportunities to produce a very high quality project with the potential to publish in a medical journal or present at a conference. During the third year, there are two SSCs. The first SSC is two weeks in length and takes place at the end of the first term. This SSC often has a range of fun topics to choose from such as acupuncture, Spanish – medical language, and teaching sex education to schools around Leeds. There is also a longer five-week SSC which takes place at the end of the year after the final examinations. Many students take this opportunity to undertake a small project of interest (eg an audit, research or literature review).
Exams	During the clinical years (years 3, 4 and 5) exams take the form of both written and OSCEs (objective structured clinical examinations). These exams are held at the end of the year. Written exams usually consist of two papers that are in the form of both EMQs (extended matching questions) and MCQs (multiple choice questions). The OSCEs are practical exams that take place over two days and consist of a number of stations where you are presented with clinical scenarios and given a limited time to perform the task in front of an examiner.

Hospital placements/academies

Depending on the clinical year placements vary in length between two to six weeks. The accommodation offered at the smaller district hospitals outside of Leeds (all the hospitals except Leeds General Infirmary and St James' hospital) is usually very basic. They usually provide a basic room with a study desk and wardrobes, communal showers, toilets and a kitchen with basic utensils, fridges and freezers. None of the accommodation has internet within the rooms but there are small computer clusters in every hospital. Airedale and Harrogate Hospital has a reputation for providing the best accommodation with modern flats and en-suite rooms. During the clinical years teaching usually takes place in small groups and therefore clinical placements usually have between two to six students each. This therefore ensures better quality of teaching and learning opportunities.

All placements in the smaller district hospitals have a good reputation for providing good clinical teaching especially Bradford Royal Infirmary and Pinderfields hospital. All district placements are very similar and are usually very quiet at night with not much to do. Placements at both Leeds General Infirmary and St James' University Hospital (as known as Jimmy's) are always the most popular placements due to a combination of the convenient locations and excellent reputation of both these large teaching hospitals within the field of medical research. St James' University Hospital is famous for being the largest teaching hospital in Europe and is a regional centre for numerous specialist services such as cardiac surgery and oncology (with the recent development of a new oncology wing housing the St James' Institute of Oncology equipped with all the latest technology). It is also one of six centres in the UK to conduct liver transplants by some of the world's most famous hepatobiliary surgeons. However, these teaching hospitals are often notoriously busy and therefore the learning and teaching opportunities are sometimes compromised.

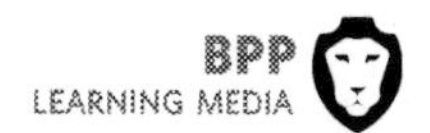

Hospitals and Travel Time from University	
Leeds General Infirmary	On campus
St James' University Hospital	10 minutes
Bradford Royal Infirmary	35 minutes
Pontefract Hospital	30 minutes
Calderdale Royal Hospital	30 minutes
Airedale Hospital	55 minutes
Harrogate Hospital	35 minutes
Pinderfields Hospital	30 minutes
Huddersfield Royal Infirmary	30 minutes
Dewsbury and District Hospital	30 minutes

The medical school

Work						Plenty of time for work and play
Facilities						Excellent medical library and numerous computer clusters
Support						Good informal support schemes set up between the senior and the lower years
Feedback						Feedback during clinical placement is quite variable

Facilities

There is a large and newly refurbished Health Sciences library within the medical school that is extensively equipped with textbooks and provides a very comfortable environment for study with many computers and private study desks. Computer facilities are not short within the medical school, with three further recently refurbished computer clusters. There are also two clinical skills labs, one at Leeds General Infirmary and one at St James' University Hospital. These are well stocked with equipment and resources to help you practise for the clinical Objective Structured Clinical Examinations (OSCEs).

Student support

There is a personal tutor scheme at Leeds, consisting of a small group of medical students from all years and a senior doctor, usually a consultant or General Practitioner, who is your personal tutor for the duration of your time at medical school. This scheme aims to provide support and advice for all students through 'personal tutor meetings'. These meetings usually occur once every term and can take the form of a formal meeting, or more often tutors like to meet up over an evening meal. Although meetings are usually held once every term personal tutors can be contacted as needed for help or support via email. This scheme can be very effective, but more often than not, many students find that they are not able to contact their personal tutors and therefore progress through medical school without this support.

On an informal basis there is also the 'MUMS' scheme, where students from the older years are linked with first year students. This scheme aims to provide first years with support and academic advice from their peers and also gives students the opportunity to socialise with students from different years. Finally, the student union and university also provides a counselling and health service if required.

Medical societies

The 'Medsoc' society is the most well-known and active society in the medical school and probably the whole university. With a history tracing back to over 150 years ago, this society is run by medical students and currently around 98% of medical students are members. This society is infamous for organising endless fun events such as summer BBQs, cocktail parties, annual spring balls and an annual Medics' ski trip to fill up the medics' social calendar. Essentially 'Medsoc' organises the social life for Leeds medics who like to 'work hard and play harder'!

Every event has proved to be a big hit for everyone year after year. There are also many well-established and popular medics' sports teams which include football, rugby, hockey, netball, cricket and badminton. The university also has many sports teams of their own and a large sports centre with a new swimming pool currently under construction.

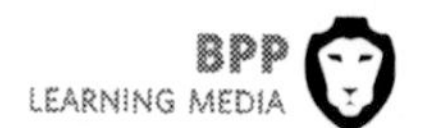

Finance

Further info: www.leeds.ac.uk/info/30500/your-finances

See scholarships: www.leeds.ac.uk/medicine/intercalated/scholarships.html

There is student aid: www.leedsuniversityunion.org.uk/helpandadvice/money/hardship

Student opinion

'Leeds medical school provides a comprehensive, well-structured and challenging course integrating patient contact at an early stage. Even in the pre-clinical years teaching is very clinically orientated through a systems based curriculum which uses a variety of teaching methods combined with an element of self-directed learning to provide a stimulating course. The clinical years consist of dedicated small group teachings thus giving you the opportunity to develop yourself professionally to become a competent foundation doctor.'

The university

Accommodation	Choice of campus or non-campus
Further Info	www.leeds.ac.uk/accommodation/

Accommodation

The nucleus of student housing for all years lies along the infamous Otley Road. There are a number of halls of residences along the road as well as on campus. My personal recommendation would be Bodington Hall. Do not be put off by the long bus journey; the bus journeys to and from nights out are absolute classics and the social scene at Bod is second to none. It also means you make friends more quickly on your course as you are not tempted to slope back to your campus room for a quick nap in-between classes.

Study facilities

The medical school has its own library, which has been recently refurbished to a very high standard. There are separate areas for both silent and group study. There are two large computer rooms inside the library complex, along with many computers dotted around in the main library. Inside the medical school itself there are around four different computer suites, so you are sure never to be without a computer. The library is well stocked with all the latest texts and has licenses to allow students access to all the main academic journals.

University sports & students' union

The union building lies only a short walk from the medical school and is used by all students at the university. Inside the uni there are a variety of places to eat to suit everyone's needs, as well as a small Co-op supermarket to pick up all those essential items, (the shop is rather wittily called 'essentials'). The union attracts some fairly big name artists during freshers' week, but the highlight on every Friday throughout the year is Fruity. This cheese night regularly sells out and soon becomes an absolute staple; a perfect time to let your hair down, grab whatever fancy dress you can find in your room and head to the terrace bar for a few drinks before destroying the dance floor. A must for any budding fresher.

The gym at Leeds is well equipped and is accompanied by two large sport halls. There is a 25-metre swimming complex and a few miles out of the campus are the university playing fields, where there are a number of astro-turfs and two new 3G pitches. There is also a large selection of rugby, soccer and lacrosse pitches. In the summer the university boasts a cricket pitch capable of hosting first class matches.

Student opinion

'Overall I can only say that my experience of Leeds University has been a positive one. Almost without exception the staff are helpful and knowledgeable. The facilities are first class, and the atmosphere is one where achievement in all aspects of life is recognised and valued.'

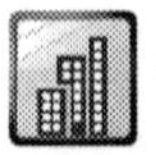

The city

Safety	🛡	🛡				As long as you are sensible, you will have no trouble
Nightlife	☽	☽	☽	☽	☽	Clubs and pubs for every type of person
Transport	🚌	🚌	🚌			Good train links to hospital placements, but a car may be helpful
Cost of Living	🐖	🐖	🐖			£59 a week is standard, and pints can cost from a £1 on a student night

Things to do

Leeds is located near several national parks and the Yorkshire dales are a stones throw away.

If you are into your rugby or football, Leeds is the place for you, with football at Elland Road and Leeds Rhinos to support. The city boasts many shopping malls, and museums, such as Harvey Nick's and the city museum, to keep you busy for hours. Other northern cities such as Sheffield are only a short journey away so visiting friends that are at university in nearby cities could not be easier.

Places to Go		
Place	**Brief Description**	**Entry Fee/Opening Time**
Halo	Converted church, Lady Gaga meets vintage glam!	£5 with student night. Monday, Friday and Saturday 10.00pm till 3.00am.
Oceana	Five-floor superclub	£4 on student night. Wednesdays for students 10.00pm till 3.00am.
Gate Crasher	Big superclub. Sometimes does a good theme night.	Student night Monday, Tuesday, Wednesday £4

Place	Brief Description	Entry Fee/Opening Time
Otley Run	Pubcrawl with option of 17 pubs ending in the centre of town. Normally done with a group in fancy dress.	Start at 3.00pm Saturday finish 3.00am Sunday. Amazing!
Student union	Best union in the country. three nightclubs inside	Fruity on a Friday night £4 with two drinks

Student opinion

'Life at Leeds is centred on a good night out. There is something for everyone, and no excuses for not getting involved. There is such a range of people that you are guaranteed to find people with similar interests. Although the weather is cold in Leeds you will get a warm welcome.'

Student's view

Pre-clinical

'The overall impression I have had from studying at Leeds is incredible. From the outset you are made to feel part and parcel of the medical school. The information pack sent out about a month before freshers' week contains all the information you should need to make the transition from studying at school to working independently at university as easy as possible. Leeds itself is an outstanding city and the nightlife is exceptional. Many students come for nights out from other universities across the northwest of England. The accommodation for first years is always of a high standard, and for the rest of your time at Leeds you will find a plentiful supply of very good and very affordable housing within a short walk of the university. The experiences you have here and the friends you will make will stay with you for a lifetime. Not only this but you have the biggest acute healthcare trust to be taught in which is a regional centre for many things including transplant and plastic surgery. I have no hesitation in recommending you the University of Leeds School of Medicine.'

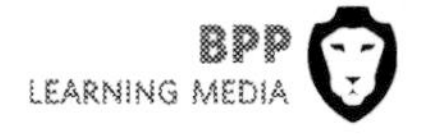

Clinical

'The clinical training at Leeds actually begins during January of year 2, consisting of hospital placements one morning a week. Clinical exposure is then gradually increased eventually becoming four days a week by the mid-third year therefore maximising clinical exposure and learning. Generally your days will begin at about 8.00 or 9.00am and finish at about 5.00pm. The days are filled with ward work shadowing doctors and bedside teaching sessions. Starting your clinical placements is one of the most exciting times of the medical course as it is the first time to interact with real patients and gain practical hands on experience such as taking blood and inserting cannulas. At the end of the third year you will sit the first Objective Structured Clinical Examinations (OSCEs). As these are practically based, preparing for these exams can be very difficult and different from any other exams you have ever done. The best advice to pass these exams with confidence is to ensure you spend plenty of time examining real patients on the ward and taking every opportunity to practise your clinical skills while on placement. The OSCE exams aim to provide you with clinical scenarios to assess your practical, communication and examination skills and places you under pressure to perform a task in front of an examiner under timed conditions.

The final year is one of the most exciting years due to the elective period, which is definitely the highlight of medical school. During this elective period students take the opportunity to undertake a clinical placement anywhere abroad while taking this unique chance to also relax and explore another country. However, soon after returning from your elective there are only six months until the final examinations held in April and therefore the stress levels are generally high among all students during this time. It can get quite busy, as you have to revise, complete SSCs, attend placements and complete a lengthy application form for employment in addition to attending interviews and writing CVs. Before you know it the year is over and finals have arrived!

Overall the medical course is an exciting, stimulating and challenging course. In addition Leeds is a great city with lots to occupy you when you're not studying.'

Once you get in...

Before you arrive, you receive a very helpful pack inviting you to become a lifetime member of the Medical Society for the bargain price of £37. This is well worth it in club discounts alone. The pack also introduces many affiliated medical societies including the rugby and football clubs as well as the medical school choir and orchestra. You don't have to be a seasoned professional to take part, being enthusiastic is normally more than enough.

The Best Thing	The best thing about Leeds in the first few years is the anatomy teaching and relatively early exposure to patients. This is not as early as at some medical schools but at least you might know your fibula from your infundibulum when you do!
The Worst Thing	Without a doubt this has to be the chronically boring social modules, which are a feature of medical schools

Student top tip

Do not buy any books before you arrive, wait and see what the library has to offer before shelling out your beer money on the latest edition of an obscure biochemistry book.

Summary Table

Positives	Negatives
Brilliant city and nightlife	The medical school looks like a Soviet prison
Great anatomy teaching and dissection	After the first year having not seen any patients, and hearing stories from other universities of regular contact
Early exposure to patients	You have to do more work than any of your other mates in halls
Two well regarded teaching hospitals on your door step	

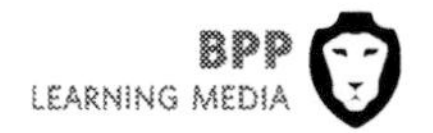

Leicester

University of Leicester Medical School
Maurice Shock Building
PO Box 138
University Road
Leicester
LE1 9HN

www.le.ac.uk/sm/ler

With a huge multicultural population Leicester offers a diverse range of living experiences from exotic cuisine, majestic places of worships, and vibrant entertainment like the colourful Diwali Celebrations and the lively Caribbean Carnival annually. Leicester is also home to the internationally renowned Leicester Tigers Rugby team and offers a wide range of recreational activities from theatres, museums and galleries to pubs, clubs, restaurants and live music gigs. The multi-building shopping complex, HighCross, offers the chance to relax with some retail therapy while Leicester market offers an authentic experience of the hustle and bustle of a traditional market. The university's excellent reputation for teaching and learning opportunities ranked it in the top ten medical schools nationally with a rating of 23/24 for teaching awarded by the GMC. Leicester Medical School's integrated course spanning over two phases within the five years ensures excellent accomplishment of competencies as a doctor and has been successful for the past 30 years.

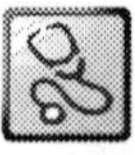

The medical course

Key facts

Course Type	Traditional	Degree Awarded	MBChB
Basic Entry Requirements	AAA	Entrance Exams	UKCAT
Year Size	Approx 180	Open Days	End of June/July Beginning of Sept/Oct
Admissions Website	www.le.ac.uk/sm/le/		

Getting in – student tips

Leicester are not necessarily interested in what type of work experience you have done (as long as it involves being within a caring environment), more what you gained from this experience. Try to use hobbies, personal experience and opinions to give weight to what qualities you think you have to be a good doctor.

The interview is intended to make you immediately feel welcome and at ease; with the two interviewers made up of an experienced NHS clinician and a final year medical student. They will wish to further explore you as a person, building on from what you have written in your personal statement – especially what you may have gained from your work experience – and aim to discuss topical medical issues with you. This may include ethical issues, such as assisted suicide.

Course details

Foundation / Pre-Med	N/A	**Graduate**	Yes
Student Population	Male: female ratio: 40:60	**Term Length**	Pre-clinical: 12 weeks Clinical: 18 weeks
Erasmus / Foreign Exchange	Erasmus exchange possible after first year in Germany and Switzerland	**Elective Period**	After finals in year 5 (May onwards). A minimum of 7 weeks' duration

Intercalation

Stage	Mostly between year 3 and 4 some between years 4 and 5, only exceptionally between years 2 and 3	**Degree Awarded**	BSc (or BA for Medical Humanities)
Requirements	Usually those passing the pre-clinical exams are considered	**Subjects**	Medical Sciences and Medical Humanities

Anatomy teaching

Leicester has a thorough anatomy curriculum taught throughout the pre-clinical years and due to the integrated nature of the course, anatomy is continually re-visited throughout the clinical years. Time allocated to anatomy studies varies according to the semester of study and thus the number of anatomy modules being taught, but on average, anatomy teaching consists of three hours of formal teaching and up to seven hours of self study per week.

Anatomy is mainly taught through lectures, small group work sessions and cadaveric dissections delivered by senior anatomy lecturers and clinical demonstrator staff. There is ample opportunity to book the dissection room for private study with staff before and during exams. In addition, throughout the course, modules have inbuilt vivas to help students assess their progress and to experience a mock OSCE style anatomy exam. There are also anatomy special study modules offered in the second year for those with a keen interest in the subject matter and an opportunity to win a university anatomy award.

Pre-clinical/Years 1–2	
Topics	***Year 1:*** Basic medical sciences – Molecular medicine, Histology, Pathology, Epidemiology, Cardiovascular and Musculoskeletal systems. ***Year 2:*** System based modules – Urinary, Respiratory, Gastrointestinal systems, Infectious disease, Psychosocial, Reproduction and Head and Neck studies. Clinical teaching half day every week.
Teaching	Traditional lectures are used alongside small group work teaching (a total of 20 hours per week). Group work aims to build on the themes covered within the lectures; questions based on clinical themes are attempted with the help of clinical demonstrators or scientists. The quality of teaching, especially within the group work, is usually of a high standard. This is mainly down to the use of clinical demonstrators, most of whom are previous Leicester students. They are more approachable and understand the structure of the work, the course, and most importantly the exams!

SSC Periods	There are two SSCs during the pre-clinical years (Phase 1); one in the second half of year 2 and another in year 3, plus a dissertation which is developed across the whole of the first two years. A broad range of modules are available, with foreign modern languages, disability in the arts, world health and faith alongside more traditional subjects such as vascular biology, neurology and pharmacology. At least one of the two must be science based.
Exams	At the end of each semester two written papers examine students covering the whole of that semester's work, plus key principles from previous modules. These focus on cross-modular links between different topics, aiming to encourage thinking similar to that of a qualified doctor. There are also two clinical exams (OSCEs), at the end of year 1 and halfway through year 3. The exams increase in difficulty as the years progress, mainly due to the increasing volume of knowledge required in later modules. This has the advantage that, although difficulty increases, you have greater experience of the exam style and the extent to which you need to work in order to pass well. Fail rates vary, but up to one fifth may have to resit that year's exams at the end of July.

Clinical/Years 3–5	
Topics	***Year 3:*** Pre-clinical subjects in the first half of the year include Neuro-anatomy and Physiology, Pharmacology, Integrative Module, Embryology and Clinical Skills. The second half of the year covers three of the following junior clinical rotations: General Practice, Orthopaedics, Cardio-respiratory Medicine, Perio-operative Care (including Surgery and Anaesthesia), Psychiatry and Gastrointestinal, Endocrine and Renal Medicine (last three as one rotation). ***Year 4:*** The first half covers three junior rotations not done in the third year out of the six mentioned above. The second half of the year covers three of the following senior rotations: Paediatrics, Oncology, Emergency Medicine, Geriatrics and Chronic Care (as one rotation), Obstetrics and Gynaecology (as one rotation) and ENT and ophthalmology (as one rotation). ***Year 5:*** The first half covers three senior rotations not done in the fourth year out of the six mentioned above. The second half includes finals, a six-week elective and foundation preparation course before commencing paid work as a junior doctor.

SSC Periods	Four SSCs are offered in the clinical years and are mainly attachments with all medical and surgical specialties in any of the Leicester teaching hospitals and affiliated peripheral hospitals. The options are vast and include every specialty and sub-specialty of Medicine and Surgery. Examples include Plastic Surgery, Ophthalmology, Vascular Surgery, Haematology and many more. The aim is allow students to develop essential experience in a specialty that interests them and can be tailored for the student. There are many opportunities to do multiple audits and mini research projects. Publication opportunities are rare and do depend on the individual SSC supervisor.
Exams	Short answer question exams. There are two main exams in the clinical years, the Intermediate Professional Exam taken in the middle of the fourth year and the Final Professional Exam taken at the end of the fifth year. Exams are marked using a threshold marking scheme. There are also clinical exams in the style of OSCEs which assess skills such as history taking, examination and practical skills. The pass rates are high and approximately 10% resit the exam, with a majority passing second time.

Hospital placements/academies

Peripheral hospitals are renowned locally for their excellent teaching. Within Leicester, the Glenfield Hospital is nationally known for its expertise in Cardiology and the Leicester Royal Hospital has Europe's largest Accident and Emergency Department. Furthermore Leicester hospitals have an excellent reputation for research. Accommodation depends on the hospital however all are satisfactory. The best accommodation is in Boston, which has en-suite rooms and a breakfast bar in the kitchen. Most students live in rented houses during the clinical years and hence accommodation obviously varies. Placements last seven weeks and up to six students go on placements peripherally. Locally, groups of 36 students can be divided and placed in one of the three Leicester local teaching hospitals. Students are paired up for placements.

Hospitals and Travel Time from University	
Leicester Royal Infirmary	5 minutes
Glenfield Hospital	15 minutes
Leicester General Hospital	10 minutes
Kettering General Hospital	45 minutes
Northampton General Hospital	1 hour
Pilgrim Hospital, Boston	1 hour 45 minutes
Lincoln Hospital	1 hour 30 minutes
Peterborough Hospital	1 hour 5 minutes
Burton Hospital	1 hour
Bedford Hospital	1 hour 30 minutes

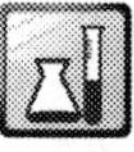

The medical school

Work						Good support and framework for learning the vast quantity of knowledge needed
Facilities						Good basic facilities such as canteen, computer suite and common room
Support						Excellent academic and personal support offered throughout the course
Feedback						Generally good feedback on written work but poor exam feedback

Facilities

Facilities include an IT suite and a clinical skills lab where practical skills and simulations take place for both teaching and exams. There are two lecture theatres connected by video link and each one is fully equipped with audio visual systems. There is also a fully furnished common room with its own cafeteria and refreshment facilities. The main library has been completely renovated with a coffee lounge, mini restaurant and a bookshop, which sells all medical curriculum books.

Student support

Leicester Medical School provides an extensive support network. A medical parent-sibling system guides freshers through their first year and helps new students build contacts in senior years. The parent system tends to provide support throughout medical school and is a popular informal method of support. Students are given their parent's details and are encouraged to arrange 'family outings' to get to know each other. Thereafter contact is dependent on the student but generally most medical parents are forthcoming and helpful. Further support is available through 'Medics Welfare', which is a society run by students for students and helps with issues such as home sickness, exam stress, personal crises and financial advice. In addition there is a chaplaincy and the university provides a nightline service run by volunteers, which offers students advice for any issue from 8.00pm to 8.00am. Students will also register with a local university GP who is available by appointment for health reasons. Help academically is provided via a personal tutor service throughout medical school.

Medical societies

The main medical society is called LUSUMA under which all socials are organised including intro and outro weeks, summer, winter and graduation balls, themed nights out, pub crawls and leisure trips such as skiing in the alps. LUSUMA organises a fun packed freshers' week, which includes the famous Leicester medics' pyjama pub crawl; probably the most exciting night in the entirety of medical school. Other societies include SCRUBS, Student Physician Society, Teddy Bear Hospital, Trauma and Acute Care Society, GP Society and many more! There are also many medical sports teams including medics' football, rugby, netball, tennis, cricket, basketball, hockey, squash and badminton. Leicester annually holds the famous medics v lecturers summer cricket match, which is always a brilliant event! These are excellent societies to meet friends and socialise as well as get fit and play competitively against other university teams.

Finance

www.le.ac.uk/study/fees/undergraduate/

Student opinion

'Sitting in the peaceful Victoria Park next to the university you can see the medics' football team practising for a summer match while others are reading in the sun preparing for an exam and thinking about how good it will be when they can finish them and concentrate on the summer ball 'Arabian Nights' costumes. Being a Leicester student is always this exciting.'

The university

Accommodation	Mainly non-campus halls of residence
Further Info	www.le.ac.uk/accommodation

Accommodation

The accommodation is mainly situated at Oadby Village, a 30-minute walk or ten minutes by a regular bus service away from the university campus. The main self-catered accommodation (Opal Court and Nixon Court) is no more than a five-minute walk from the university. Many find Oadby Village is an excellent place to live and socialise for their first year, with sports facilities (including a gym) close by.

I fully enjoyed my time there, with the majority of freshers living nearby it gave me a brilliant social experience, and being a little away from campus gave me an escape from the university and all its lectures! Obviously the best halls come down to personal preference, although general consensus says that both Beaumont Hall and Gilbert/Murray/Stamford are very good. The main student area resides in Clarendon Park, adjacent to the university campus.

Study facilities

The David Wilson Library on campus provides students access to a first-rate resource. It contains a large number of computer rooms, together with quiet zones in which to study and seminar rooms (where flat screen monitors and computers can be used to aid learning) – helping to meet any student's needs. It is regularly used by medics because of its nearer proximity to accommodation than the clinical library, based at the Leicester Royal Infirmary.

University sports & students' union

Easily accessible across from the medical school, the union houses a gym, shop, admin offices and the SU club (open Wednesday and Friday nights). Much of the time spent on campus is within the medical school, but the student union is regularly used by medics (especially for events) throughout the year. Live music can also be found at The Venue, with past acts including Feeder, Pendulum and The Arctic Monkeys.

Anyone who is interested in using the two university gyms or the sports facilities at Manor Road (next to Oadby Village) must buy a sports card, priced at around £60. Fortunately this is a one off cost, and gives you free rein of the good facilities at Manor Road including a medium sized gym, football cage, astropitch, and numerous tennis courts. The sports pitches nearby are kept in excellent condition, and this is definitely one of the attractions of playing sport for the university. The sports card also covers you for any insurance needed to join a sports team, although it won't pay for your membership fee!

Freshers' week festivities begin in early October, continuing for two packed weeks. The main event is the freshers' fair held over the first week, where all of the university societies set up stalls under one roof – including all sports socs, charities, and one of the largest Hindu societies in the whole country. Events are run throughout the two weeks by different societies and the university as a whole – all you have to do is sign up and get involved!

A further attraction of Medicine at Leicester is that it holds a separate 'Intro week', organised by LUSUMA (the medical society), starting a week earlier than the rest of the university. This is a brilliant way to get to know the city and other medics before the masses descend, with events such as Sports Night, meeting your medic parents, nights out and bowling arranged throughout the week. Particularly infamous is the 'PJ pubcrawl', a night where every year of the med school (and some stealthy doctors) don all kinds of fancy dress through the streets of Leicester, with first years wearing pyjamas!

A separate medics freshers' fair also gives you an opportunity to get involved with the many societies linked with the medical school, such as medic's sports teams, charities and SCRUBS (the surgical society). Introductory lectures in medical school and group activities throughout the week help to ease you into medical school life too, with students on hand to a nswer any burning questions you may have.

Student opinion

'From the open spaces of Oadby Village and the university campus, to the unmatched camaraderie with other medics from the outset, you immediately feel at home in this vibrant and colourful city.'

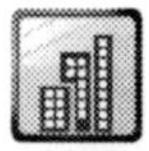

The city

Safety						A safe city overall
Nightlife						Generally good but not as much variety of clubs as other cities
Transport						Parking can be a problem around university. Traffic is also bad, Leicester can be congested. You do not need a car for pre-clinical years as there is a free hospital hopper but clinical years can be a problem
Cost of Living						Rent costs approximately £200 a month. Taxi costs less than £5 into the city centre and costs approximately £15 for a night out

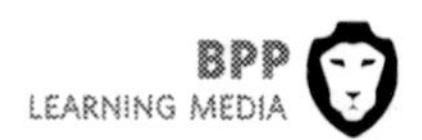

Things to do

Leicester's greenery means there are lots of nice parks to relax in and enjoy the sun in the summer. HighCross offers excellent shopping experiences and there are plenty of fancy restaurants providing a wide range of cuisines. There are three major cinemas including Cinema de Lux, Odeon and Warner Bros as well as Bollywood cinemas.

Furthermore there are plenty of bars, pubs and clubs to keep students entertained at night with good cheap prices and a popular 'Jonglers' in town which is an excellent place for a good laugh. The Leicester student union venues are also popular places for experiencing live music and great nights out. The downfalls are that after a while some of the clubs can become boring as there aren't as many as in other cities and walking through Victoria Park alone at night to get back to student accommodation can be risky because of the poor lighting there.

Places to Go		
Place	**Brief Description**	**Entry Fee/Opening Time**
Liquid	Popular club for all	£2, Wed and Fri 10.00am–3.00am
Revolution	Night club/bar in the city centre	£2–3, Thurs 10.00am–2.00am
Life	Popular club	£2, Tues 10.00am–3.00am
Zanzibar	Club opposite St Margaret's Bus Station	£2, Mon and Fri 11.00am–2.00am
The Loaded Dog	Popular student pub	£Free; Mon-Sat 6.00pm till late
Landsdowne	Posh student bar in the city centre	£Free; Mon-Sat 8.00pm till late
Time Bar	One of the pub crawl stops, popular bar	£Free; Mon-Fri 6.00pm till late

Student opinion

'Sitting outside the Landsdowne Bar in the evening you see students hurrying down into town for a student night offering cheap drinks all night. The air is filled with the smell of Indian curry from the nearby restaurants and the smoke of shisha from the café. It's a great experience for any student, the city is truly alive.'

Student's view

Pre-clinical

'I found the structure of the timetable over years 1 and 2 was organised very well. My basic day would consist of half a day of lectures and group work, with a little time to socialise in between, leaving the rest free to sleep, work and/or relax. This is a great deal better than travelling in and out of university all day, with lectures or seminars scheduled hours apart from one another! Another advantage of this timetable was that it gave me free time almost every Wednesday afternoon, giving me the opportunity to play university sport without having to miss timetabled work.

I was attracted by the welcoming and relaxed atmosphere of the university, combined with a medical school that offers a good, strong reputation and the advantage of being able to intercalate (either into lab or clinically based research). I was also an admirer of the overall course structure, organised so that I could develop knowledge of essential anatomy, physiology and pathology before beginning my clinical teaching in year 2, led by an experienced clinician in one of the three main hospitals for half a day each week.

The exam questions can be difficult to understand and as with any medical exam it can be stressful, but I have found that most of those who put in the work pass well. To help with revision for many of the exams, there are a number of peer-assisted teaching sessions run by the older years, such as practising exam style questions (ESA Insight) and anatomy teaching from SCRUBS. I have found these invaluable in helping to cover the key topics, many of the themes running between modules, and give me confidence in answering the type of question used in Leicester exams. In addition, we can now get feedback on each of our exams. I have discovered that not only is it important in giving you a rough idea of your performance, but it also gives a strong indication of how to improve your performance in future exams.

I have many and varied highlights of my first few years here at Leicester. Of most importance to me are the friends I have made over Intro Week, enjoying the multicultural vibe of the city, and having the half days free to pursue other interests outside of the medical school. The medical societies, especially medic's hockey, have also given me a great opportunity to socialise with a broader group of people and keep fit. I couldn't fault anything of my experience so far, and I have no doubt that this will continue!'

Clinical

'Personally these are the best years of medical school. A typical day begins with a morning ward round followed by teaching and lunch in the canteen. Afternoons usually consist of theatres or clinics and an opportunity to do some private study. Often there are bedside teaching sessions arranged for students by a range of medical staff. As the years go by, you begin to feel like a true member of the medical team and most teams are very pleasant and supportive. The true experience of clinical medicine is during night shifts and on calls where you can be thrown in the deep end and expected to clerk and initially write up a basic management plan. The wide range of hospitals means that each placement is exciting and a new living experience including a chance to experience new clubs, pubs and restaurants! The best aspects are the chance to gain valuable experience of being a junior doctor, experiencing good team working and both formal and informal teaching. The worst aspects can be travelling long distances away from Leicester, which can be a problem without a car and having to continually re-settle at different placements.

Personal highlights would be all the students gate-crashing the doctors' mess at each new placement, the orthopaedics placement at Kettering General Hospital which was truly a barrel of laughs and doing the Accident and Emergency rotation in Europe's largest A&E in the Leicester Royal which was an experience beyond my expectations! My main advice is to work slowly but continuously through the rotations to put you in good stead for the exams in the clinical years and to relish the social life at all the different placements.'

Once you get in...

Once accepted, the university sends out useful information regarding accommodation, university sports teams, and forms to order your sports and library cards. The medical school also sends you a reading list (but wait until you ask the older years in your first week before buying any!), information regarding your medic freshers' week, and how to join LUSUMA – the med soc.

It may seem like a bore, but try to sort all this admin out before you turn up to Intro Week – it'll save you a lot of hassle and give you more time to do what the week's meant for, having fun and settling in. It's a great way to meet loads of new people, many of whom you'll still be speaking to five years later, so seize the opportunity to talk to a countless number of new faces and get involved in as many events as you can handle! There's no doubt it will be one of the best weeks you'll have ever had.

The Best Thing	Excellent student experience and atmosphere
The Worst Thing	Lack of information about the course structure and not much forewarning given before important deadlines

Student top tips

- Enjoy freshers' week as much as possible and dive into all the opportunities provided, it will truly be an experience of a lifetime!
- Do all the form filling before you arrive at Leicester such as ID badges, society forms and health forms to save you time and help you adjust better when you arrive.
- Research accommodation halls and attend open days to get a feel for the city and university so that you make an informed choice about studying at Leicester.
- Take time deciding what societies to join as they are hungry for your money on the day you arrive!

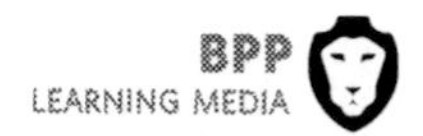

Summary Table

Positives	Negatives
Excellent and unique student lifestyle	Poor prior information given about the course
Brilliant teaching	The intensity of workload including lots of written components
Lots of academic opportunities to make you shine	Competitive ethos fostered during exams
Great student support services provided	Poor parking facilities for students
Relatively cheap living costs	Ignored comments on how to improve aspects of the course

Liverpool

School of Medicine
MBChB Office
Cedar House
Ashton Street
Liverpool
L69 3GE

www.liv.ac.uk/sme/

The home of The Beatles, a rich maritime history, two cathedrals and, of course, two of Europe's most successful football teams, Liverpool is one of the UK's most exciting and expanding cities. Previously the European Capital of Culture 2008, the city is a 24-hour hub of activity with a student population of over 60,000. The Liverpool ONE complex dominates the city centre and it includes designer shops, bars, restaurants and a cinema.

A member of the Russell Group of research universities, Liverpool is the original redbrick university – the name being inspired by the impressive Victoria Building completed in 1892.

As well as the city, the university has benefitted from considerable investment, boasting new library and sports facilities. The medical school has also been refurbished, including new lecture theatres, computer centres and a state of the art Human Anatomy Resource Centre.

Liverpool Medical School prides itself on a modern, PBL-based course with early patient contact, and traditional lectures. Against a backdrop of a culturally rich and upcoming city, the University of Liverpool is welcoming and is an inspirational and dynamic place to study.

 *The medical course*

Key facts

Course Type	PBL	Degree Awarded	MBChB
Basic Entry Requirements	AAA	Entrance Exams	N/A
Year Size	Approx 300	Open Days	Throughout year
Admissions Website	www.liv.ac.uk/medicine/prospective/index.htm		

Getting in – student tips

The interview panel at Liverpool consists of two trained interviewers, including university academic staff, NHS clinicians, local GPs and members of local NHS trusts. Interviews are semi-structured, and last approximately 15 minutes. There is an informal, relaxed atmosphere, and questions are typical of what might be expected at a medical admissions interview. Why do you want to be a doctor? Have you always wanted to study Medicine? What has attracted you to Liverpool? An ethical scenario is also usually discussed at the end of the interview, along with selected points from your personal statement.

Interviewers are looking for a real interest in Medicine, awareness of current medical issues, good communication skills, enthusiasm and confidence.

Course details

Foundation / Pre-Med	N/A	Graduate	Yes
Student Population	Male: female ratio: 50:50	Term Length	Pre-clinical: 12 weeks Clinical: 16 weeks
Erasmus / Foreign Exchange	Erasmus European exchange possible in year 5 to Angers, Ulm, Pavia, Salamanca, Linkoping, Thrace	Elective Period	End of Year 3, 5 weeks, mid June–mid July (but can be extended with permission)

Intercalation

Stage	Between year 4 and year 5	**Degree Awarded**	BSc; MSc; MPhil or MRes
Requirements	Evidence of high grades may be required for acceptance on to some courses. Students can also apply to courses outside of Liverpool	**Subjects**	Medical Sciences, Humanitarian Studies and various others

Anatomy teaching

There are no taught anatomy sessions at Liverpool. In the first year, two hours of time per fortnight is allotted for students to attend the state of the art Human Anatomy Resource Centre (HARC). Cadaveric prosections, anatomical models, microscopy stations and radiographs are available for students to use as they please to support their PBL learning. Technicians are available to help with any queries.

In subsequent years, the HARC is open 9.00am–5.00pm every weekday and students can 'drop in' at hours to suit them. Attendance of HARC is optional in all years, but is recommended to support learning.

Dissection is not performed at Liverpool, but the prosections are well prepared, and are excellent learning tools. There are opportunities to take SSMs in dissection during the course, for those students who have a keen interest.

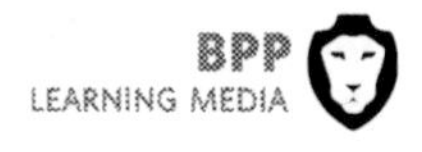

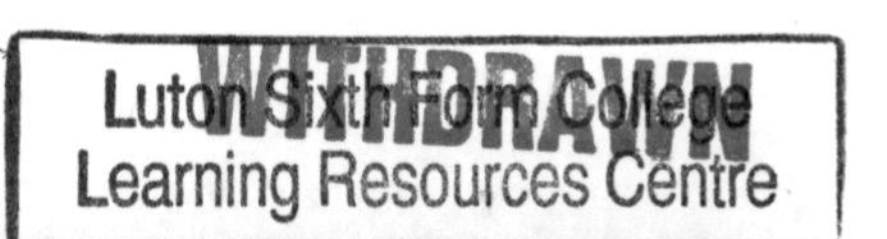

Pre-clinical/Years 1–2	
Topics	***Year 1**:* In 11 two-week PBL modules, all major systems of the body are covered. Basic molecular and cellular medicine, basic embryology, child development milestones, ethics, patient psychology and statistics are also covered. In addition, there is a community GP placement in the spring. ***Year 2**:* Pathology is introduced in the second year. Fifteen two-week PBL modules cover a different presenting complaint, such as chest pain, shortness of breath and jaundice. Basic anatomy, physiology, ethics, psychology and statistics are also revisited from the first year. Clinical placements are also started in this year, including spending two days a week in one of Merseyside's four large teaching hospitals.
Teaching	Lectures, PBL group sessions, clinical skills sessions (year 1), communication skills sessions, community care sessions, hospital consultant teaching (year 2), self-directed HARC sessions.
SSC Periods	At Liverpool, these are known as SSMs (Special Study Modules). In the first year, there is one SSM period lasting four weeks after the Christmas break. A project is chosen from an extensive catalogue (usually around 100 projects), covering a great deal of medical and surgical specialties. Over the period, a 3,000 word report must be completed on the chosen project, in a style often specified by the module convenor. SSM2 and SSM3 take place in year 2, each lasting four weeks. There are six SSMs in total which must be completed over the five-year course.
Exams	Formative (mock) exams in January and summative exams in May/June. Multiple Choice Questions (not negatively marked), True or False Questions, Extended Matching Item Questions, Short Answer Questions, OSCE. Pass mark for written exams – 60%. Pass mark for OSCEs – 80%. Resits in August.

Clincal/Years 3–5	
Topics	***Year 3**:* The third year covers specialties, with rotations in obstetrics and gynaecology; paediatrics; psychiatry; disability and pharmacology. Subjects are taught through a mixture of hospital attachments, lectures, problem-based learning and group projects. ***Year 4**:* In the fourth year, students are places in a hospital for four days a week, moving through rotations in medicine, surgery and the specialties. Problem-based learning continues to support hospital led teaching including lectures, bed-side teaching and tutorials from doctors in the specified fields. Students are able to practise clinical skills such as blood taking and fitting nasogastric tubes. This year is about fine-tuning history and examination skills and understanding appropriate investigations and management plans in preparation for the final examinations in June. ***Year 5**:* Fifth years spend seven weeks on each of Accident and Emergency, GP, a ward attachment where they shadow a newly qualified F1 doctor, and two 'Selective in Advanced Medical Practice' (SAMP) which is what Liverpool calls its clinical attachments and are chosen by the student in an area of their interest.
SSC Periods	Two Special Study Modules are completed in the third year, the first during a dedicated four-week period and the second as a longer project, one day a week for 16 weeks. SSMs are based on laboratory work, literature reviews, audits or statistical analysis of data, and may include clinical contact and presentations. All students must submit a 3,000 word write-up at the end of the SSM period. Subjects range from 'Resuscitation' and 'Obstetric Audit' to 'Molecular Origins of Cancer' and 'Pain Management'. The final SSM is done after exams in the July of fourth year, and may be chosen from the SSM catalogue or arranged by the student in a field of their choice. SSM is a chance to demonstrate skills in both research and presentation, and several students reach such high standards as to be invited to present their work to hospital subgroups and at national conferences.
Exams	Extended Matching Questions, Short Answer Papers, OSCE and in fourth year LOCAS. There is lots of help with revision in the run up to exams. The final exams are sat in the fourth year; progress in the fifth year is assessed through portfolio work and regular meetings with academic supervisors.

Hospital placements/academies

In Liverpool, students generally live in their own rented accommodation as most hospital placements are within a reasonable distance. Some hospitals further away offer accommodation if students choose to move there during the fourth year, though others require students to arrange their own accommodation. Hospital undergraduate teams oversee the wellbeing of students placed in their centres, numbers of whom can range between 10-40 per clinical year at a time. Most hospital sites are equipped with medical libraries, clinical skills and simulation suites, and undergraduate teams help organise bed-side teaching and lectures with specialists from the hospital. Rotations in specialties in the third year last around six weeks; in the fourth year students are placed in a hospital four days a week for the whole year, with the remaining one day spent in General Practice. Rotations in the Liverpool Women's Hospital and Alder Hey Children's Hospital are particularly rewarding, being specialist centres at the forefront of research. Students are encouraged to get involved in research projects, especially audits, which often begin as Special Study Modules.

Hospitals and Travel Time from University	
Royal Liverpool University Hospital	<5 minutes
Liverpool Women's Hospital	10 minutes
Arrowe Park Hospital	25 minutes
Alder Hey Children's Hospital	25 minutes
Aintree University Hospital	30 minutes
Whiston Hospital	40 minutes
Warrington Hospital	50 minutes
Southport Hospital**	50 minutes
Chester Hospital**	1 hour
Blackpool Hospital**	1 hour 30 minutes
Lancaster**	2 hour
Barrow in Furness**	2 hour 15 minutes

***Only used in the later years, students generally move there in the fourth year for the year.*

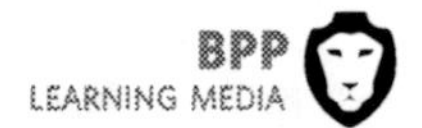

The medical school

Work	●	●	●			If you are motivated and suited to self-directed learning the work is easily manageable
Facilities	●	●	●			Most facilities are up to date and are easily accessed
Support	●	●	●	●		There are several support mechanisms in place as described and Faculty is approachable and understanding if students have any concerns or problems
Feedback	●	●	●	●		Students receive individual feedback on OSCE exams and overall feedback on written papers. Progress is also monitored by the number of patient cases and clinical skills logged online and fed back by hospital undergraduate teams

Facilities

The school's facilities are all located within close proximity on the main university campus. The modern Sherrington Building houses two large lecture theatres, IT suite, Madison's coffee shop and the Human Anatomy Resource Centre, which can be accessed throughout the week. Opposite this, Cedar House accommodates the medical offices and further IT facilities, and is the venue for PBL from the first to the third year. There is also a Clinical Skills Lab used for teaching and drop-in. Further facilities can be accessed on placements with hospital libraries, clinical skills labs and simulation suites on several sites.

Student support

During the first week at Liverpool students are assigned a 'personal tutor', usually a researcher or lecturer within the health sciences, who they are encouraged to meet up with regularly throughout their time at Liverpool to discuss any concerns or difficulties they are experiencing. Around the same time, the Liverpool Medical Students Society runs a Mentor-Mentee event where first year students are assigned second year mentors, who are there to help with advice ranging from book choices to which sports teams to join. Faculty are very approachable for students experiencing any problems, academic or personal. There is also further support available in the university with the Student Heath Service and a counselling service should it ever be needed.

Medical societies

The Liverpool Medicine Students Society (LMSS) is the second largest society in the university, hosting regular social events from fashion shows to four annual dinner-dances, and organising student-led lectures to help supplement learning. Sports teams include rugby, hockey, netball, swimming, squash and cheerleading, with the larger teams competing annually at NAMS. Aside from sport, students can get involved in medics' choir or language groups, write for the termly magazine, 'Sphincter', and join 'Artefacts', the medics' theatre company, who encourage budding actors, singers, instrumentalists and technical folk to take to the stage in productions such as Pirates of Penzance and FAME: The Musical. Other medical societies include Surgical Scousers, Physician's Society, Wilderness Medicine and Sports Medicine, which allow students to develop their interests in these specialties.

Finance

www.liv.ac.uk/study/undergraduate/finance/

www.liv.ac.uk/study/postgraduate/finance/

A small hardship fund is available for home students experiencing financial difficulties. Students may be eligible to apply for further scholarships and bursaries through the university.

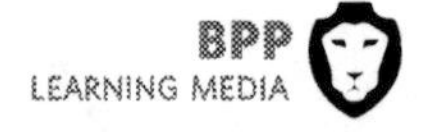

Student opinion

'Learning Medicine as an integrated course, in a friendly and highly encouraging environment, in a city as vibrant and up-and-coming as Liverpool has been so much fun and has only served to further my love of the subject.'

The university

Accommodation	Non-campus halls of residence
Further Info	www.lgos.org/ www.liv.ac.uk/study/ www.liv.ac.uk/accommodation/

Accommodation

Most first years live in either the Carnatic or Greenbank halls of residence. These are around three miles away from the university campus. Walking takes a good 40 to 50 minutes, but buses leave frequently from right outside the halls. There is some accommodation next to the campus, but these are less popular with first years, and are often reserved for post-graduates and international students.

Both sites include a number of different halls with catered and self-catering rooms. Carnatic and Greenbank are both in parkland settings with a great deal of green space, which is open for students to use however they please. Barbequing in the summer is definitely a highlight.

Study facilities

There are two libraries on campus – the Harold Cohen and Sydney Jones libraries. The Harold Cohen is the main library for the sciences, engineering and medicine, while the Sydney Jones deals with the arts. Both are open 24 hours a day during term time. The HCL and SJL have just been refurbished in a multi-million pound project including new buildings and computer facilities. Medics will find the HCL very useful, as the medical library spans two floors, while the SJL houses a number of books which aid in the sociological aspects of the course.

University sports & students' union

The students' union at Liverpool is known as the Guild of Students. It has the largest student union building in the UK and second largest in Europe, which is located in the centre of the campus. The large Saro Wiwa bar is a great place to meet, and serves food and drink at more than reasonable prices. Other facilities include a mini supermarket, hairdressers, meeting rooms, computer facilities and more bars. The Guild is also home to the Mountford Hall, which is used for balls, club nights and live music among other things. Recent visitors to the Guild include the likes of Kasabian, Bloc Party, Dizzee Rascal and Pendulum. The Guild has excellent welfare facilities and is a great live music venue, but most students prefer to centre their nightlife around the Concert Square area of the town centre.

A student membership for the university sports centre costs around £110 for a year. This grants access to the gym, swimming pool and allows booking of courts and pitches free of charge. Classes are also available, such as 'boxercise' and aerobics. The gym is adequately sized, but can get busy at peak times. It offers a full range of cardiovascular and weight training equipment.

Wednesday afternoons are reserved for sport and teams train at a wide variety of venues across the university. University and medical school teams are available to join at all levels. The medics' hockey and surf clubs are particularly popular!

Events throughout the freshers' week include balls, club nights, fairs and society meetings. The freshers' fair often takes place during the first weekend after moving into halls. Every university society is represented there, as well as other organisations from around and about Liverpool trying to promote their services, including hairdressers, clubs and restaurants. Medicine is well represented at the fair, with the LMSS (Liverpool Medicine Students Society), Surgical Scousers (surgical society) and Wilderness medicine society always in attendance, as well as the medics' sports teams. The fair is well worth attending, as it is a great way to find out more about what's going on at the university – and for the free stationery!

There are also a great deal of medics' events over the course of the first few weeks. Particular highlights include the first year bus tour, which is a must. Buses collect students from halls, and then take them on a tour of Liverpool's finest pubs and bars, finishing with a club night in the Guild.

Student opinion

'Liverpool is a vibrant and bustling city with an incredible amount of things to do. The new Liverpool ONE centre is great, especially the open air park on the top floor and I love to visit the stylish Albert Dock. You can't escape the culture of the place, not least The Beatles, which really immerses you into the atmosphere of the city and makes you feel absolutely at home. The university is extremely friendly, and the balance between work and play is always struck. I am very proud to call Liverpool my home.'

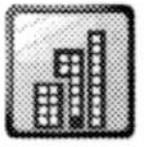

The city

Safety						Liverpool city centre is statistically one of the safest in the country, but like all cities, extra care should be taken in non-student areas
Nightlife						There is a wide range of clubs to cater for all tastes, most located in the Concert Square area of the city centre
Transport						Public transport is excellent, but parking can be very difficult. A car, however, is not necessary
Cost of Living						Expect to pay around £55–60 per week rent, £4–6 for a taxi to the city centre, and £20–30 for a night out

Things to do

Liverpool is an incredibly vibrant city with a rich history. The city centre is large, and is dominated by the Liverpool ONE complex. Nothing is far away, and all amenities including shops, restaurants, bars, cinemas and tourist attractions are within easy reach. There are also a number of music venues such as the famous Everyman and Empire theatres, the O2 Academy and the new Echo Arena.

The parkland areas of Liverpool come alive during the summer months, especially Sefton and Greenbank parks near the university halls of residence. West Kirby and Formby beaches are also within travelling distance on public transport, and are popular days out. Students use all areas of the city to socialise, and there is a real feeling of camaraderie wherever you go.

In terms of nightlife, there is a student night almost every evening during the week at various venues around the city. All music tastes are catered for in the variety of bars, pubs and clubs Liverpool has to offer, and discounts are common. The city centre is extremely safe on nights out, with a good police presence at all times.

Places to go		
Place	**Brief Description**	**Entry Fee/Opening Time**
Mood	Popular club in Concert Square	£5–6; Mon–Sat 10.00pm–3.00am
Nation	Superclub, huge Wed nights	£5 Wed 9.00pm–Late
Heebie Jeebies	Alternative indie/jazz bar	£Free, Mon–Sat All evening
The Raz	Underground medics favourite	£2 Mon–Sat 10.00pm–3.00am
CaVa	Student favourite tequila bar	£Free Mon–Sun All evening

Student opinion

'Student life in Liverpool is academically challenging and socially dynamic in equal measure, and in light of the current regeneration of the city, there is no more exciting place to be.'

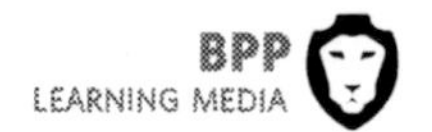

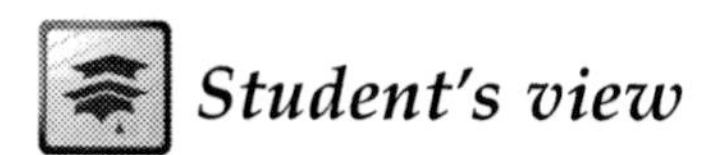

Student's view

Pre-clinical

'The first year is a whistle-stop tour of the normal human body and provides a good foundation for the following years. The workload from PBL can seem intense, but as long as you keep on top of all your learning objectives, you will have no problems at all. There are also many clinical skills to learn, which can make the OSCE a daunting prospect. Again, however, grasping these skills early on make the following years a great deal easier. There is still plenty of free time though, with only a couple of hours of each day taken up by compulsory sessions.

A typical day begins with the journey to university, more often than not by bus. A yearly pass for the Arriva buses is essential! There is a one-hour lecture every morning at 9.00am, which can be difficult at first, but is certainly worth going to in order to support PBL objectives. This is often followed by PBL itself, clinical skills, communication skills or HARC. Some days, however, you may be free for the rest of the day!

The second year changes quite radically. Two days a week are spent on hospital placements and one on a community attachment, in a GP surgery for example. Only Mondays and Fridays are spent in university – either lectures or PBL. There are no longer clinical skills, communication skills or timetabled HARC sessions, as you should have all the material you need from the first year. Self-directed learning is encouraged at Liverpool and I learned very quickly that time management is an essential skill!

Examinations can be tough, especially with OSCEs often being in the same week as the written exams – sometimes even the day after if you are unlucky! However, there is no negative marking in the exams, unlike some other medical schools, which takes the pressure off a little bit!

Life at Liverpool in the first two years is a great mix of work and play. There is plenty of time in the first year to socialise, find your bearings and have a great time, provided you keep on top of all the

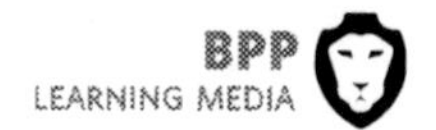

learning objectives. Highlights of my first two years include the wild medics dinners, annual smoking concert (which is a must!) and having barbeques with friends at Roscoe and Gladstone Hall!'

Clinical

'As a fourth year, my day typically begins at 9.00am with a ward round, following the team and receiving teaching on interesting cases. The morning is then spent taking patients' histories and doing examinations in preparation for the final examinations. After lunch, I can attend a clinic or theatre session for a few hours, then have a lecture or PBL session before going home. In Liverpool, the later years are highly integrated so that although learning is guided by PBL, students learn a lot through seeing patients and receiving teaching on these cases. The workload does increase in the later years, as students gain more responsibility and near final exams, but the wide range of activities and weekly socials with the LMSS have helped ease any stress. Exams themselves are always daunting but there's always something to look forward to – be it elective in the third year or just the fact that this set of exams will be your last in the fourth year! I have thoroughly enjoyed doing the integrated PBL course at Liverpool. PBL enabled me to learn in a way that suited me, and allowed me to avoid 9.00am–5.00pm lectures, which are certainly not my cup of tea! Seeing patients from an early stage brought to life what I was learning in books, and improved my confidence tremendously. Of course, Liverpool isn't for everyone – for PBL to work you need to be quite motivated, but this is something which will be essential later on as a doctor furthering your career, so it is a good skill to learn early on. I feel as though the course at Liverpool has equipped me well with the knowledge, clinical skills and confidence I will need as a newly qualified doctor, and, thanks to PBL, if there's something I don't know, I'll know where to find it!'

Once you get in...

The medical school will send you a large pack of information, as well as the university itself. Expect to receive a pack containing information about accommodation first, which is a big decision. The university will provide all the information you need to make an informed choice. All accommodation arrangements are made online, through the university's SPIDER application. You will also receive information about the sports centre, and how you can join university sports teams. It is well worth signing up for the gym online, saving a great deal of time when you get to Liverpool. The freshers' fair is the place to sign up for teams. A freshers' week timetable will also be enclosed, explaining what events will be happening over the first two weeks of term.

The medical school will send you a pack containing a welcome letter from the LMSS President and whole host of useful information, including a reading list, items you will need to bring with you, overview of a typical day at university and a list of the most popular medics' nights out. You will find it hard not to escape 'The Raz!'

Once you have chosen your accommodation, you will receive an information pack from your hall, giving details of when you can move in, and events that will be taking place during the first few weeks. As usual, there will be some forms to sign and send back.

The university will also ask you to send them a number of passport photos in order to have your ID card ready for you when you arrive.

The Best Thing	Early patient contact with modern PBL teaching
The Worst Thing	Lack of taught anatomy sessions

Student top tips

- Get your Welcome Week wristband, gym membership and LMSS membership pack online before you arrive to save time.
- Go to the freshers' fair to see the societies the university has to offer, as well as local businesses who are looking to give away vouchers and merchandise.
- Be sure to get an Arriva bus pass for the year if you are living in halls of residence. It will save you a great deal of money.
- Keeping your door wedged open in halls of residence is a great way to meet new people when you move in!

Summary Table

Positives	Negatives
Modern PBL based course	Lack of anatomy teaching
Enthusiastic medical society	Tough OSCEs
Excellent sport facilities	Distance of travel to some placements
Great student areas and amenities	Halls of residence not on campus
Regenerating and exciting city	Lack of parking

London: Barts and the London School of Medicine and Dentistry

Barts and the London School of Medicine and Dentistry
Garrod Buildings, Turner Street
Whitechapel
London
E1 2AD

www.smd.qmul.ac.uk/

Nestled deep in the heart of London's east end Barts is a medical school encapsulated by extremes of wealth and culture. The medical school prides itself upon training communicative and culturally aware doctors and places a strong emphasis on these skills in the course material. The location of the college and it's incredibly diverse population makes this a perfect place to learn those skills, and to be exposed to a rich variety of clinical conditions. Barts also provide an exciting mix of modern teaching techniques set within a prestigious and prosperous medical school steeped in history and tradition.

The medical course

Key facts

Course Type	PBL	Degree Awarded	MBBS
Basic Entry Requirements	AAA	Entrance Exams	UKCAT
Year Size	Approx 280	Open Days	Late Aug/Sept
Admissions Website	www.smd.qmul.ac.uk/admissions/index.html		

Getting in – student tips

Your personal statement has to be written in a way to make it distinctive yet at the same time portray a serious and mature tone. It is very important to be truthful since you will be asked questions about it in the interview. A good personal statement will reflect your individuality and it is better to talk about a few good points in depth rather than listing everything you are interested in.

An article is issued approximately a week before the interview date. This is based on a study, for example, Kate Jones, a 13-year-old patient who has cardiomyopathy and has had enough of all the surgeries and wants to die at home with friends and family. This is similar to the type of PBL (problem-based learning) scenarios you will get in your studies so they want to see how you approach a case like this. The main focus is on the ethical issues and remember there is no right or wrong answer it is more how you answer and back up your rationale.

Course details

Foundation / Pre-Med	No	**Graduate**	Yes
Student Population	Male: female ratio: 60:40	**Term Length**	Pre-clinical: 11 weeks Clinical: 14 weeks
Erasmus / Foreign Exchange	N/A	**Elective Period**	Year 5 – 6 weeks

Intercalation

Stage	Following year 2, 3 or 4	**Degree Awarded**	BScMedSci (Hons)/ BSc
Requirements	130 places available, good to excellent performance in exams	**Subjects**	Medical Sciences

Anatomy teaching

Once a week you will have a scheduled time of two hours to visit the anatomy lab to examine prosections and models. You will be issued with a booklet in advance, which allows you to prepare and read up on the topics. Once inside the lab you have to answer questions within the booklet. There will be demonstrators available to explain concepts and expand on your existing knowledge. The labs are also available Monday to Friday for self-directed learning; the information will remain posted for a week after the demonstration. The anatomy is also covered in lectures to reinforce the content you need to know.

Although dissection is not part of the main course structure it is available as an optional module. In the first year you will dissect the limbs and the remainder of the body will be covered in the second year.

Anatomy is examined as MCQs which are not negatively marked. The exam is computer based and will also contain the microanatomy and data interpretation elements of the course.

Pre-clinical/Years 1–2	
Topics	***Year 1:*** Fundamentals of Medicine, Human Development, Cardio-Respiratory, Metabolism, Locomotor, Brain & Behaviour. ***Year 2:*** Cardio-Respiratory, Brain & Behaviour, Human Development, Human Sciences & Public Health, Locomotor, Metabolism.
Teaching	The first two years will mainly be lectures and later you will be more exposed in the hospitals. There are also PBLs, which you will eventually have twice a week, and Medicine in Society (MedSoc) fortnightly where you will visit GP practices.
SSC Periods	In each year you will do two SSC modules during February and April in the first year and December and February in the second year. There is a wide range of SSCs to suit everyone's taste. You can choose modules in medical hypnosis, history of medicine or if you have a particular interest you can do a self-directed SSC but by far the most popular is the dissection SSC. It is possible to arrange your own SSC including audits of a GP surgery. Some students can further their work during the SSC and try to publish their findings, for example, one student experimented with the best way to teach fundoscopy for a medical education SSC. There is also another component of SSC in the first year, which involves group work to produce two academic posters to present to the doctors and researchers and possibly the Dean of the medical school.
Exams	There is a multiple choice exam (MCQ) and then a short answer question paper (SAQ) testing your PBL and lecture knowledge. The anatomy will be tested with pictures on a computer and will also be multiple choice.

Clinical/Years 3–5	
Topics	***Year 3:*** General hospital medicine and surgery: Cardiology, Respiratory medicine, Gastroenterology, Endocrinology, Urology, General surgery, Breast surgery, Metabolism, Community placements. ***Year 4:*** Specialities: Neurology, Psychiatry, Obstetrics Gynaecology, Paediatrics, Dermatology, Heath Care of the Elderly, Musculoskeletal, Community placements. ***Year 5:*** General hospital medicine and surgery, Urgent & Emergency Care, GP placements, Acute and critical care, Elective.
SSC Periods	***Year 3:*** Two SSC periods within the year within hospital placements. One is a written piece on a subject agreed with, and marked by a consultant. The second is a full patient clerking and write-up, includes an audio recording of the history taking. You will meet a patient and gain their consent to take a history and examine them, this is written up and then further discussion of relevant ethical, psychosocial and communication details are written up too. ***Year 4:*** Dissertation (6,000-8,000 words) on a subject of student's choice. A list of subject titles is given by the medical school but students are encouraged to self-organise an essay title. ***Year 5:*** Two four-week periods which can be spent in clinical placements of the student's choice. Again, the medical school provides a list of possible placements but students can self-organise. It is possible but not usual to have one of these SSCs abroad.
Exams	Exams at the end of the third and fourth years. Finals are taken midway through the fifth year so that anyone who fails has time to resit before the year ends. Third and fourth year exams consist of two written papers and a practical paper (includes five- and ten-minute stations examining practical and clinical skills and communication skills), students must attain 50% minimum to pass. Finals involve one written paper and three practical papers on communication skills, practical procedures and clinical skills.

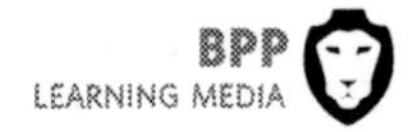

Hospital placements/academies

There is a great choice of hospitals for placements in the clinical years. 'Out' firms, such as Southend or Colchester, are those which provide accommodation as you would normally reside within the hospital's property for the duration of the placements. These hospitals offer a lower consultant:student ratio and so are great learning experiences. The 'in' firms, such as Barts or The Royal London, do not provide accommodation. They are big teaching hospitals and offer students the chance to see a huge variety of patients, some with rarer pathologies. The Royal London is currently undergoing major refurbishment to become the largest hospital in Britain with the country's leading trauma centre and largest renal service. It is also home to HEMS, the London helicopter emergency medical service (as seen on BBC's *Trauma*).

Each hospital has an undergraduate co-ordinator who organises the teaching during placements and there is variety between the trusts as to the amount of consultant-led verses lecture based teaching. In every case the hospitals provide excellent teaching and hands on experience.

The length of placements varies widely during the third to fifth years. Broadly speaking the third year is about learning the general medical and surgical topics and getting up to scratch with patient examination and interaction. The fourth year has more placements but in specialist areas and is generally considered to be the hardest year. The fifth year has placements in other areas but is about learning to practise independently and gaining more experience in preparation for becoming and FY1 doctor.

Hospitals and Travel Time from University	
Barts	10 minutes
Newham	35 minutes
King George, Essex	60 minutes
Colchester	85 minutes

The medical school

Work						Good work life balance
Facilities						Several big libraries most of which are open 24 hours. Lots of computer suites available, however they can be temperamental
Support						The medical school is keen to help and support its students
Feedback						Possible to get feedback on PBL work but can be harder when it comes to exams

Facilities

There is a big medical library on the Whitechapel campus with lots of computers. The library at Barts is smaller but is generally preferred by students as it is the original medical school library on the Barts site (Oak panelled etc!). There is also a big library at the Mile End campus of Queen Mary University which is available to medical students. There are several computer suites available to students across the campuses, although the IT can be frustrating with lots of computers not working. Barts has a large clinical and communication skills suite which is available to book throughout the year. This gets very busy near exams but the staff are very accommodating and keen to help.

Student support

There is a whole host of services available to students who need support. The medical school makes a point of letting the students know that help is available and how it can be accessed, which is very easy to do. There are academic year tutors, pastoral support, financial advice services and careers advice available to medical students. The Dean and Deputy Dean for students are very accessible if anything comes up during the year. There is an occupational health service, which is part of Queen Mary University, who are there to help with health concerns and any vaccinations required.

Medical societies

Barts and The London Medical School has its own student association. As a medical student you can use this or the main Queen Mary University union. Both have undergone a large refurbishment in recent years and have great bars and other facilities.

The medical students have their own sports clubs and compete with other medical schools. The highlight of the year is the Merger Cup, when Barts teams play teams from Queen Mary. It comes from when the medical school merged with the main university.

There are many, many societies which students can join from the Tamil Society to Barts and The London Emergency Medical Society. There is a great atmosphere at the student's association and everyone is keen to get involved.

Finance

A QMUL bursary is available to all means assessed students (up to £1,000 pounds). The Dean's beneficiary fund is also available for students experiencing hardship through study, awards based on application and need.

Student opinion

'The medical school campus is located next to The Royal London Hospital away from the main university campus. With its own students' union too, you feel like you're part of a distinct community, part of the hospital one. The medical school is located in some of the poorest boroughs in the UK with a very diverse community, allowing you the chance to see pathology and meet patients which no other medical school can offer.'

The university

Accommodation	Choice of campus or non-campus university
Further Info	www.smd.qmul.ac.uk/ www.bartslondon.com/

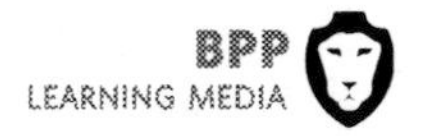

Accommodation

Accommodation choice at Barts is varied and it is very much a personal choice. The main choice is between Dawson House, Floyer and Mile End campus, all of which are within easy walking distance of tube stations. Dawson House is for medical and dental students and is situated in central London. Floyer House is also for medical and dental students and is located at the Whitechapel campus, which is convenient as it is within a couple of minutes to the library and the main lecture theatre. The Mile End campus has a student village, which is modern and provides a great social environment as there are a number of events such as resident's roast, where you can get a full meal for a few pounds, and you can buy cinema tickets at a concessionary rate. It is shared with students from other disciplines, so it is good opportunity to have a range of social networks.

Study facilities

There is a specific medical library at both Whitechapel and Charterhouse (near Dawson Hall), with a number of copies of the recommended texts. There are also a few books available at Mile End main library. As a student at Barts it is possible to use any one of these, but the medical libraries are usually the quietest and the busiest throughout the year. The library at Whitechapel is an old church making it a nice place to study and the stain glass windows have medical illustrations adding to its character.

University sports & students' union

The gym on the Mile End campus has all the facilities of a high street gym but at much cheaper price and you can join from as little as £15 per month. The gym also contains squash courts and holds aerobic and exercise sessions. It also has a separate female only section. There are many facilities around the area which different societies use and you can find rock climbing centres and tennis courts close to the university. There is also a leisure centre at Mile End which has swimming facilities and a running track as well as a gym available to the public.

The union is the social centre of the medical school and is a cheaper alternative to going out in London. During lunch many students take their food and eat at the union, where it also offers great lunch deals. Society meetings are held at the union, as there are lots of free rooms and there is also a union shop where you can buy Barts merchandise.

Student opinion

'I stayed in Pooley House and enjoyed the campus community. Meeting students from all subjects gave me a wider view of university.'

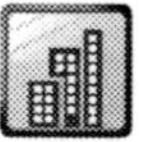

The city

Safety	🛡	🛡	🛡			Being a big city do be careful but generally is safe
Nightlife	☾	☾	☾	☾	☾	Endless amount of clubs and bars
Transport	🚌	🚌	🚌	🚌	🚌	With the underground and bus routes transport is very good and parking in London makes having a car too expensive. Also keep in mind congestion charge
Cost of Living	🐷	🐷	🐷	🐷	🐷	Rent may start around £100 per week. Taxi would be £20 into central London but taking the tube would be much cheaper

Things to do

In London there is something for everyone and exploring the city will never bore you. There are the usual tourist attractions and lots of nights out which other cities would struggle to provide. You can visit the west end theatres or shop on Oxford street. To relax London has Hyde park but even closer is Victoria park.

London is a great place to live. Events will come to you rather than you going to travel to see bands or shows. The O_2 arena hosts many concerts and sporting events if Wimbledon isn't enough for you.

Being a student in the city provides you with many places to eat and go out with friends and there will never be a Starbucks out of reach. On the other hand, your costs can spiral if you're not careful or you may even drift away from studies. It is possible to keep to your tight student budget with student discounts and limiting your shopping sprees.

You will really feel you are at the centre of the world and everything you need is at your doorstep. London has its charm and many who do live here never want to move away, so you have been warned!

Places to go		
Place	**Brief Description**	**Entry Fee/Opening Time**
Tiger Tiger	Stylish club with five areas	£5, Mon-Sat 11.00am-3.00am
Fabric	Guest DJs playing Drum&Bass/Hiphop/Funk	£10, Fri-Sun 10.00pm-5.00am
Ministry of Sound	Super-club with three huge dance floors	£15, Fri-Sat 11.00pm-7.00am
Funky Buddha	Popular nightclub in Mayfair	£20, Tue-Sat 10.00pm-3.00am

Student opinion

'London is an amazing place to be a student. The buzz and endless variety and opportunity of the big city never gets tiring. Being part of Barts and The London you get to see a side of London which most people don't.'

Student's view

Pre-clinical

'In the first year you will learn about the normal structure and function of the body. Along side this you will learn in detail disorders through the PBL part of the course making the knowledge

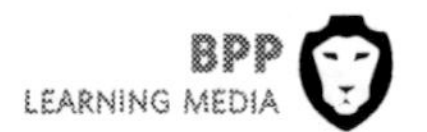

you learnt in lectures relevant and more interesting. The lecturers are light hearted and friendly making it easier to digest the vast amount you are expected to learn. You will be advised that it's a good idea to do three hours a day and then you won't need to do last minute cramming. If you do keep up with work and attend lectures you will have no problem passing the exams and this is one thing I now recommend.

A typical day would start from 9.00am and finish at 5.00pm, and twice a week you would meet with your PBL group.You will get to know this group well and some even study together making life less lonely. Once every two weeks you will be travelling to your allocated GP to hone your patient-doctor skills and being dressed formally really brings out the professional in you.

There is a lot of history associated with the medical school. It is one of the oldest in the country and the Royal London Hospital founded in 1740 gives you a long list of famous predecessors. You may even get to meet the skeleton of 'The Elephant Man' Joseph Merrick kept in the museum of the Garrod Building and not publicly exhibited. The history is only beginning as The Royal London has been granted a £1 billion redevelopment making the hospital the leading trauma and emergency centre in London.

The course is intense but manageable and it does certainly stretch your abilities, particularly during the Brain & Behaviour module. The pile of books on your desk will become a safety hazard. Nevertheless, the support and help offered is excellent such as the extra lectures run by MESS. This is a peer-to-peer teaching group that is internationally accredited and so the quality is high. In later years you will have the chance to become a MESS teacher as I've done and help your more junior members of the medical school.'

Clinical

'I have thoroughly enjoyed learning clinical medicine. It can be a scary moment when the Consultant asks you to talk to and examine a new patient in order to present to them but it's very rewarding seeing how much the patients trust you, even as a student. I much prefer the bedside teaching of the clinical years than the heavy lecture based teaching in years 1 and 2.

A typical day involves morning ward round at 8.00am or 9.00am, this can take anything from 30 minutes on a surgical firm to four hours on a medical one. These can be great learning experiences but only if the Consultant is in the mood! The rest of the day can be taken up with teaching, outpatient clinics or operating theatre time if you are on a surgical firm. I have always found the FY1s to be really keen to help teach and get students to do procedures (taking blood, inserting cannulas, taking arterial blood gas samples etc). The trick I've noticed with clinical teaching is that you have to put in the effort in order to get the most out of it, the opportunities have to be found and are not presented to you on a plate.

My favourite moment so far was when I got to assist with a facial reconstruction. I had waited all day and finally after eight hours of standing around the Consultant got me to scrub in and help. It was worth the wait!'

Postgraduate

'A typical day is BUSY. Mondays are typically 9.00am until around 4.00pm with minimal gaps in between with the rest of the week varying to make up to around 25-30 hours a week of contact. I found the majority of the lectures to be of excellent quality and generally the notes provided are great and really guide you towards the important aspects of the PBL scenarios.

The stress of examinations is quite high on the graduate course but it never got in the way of my enjoyment, and the feeling of overwhelming joy/relief when I finally received my pass at the end of the year was really rewarding.

Another massive plus for me is the location of Barts, as the often impoverished and diverse population means that clinical firms can be exciting and the opportunity to see new or interesting cases or disease presentations is always present. I also like the fact that Barts is a well respected research institution, with world famous oncology centres within the university grounds and the new centre for the cell at Whitechapel. This means you really feel like you are at the cutting edge of Medicine while studying here.

As a Barts student you are expected to become a well-rounded clinician so extra-curricular activity is heavily encouraged,

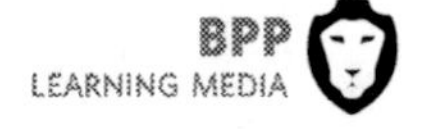

something I was very relieved to learn when I arrived. There is a freshers' fair at the beginning of the year at which all the different societies and clubs attempt to gain your membership. There really is something for everyone at the school, be it jumping around on stage with the dance society, walking and climbing with the alpine club, or getting naked and singing with the rugby boys at tables!'

Once you get in...

Before you go out and celebrate your offer there are many things to sort out. Luckily, this is very easy as much of it is done online, like choosing your accommodation and paying your deposit. You will need to send in your certificates by post and collect them once you get there. You will get a handy book made by the medical school which provides a guide to freshers' week outlining all the events and tips about eating in the area etc.

During your first week at medical school there will be the usual introductory lecture and you will be issued with a folder containing information about the course, examinations and procedures as well as important contacts and dates for the year. It is important to keep this safe as it contains your PBL scenarios and handy paperwork. There is a list of recommended books, but before spending your money buying them all, take time to see which ones you use the most, or borrow them from the library – there should be many copies.

At the beginning try to enjoy yourself and don't be too keen to start working towards exams otherwise you will run the risk of burning yourself out.

The Best Thing	The friendly attitude of the medical school towards its students and the close knit community this promotes
The Worst Thing	Anatomy teaching could be improved

Student top tips

- Keep an eye out for celebrities on your walk into university, the achingly chic Shoreditch and Brick Lane area seems to be full of them!
- Take advantage of the cheap local cuisine, Brick Lane is ten minutes' walk from the union and provides cheap, great tasting Bangladeshi cuisine all night!

Summary Table

Positives	Negatives
Being in London	High cost of living
Personable staff	Daunting to live in a big city
Lots of facilities	Too many students on some firms
Medical school has its own campus and union	Separate campuses
Plenty of opportunity for sport	Anatomy teaching is slightly weak

London: Imperial College

Imperial College Medical School,
Sir Alexander Fleming Building,
South Kensington, London, SW7 2AZ

www.imperial.ac.uk/medicine

Imperial College School of Medicine (ICSM) recently celebrated its decennary. Within that time it has amassed an abundance of achievements and international recognition. Situated in the heart of the capital, ICSM is one of the leading institutions on the continent, offering a traditional curriculum incorporated within a contemporary framework in accordance with the GMC's *Tomorrow's Doctors*. Not only will you be taught by international experts in Medicine and Surgery, you will also have plenty of opportunities to learn in one of the largest UK healthcare trusts.

The university campus holds state of the art facilities and amenities including a multi-storey gym and refurbished halls of residence next to Hyde Park and the Royal Albert Hall, all just a stone's throw away from each other. Nevertheless, it takes a lot more to be a doctor besides medical school. ICSM consists of a multi cultural student body with a vast range of interests and talents. You are bound to find life-long friends to accompany you in your unique journey through a challenging medical course.

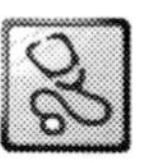

The medical course

Key facts

Course Type	Traditional	**Degree Awarded**	MBBS, BSc (hons)
Basic Entry Requirements	AAA	**Entrance Exams**	BMAT
Year Size	Approx 280	**Open Days**	June/July
Admissions Website	www.imperial.ac.uk/medicine		

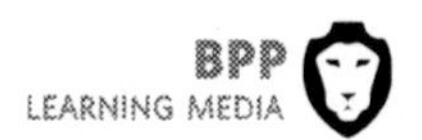

Getting in – student tips

At Imperial College a good personal statement, more often than not, can decide whether an applicant 'makes-it-or-breaks-it' in their quest to secure an interview. What the admission panel looks for is whether you have shown a genuine interest in Medicine, for instance, demonstrating evidence of reading articles on Medicine, attending a first-aid course or undertaking work experience placements at your local GP or hospital. It is important that you are able to describe your practical experience of Medicine in detail, which could include what you learnt and gained from the placement, which aspect you enjoyed the most or what you found difficult. Therefore, it might be worthwhile keeping a diary of your experiences. Furthermore, a section of the personal statement should be devoted to your involvement in the local community, such as volunteering to help out at charitable organisations or care homes.

All students will be interviewed for a place at Imperial College. If selected, you will be required to attend a 15-minute interview which will take place at the South Kensington campus between January and April. Generally interview panels consist of a chairperson, two members of the selection panel, a senior medical student and frequently a lay observer.

The interviewers at Imperial often ask typical questions, such as 'Why do you want to become a doctor?', 'What have you done to show your commitment to Medicine and to the community?' and 'Why have you applied to Imperial?'. Intertwined with these will be questions to assess your ethical reasoning and knowledge of Medicine, along with a discussion on your personal statement, with a particular emphasis on the work experience section.

Gap years are becoming increasingly popular and can add considerable weight to your application provided that you can show that you used your time sensibly and took part in activities which are likely to favour your medical application.

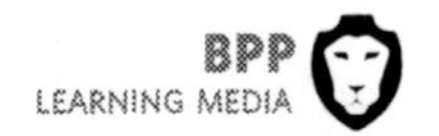

Course details

Foundation / Pre-Med	N/A	Graduate	Yes
Student Population	Male: female ratio: 50:50	Term Length	Pre-clinical: approx 11 weeks Commencing: early October Clinical: 37–52 weeks Commencing: between early July and mid September
Erasmus / Foreign Exchange	Usually available to BSc students to do research in Tanzania or Japan. European (EMSA) and Asian (AMSA) medical student associations organise group exchange programmes	Elective Period	Between July and February 7-9 weeks

Intercalation

Stage	Year 4	Degree Awarded	Student BSc (hons)
Requirements	Compulsory	Subjects	A variety of medical science subjects while also offering History of Medicine, Humanities and Global Health

Anatomy teaching

In the first and second years there is three-hour block of anatomy teaching each week split up into a lecture, a living anatomy session and examining cadavers in the dissection room, all an hour each. Anatomy is taught with regard to the other modules being learnt allowing students to integrate their knowledge across the syllabus.

The lecture opens the proceedings by giving the necessary background teaching and theory to go with the more practical

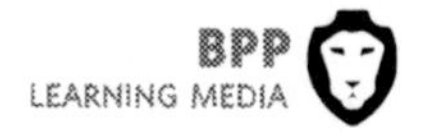

anatomy sessions later on in the day. Depending on rotations, you then either attend the living anatomy session or head towards the dissection room. The living anatomy session is interactive and enjoyable and involves understanding the clinical aspects of the anatomy. In the dissection room, the cadavers allow students to examine the anatomy close-up. Students are split into groups of ten and well-qualified demonstrators teach the relevant anatomy. This session allows you to observe everything you have learnt during the day. The practical side of dissecting is also a valuable experience with many students finding this the best method to learn anatomy.

Pre-clinical/Years 1–2	
Topics	*Molecules, cells and disease* includes molecular and cell biology, genetics, blood and blood-forming tissues, metabolism, infection, immunity, cell pathology, and carcinogenesis and cancer as a disease. *Life support systems* include the skin, cardiovascular, respiratory, alimentary and urinary systems, and the anatomy of the thorax, abdomen, pelvis and perineum. *Life cycle and regulatory systems* includes human life cycle, neuroscience and mental health, the endocrine and musculoskeletal systems, the anatomy of the head, neck, spine and limbs, as well as pharmacology and therapeutics. *Foundations of clinical practice* include communication skills, sociology, ethics and law, epidemiology in practice, and information technology. The patient contact course, which offers the earliest clinical experience, is also integrated into this theme. *Integrated body function and dysfunction* includes modules on water and electrolytes, physiology of infection, exercise, drugs and the hospitalised patient, and nutrition.
Teaching	Teaching consists of lectures, clinical demonstrations, tutorials, seminars, computer workshops, laboratory practical and clinical skills classes, and some problem-based learning.

Exams	Extended Matching Questions, Single Best Answers and Short Answer Questions. Certain examinations also demand essays. Exams in the first year take place in June, while those in the second year take place in April and June. Formative (mock) examinations occur in January for the first year students to assess their progress. Computer-based self-tests are made available throughout the year as revision aids. The pass mark is 50%.
SSC	A number of SSC periods are available during pre-clinical years.

Clinical/Years 3–6	
Topics	***Year 3:*** Hospital Medicine and Surgery firms, General Practice, Anaesthesia, Clinical Pharmacology and Therapeutics as well as a BSc Foundation course. ***Year 5:*** Pathology and rotations in ten clinical specialities: Dermatology, GP, Infectious diseases, Neurology, Obstetrics & Gynaecology, Oncology, Orthopaedics, Paediatrics, Psychiatry and Rheumatology. ***Year 6:*** Cardiology, Electives, Emergency medicine, ENT, GP, Hospital Medicine, Practical Medicine, Ophthalmology, Radiology, Renal Medicine, Special Study Courses (SCC) and Surgery.
Elective	Any medical institution in the world for at least seven weeks. Funding, although available, is very competitive and the best report is awarded a prize.
SSC Periods	Two-and-half-week period during the final year. This is an amazing opportunity to explore any speciality with over 40 medical and 12 surgical options on offer. Otherwise, you can always organise one yourself! Students are actively encouraged to contribute to research projects, journal publications and audits.
Exams	Pre-clinical: MCQ & SAQ; Clinical: EMQ, SBA, OSCE & PACES; BSC: essay and coursework. All summative exams are during summer and are challenging. People who fail may resit in autumn and discuss any extenuating circumstances with their Tutors, Head of Welfare and the Examining Board.

Hospital placements/academies

Each year consists of multiple placements with varying durations. In the third year, there are one six-week and two ten-week attachments. In the fifth year, each firm (with some clinical specialities combined) consist of nine-week blocks. Each firm is then reduced to approximately three weeks in the final year.

Groups of up to five students on any attachment are given a timetable that is divided into time on wards, in operating theatres, in outpatient clinics and in multi-disciplinary team teaching. Students will be taught by renowned physicians and surgeons and their teams in famous hospitals such as Chelsea & West Minutester, St Mary's and Charing Cross just to name a few. Furthermore, depending on your level of enthusiasm, there is time to participate in on-going research projects and audits.

Undergraduate Teaching Co-ordinators are present in every hospital to sort out timetables, offer advice and deal with any concerns. Short-term accommodation is only provided in some District General Hospitals besides the usual on-call rooms. All sites are accessible.

Hospitals and Travel Time from University	
Royal Brompton	5 minutes
Chelsea & Westminster	6 minutes
St Mary's	7 minutes
Charing Cross	8 minutes
St Charles	11 minutes
West Middlesex	12 minutes
Hammersmith	13 minutes
Central Middlesex	17 minutes
Ealing	23 minutes
Hillingdon	28 minutes
St Peter's & Ashford	36 minutes
Northwick Park & St. Mark's	36 minutes

The medical school

Work						Good work ethic is needed
Facilities						A newly refurbished spacious Central Library with a café and PC clusters
Support						Each student is assigned a tutor and a 'mum and dad' from the year above
Feedback						Regular discussion with tutors

Facilities

The Central Library is situated on the main campus at South Kensington and is open for 24 hours during exam periods (usually during summer). Every hospital has its own library and PC clusters specifically for ICSM members. Hospitals also have student common rooms, changing rooms and lockers. There are weekly sessions held in the clinical skills laboratory on site with excellent training facilities and equipment. Moreover, St Mary's Hospital also has virtual surgical simulators and a Virtual Operating Room that simulates critical scenarios to improve non-technical skills such as teamwork, leadership and communication.

Student support

Problems are naturally unavoidable in life but ICSM has an effective support system to counteract any unforeseen circumstances. Students are given contact details for their tutors (staff), the Head of Welfare at ICSM (staff) and the ICSM Student Union Welfare Officer (one student elected each year). One of the freshers' fortnight events, 'Mums & Dads night', is when new students are introduced to senior students and adopted. Mums and dads look after and support the freshers and both eventually develop a bond of trust and friendship.

ICSM is proud to consist of a multi-faith community and has a chaplaincy and Muslim prayer rooms. Students who seek counselling are given several sessions for free and all information is kept strictly

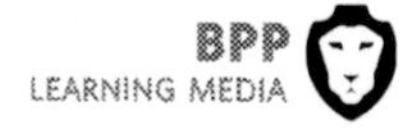

confidential. Every new student must pass a health assessment by the Student Occupational Health Centre, which also provides vaccinations, advice and safe travel packs for electives abroad.

Finance

Scholarships for sport, music, drama and academic achievement are granted on interview performances. Also, hardship funds are available to all students, provided that all other alternative fiscal resources have been exhausted.

Student opinion

'There is so much to do here! I have had the opportunity to explore various avenues within charities, sports and societies and also contributed in running nationwide events with other universities. In fact, the best thing was working with my friends and making many more through these events. You feel supported here and I really like the new facilities, libraries and computer labs.'

The university

Accommodation	Non-campus halls of residence
Further Info	www.union.ic.ac.uk/medic/ www.ulu.co.uk www3.imperial.ac.uk/accommodation/

Accommodation

The majority of first years live in the halls of residence near the campus in the South Kensington area. Imperial College has one of the best selections of accommodation on offer for its students. The more popular halls, such as Beit, Southside and the newly built Eastside, are within a five-minute walk to the main campus. Other halls like Bernard Sunley, Fisher and Southwell are housed together in the Evelyn Gardens complex, which is a 20-minute walk to the campus. The more distant halls such as Wilson House and Orient House require a bus or tube journey or a pleasant walk through Hyde Park on a fine summer's day. Each hall, however, brings with it its own charisma and character making it an enjoyable year living out for freshers.

Students in the second year usually rent properties most commonly in the Hammersmith, Baron's Court and West Kensington area, which are slightly further out (and cheaper!) from South Kensington, home to some of the most expensive land prices in the whole country.

Study facilities

The Central Library at the South Kensington campus has seen it transformed into a high-quality environment to study. With a large collection of textbooks, journals and audio, the resources available to students are second-to-none. During the exam period, the library becomes a 24-hour haven for those wishing a permanent place to revise. Imperial College is also fortunate to have departmental and campus libraries. Medical students have the pleasure of studying at the Charing Cross campus library, which is specifically tailored to Medicine and has all the latest medical textbooks and journals to aid their revision.

There is no shortage of computer facilities at the medical school. The computer lab in the Sir Alexander Fleming building has generous opening hours, and is available seven days a week. On the rare occasion when students cannot find a spare computer, the nearby Central Library is bound to have one free in its IT suite.

University sports & students' union

The Reynolds Bar, at the Charing Cross campus in Hammersmith, is the spiritual heart of the medical school and the venue for all the freshers' events, much of RAG and the infamous themed Bops. It also houses 'Sports night' on Wednesdays where all the teams return from playing to celebrate or drown their sorrows. The main union at the South Kensington campus is also a great place to head for lunch or a drink after lectures; sprawled out on the conveniently located courtyard during the summer or huddled in the warmth of one of the bars during the winter. There are regular quiz nights, gig nights and jazz and rock groups playing at the union keeping the calendar busy.

Arguably the best thing about being at Imperial is its free subscription to Ethos, the college's flagship sports centre based in South Kensington. The centre has an extensive range of facilities from a fitness gym and swimming pool to a climbing wall and squash courts. Students can also choose from a variety of classes at an additional, but subsided, cost. However, the fact that the whole college has free access to the gym means that it can get very busy during peak times.

Wednesday afternoons are kept free for sport and the vast grounds at Harlington and Teddington support an extensive programme of training and matches involving Imperial College. There is a strong sporting culture at Imperial and the medical students are encouraged to take part regardless of their abilities. The university is reputable for fielding strong rugby, cricket and rowing teams and has gained a lot of success over the years.

Student opinion

'Being at university is such a brilliant life experience and nothing else can compare with it. If it's not the independence and the fun in living out, it'll be meeting people from different backgrounds and making life-long friends or taking part in clubs and societies. There really is something for everyone, but it really does depend on the individual to make the most of the opportunities presented to him or her.

I lived in Beit Hall, which many say is the most sociable halls to live in. The fact that the union bar was located next door made for some memorable student nights, and the beautiful quad offered a great place to sit out on the grass with friends on a warm summer's day. The lecture theatre was only a five-minute walk from my halls so there were no excuses for being late to 9.00am starts!'

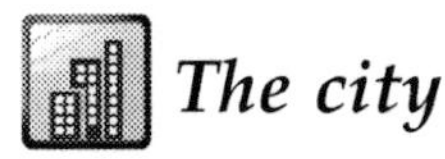

The city

Safety	⛨	⛨	⛨	⛨		London is safe as long as you act sensibly and are aware of your surroundings
Nightlife	☽	☽	☽	☽		You will be in the heart of Central London with all the world-famous clubs and bars. You are definitely spoilt for choice!
Transport	🚌	🚌	🚌	🚌	🚌	There is hardly any need for cars since parking and fines can be a pain! Fortunately, all sites have excellent access thanks to copious public transport links
Cost of Living	🐖	🐖	🐖	🐖	🐖	Expensive but worth it!

Things to do

You can only imagine how much there is to do in the heart of London, both in and out of university. It can take an entire lifetime to familiarise yourself with the city, so you might as well start exploring as a student. All tastes are fully catered for, whether you enjoy going out clubbing and pubbing, or exploring the historic landmarks, galleries and museums. In spite of all city attractions, ICSM student union puts a great deal of effort into running events only for medics across the years. Themed bops at the end of firms are always something to look forward to at our very own and exclusive Reynold's Bar tucked behind Charing Cross Hospital. There are also student nights organised with other London universities.

More specifically, the main university campus is located in South Kensington, just between the Natural History/Science Museums, Royal Albert Hall and Hyde Park. The halls of residence, central library and Ethos gym are all literally minutes away. If you tire from studying sciences, walk around the corner to explore your artistic side at the Royal Colleges of Music and Art, which are accessible by university students.

It can be pretty expensive to live and study in London, but make sure you keep looking out for student discounts everywhere you go. Do not worry if you are compelled to dig into your overdraft, which is very much expected as a medical student regardless where you study. As long as you try to stick to a budget and know your limitations, you are bound to have a great time out and about. London is fairly safe, as long as you stay away from dark alleys and do not accept candy from strangers.

Places to go		
Place	**Brief Description**	**Entry Fee/Opening Time**
ICSM bops	Reynold's Bar, Hammersmith	£3, from 8.00pm 'til late
Roof Gardens	London's only rooftop nightclub	~£15, Friday and Saturday
Cafe de Paris	Posh club in Leicester Square	~£10-15 on weekends
Fabric	World famous nightclub in Smithfield	Students £5-10, Friday-Sunday

Student opinion

'It has been a once in a lifetime opportunity to live and work in one of the best cities in the world! With lots of people around and endless number of things to do, there is not a single dull moment. It is an amazing experience to be educated at one of the best medical schools around.'

Student's view

Pre-clinical

'The first year, especially the first term, helps bridge the gap in knowledge between A level science and the Medicine to come in the following years. The opening term gently eases the freshers into the medical school with a recap of the Biology learnt at sixth-form. This module is known as "Molecules, cells and disease" and is very science-oriented. The "real" Medicine begins in the subsequent terms where students are taught about the different body systems, such as cardiovascular and respiratory, with clinical

aspects integrated into the course. This helps the students to start appreciating patient-care at an early stage.

The anatomy, especially in the first year, is enjoyable with many students coming face-to-face with a cadaver for the first time. This can be a surreal experience for some, with students initially feeling light-headed or faint by the idea of having to explore the human body. In hindsight, they realise that dissection is actually the best way to learn anatomy, especially since they were able to answer the exam anatomy questions based on what they saw in the dissecting lab.

A typical day lasts from 9.00am to 5.00pm, Monday to Friday, with Wednesday afternoons kept free for sport. It really is a full-time commitment since there is so much content to cover, and you will soon realise why there is such a strong camaraderie at the medical school with the students spending a lot of time together. But don't let this put you off. The old saying 'work-hard, play-hard' really couldn't be any truer with the medical students having a real reputation for partying and socialising.

The day typically consists of several lectures split into morning and afternoon sessions, interspersed with tutorials or practicals. Each lecture lasts 50 minutes with ten minutes spared for students to ask the lecturer anything they did not understand. The lecturers are really helpful and are always willing to help answer your queries. In the first year, there is a patient-contact course, which helps students think about the clinical aspects of Medicine. I found this module enjoyable, which consisted of following a patient through their illness and learning about the wider implications of Medicine. This is followed up in the second year, where students are given a four-week clinical attachment at a hospital. This is the first time students sample life on the wards and they are given ample opportunity to practise their history-taking skills. One of the good things about being at Imperial is there emphasis on early integration into clinical Medicine.'

Clinical

'Clinical attachments are perhaps the most enjoyable part of medical school. Patient contact is certainly why I wanted to study Medicine. Imperial College (part of North West Thames Deanery) controls

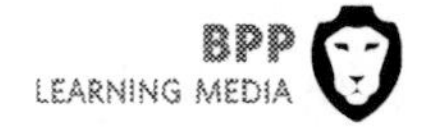

one of the largest healthcare trusts in the country with over 15 associated central and District General Hospitals and residency periods all over the UK. Holidays do not really exist in the final two years but the elective is a rejuvenating experience if you make the most of it.

There is no such thing as a normal day! Students start by attending an 8.00 or 9.00am ward round followed by either ward work or outpatient clinics. However, teaching is very good and students will attend weekly teaching sessions with different members of the healthcare team. Weekly or pre-firm lectures will give you a good idea on what to expect on the wards.

You can only imagine how busy doctors can be, so there may be a lot of waiting around on the wards or in the corridors for scheduled teaching sessions. However, if you decide to be productive and do some revision while waiting, it makes the time go faster and you will be more prepared for the grilling that awaits you by the Consultant.

You will be expected to be keen and actively participate within your team. You may have to present patients on ward rounds, after having performed their histories and examinations, and discuss their management with the Registrar/Consultant or you may be asked to present patient cases at grand rounds. These skills are instilled within us from early on since they are vital towards becoming a competent and confident doctor. There are also plenty of opportunities to contribute to research projects and case studies with the hope of being published in international journals.

Finally, the summative exams take place in the summer, usually consisting of written papers and practical scenarios. Exams are undoubtedly the toughest element of the year but once you reach the end other end, saying that there is an intense feeling of both relief and satisfaction is an utter understatement. What does not kill you may make you stronger, but you only truly appreciate clichés once you live them! The first three summer holidays are around three months long in which you can travel or just relax at home. It gets more hectic towards the end, especially in the 50-week fifth year! However, things are bound to change by the time you enter medical school.'

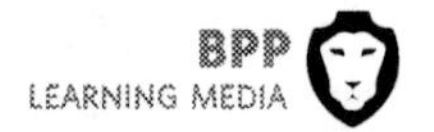

Once you get in...

Once you have met the requirements of your offer be prepared to receive a whole host of paperwork from the university. The confirmation letter is your wake-up call that you will soon be starting medical school, and this means sorting out a range of different things before term begins. Therefore, organisation is important and a folder would be handy to keep all related paperwork in it.

You will receive a pack about accommodation, which will provide information on the different halls of residences available. After reading each description, you will be required to submit a choice of five, in preferential order. You will also receive information on the facilities at Imperial, for instance Ethos, the sports centre, and other important places on the campus. The Registry and the Student Hub are popular places during the first weeks of term. Here, students can sort out problems regarding accommodation, tuition and other financial fees. If you are planning to apply for a student loan, you will need to send off your application to an external organisation ('Student Finance England'). However, Imperial does offer bursaries or grants for students in financial hardship so be careful to read the information pack thoroughly.

The union will send you a booklet on the clubs and societies that are available to join. This will help you filter out the ones which you are interested in, making the freshers' fair day a more meaningful and enjoyable one. The campus map will be invaluable to you during your first few weeks at university. Make sure that you are familiar with it as you will be required to go from the lecture theatre to Occupational Health for your immunisations or to the union for freshers' fair.

Also worth recommending is booking your induction at the gym as soon as possible. Try to get this out of the way so you can use the facilities of the sports centre straight away. Remember that gym subscription is free so naturally there will be a mad rush to book an induction appointment at the earliest date.

Furthermore, the fact that you will be living in London means that travel costs are bound to be expensive. It is definitely worth applying for the student Oyster card, which entitles you to a 30% discount. The lectures in the first and second years are split

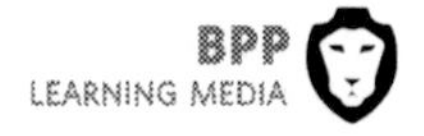

between the South Kensington and Charing Cross (Hammersmith) campuses so will involve travelling on the public transport. The NUS card is also a fantastic way to get discounts at several stores and is certainly worth its annual subscription fee. There really are many advantages of being a student in London!

The Best Thing	Everything is possible at Imperial College! Your imagination is your limitation. You will feel right at home in a friendly multi cultural community
The Worst Thing	It is a demanding course and you will be expected to work hard, especially during summer exams. Also, keep an eye on your money, it can disappear quickly

Student top tips

- Make sure you apply for your Freshers' Fortnight Passport early and attend as many events as possible. You will enjoy meeting and mingling with your classmates and with people from across the years.
- Definitely attend the freshers' fair and sign up to anything that catches your attention. You can always decide not to commit later if your expectations were not met. There will always be free taster sessions, so there is no hurry to pay membership fees until and unless you really want to join a society.
- Get stuck in! Run for committee positions, take up a new hobby and try something different. How else are you going to find out what you are good at?

Summary Table

Positives	Negatives
Good teaching and libraries	Feedback on exams
Huge free gym	Support during exam periods
Inter-year social events and Varsity	Large workload
Extremely good transport access	Lack of parking
Heart of the city	Competitive

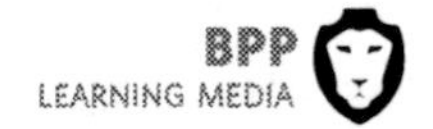

London: King's College London

King's College London School of Medicine
First Floor Hodgkin Building
Guy's Campus
London
SE1 1UL

www.kcl.ac.uk/medicine/index.aspx

Founded in 1550 as St Thomas' medical school, King's College London is now one of the largest medical schools in Europe. To give it's full and somewhat long-winded title; 'King's College London School of Medicine at Guy's, King's and St Thomas' is a medical school based over several world-renowned south/central London hospitals and campuses, offering a traditional course which has a distinct pre-clinical period which boasts excellent anatomy teaching, followed by three years of clinical Medicine in some of the most well known hospitals in the UK.

Famous people associated with what is now King's medical school include the poet Keats who trained as an apothecary, Professor Joseph Lister, the father of the antiseptic technique, and Florence Nightingale who founded the world's first School of Nursing at St Thomas's hospital in 1860.

Located in the heart of London, it is surrounded by all that the nation's capital has to offer; with world famous shops, theatres, nightlife, and art among other things.

If you are interested in a traditional course set in a friendly environment, along with the opportunity to experience one of the most exciting cities in the world, King's College School of Medicine is certainly worth a look.

The medical course

Key facts

Course Type	Traditional	Degree Awarded	MBBS
Basic Entry Requirements	AAA	Entrance Exams	UKCAT
Year Size	Approx 300	Open Days	By request
Admissions Website	www.kcl.ac.uk/medicine/index.aspx		

Getting in – student tips

King's College London looks for students who are able to demonstrate a realistic commitment to Medicine, with a genuine dedication to helping others and an understanding of what a career in Medicine entails. Applicants can demonstrate this through work experience in a clinical setting, voluntary work in caring environments and also through research into the current pathways through which those in the profession pass.

The interviews generally last about 20 minutes and begin with a discussion of an ethical scenario which applicants are given to read about 30 minutes before the interview. Aside from the case discussion, interviewers tend to ask typical questions, for example, why Medicine? Why Kings College? What did you learn during your work experience/voluntary work?

The most important thing to keep in mind when applying is that the medical school are looking for future doctors. It is not so much a university application as it is a job interview for a career in Medicine.

Course details

Foundation / Pre-Med	Yes	Graduate	Yes
Student Population	Male: female ratio: 40:60	Term Length	Pre-clinical: 12 weeks Clinical: 13 weeks
Erasmus / Foreign Exchange	Yes	Elective Period	In between year 4 and 5 – 10 weeks

Intercalation

Stage	After year 2, 3 or 4	Degree Awarded	BSc
Requirements	To have passed years 1 and 2	Subjects	Medical Sciences

Anatomy teaching

Anatomy is taught extensively throughout the first two years of the degree. This is achieved mainly through lectures which are augmented with dissection sessions lasting two hours.

Dissection room sessions consist of small groups of five to eight students dissecting a cadaver under the guidance of trainee-surgeons and academic anatomists. While some medical schools use pre-prepared prosections, King's College allows the students to actively dissect the cadavers, revealing important structures and systems for themselves.

King's is lucky enough to have Dr Alistair Hunter and Professor Susan Standring (editor-in-chief of *Gray's Anatomy*) in charge of pre-clinical anatomy teaching. Both are extremely knowledgeable teachers and gifted lecturers who do their very best to ensure an interactive and enjoyable learning experience.

Pre-clinical/Years 1–2	
Topics	***Year 1:*** Basic human sciences and physiological processes including the cellular basis of medicine are covered in the first term of year 1 ('Phase 1'). There is little clinical teaching as it serves as logical step between A level science and the more clinically relevant teaching of 'Phase 2' which begins after Christmas in the first year and continues until the end of year 2. This is taught through clinical scenarios in which a common clinical case is described, with subsequent lectures covering the relevant anatomy, physiology, biochemistry and pharmacology. There are 36 scenarios in total, 13 of which are taught in year 1. They cover all systems and the common conditions affecting each system. ***Year 2:*** A continuation of year 1, covering scenarios 14-36.

Teaching	Lectures, dissection sessions, small group tutorials, practical sessions, histology/microscopy sessions, GP and hospital visits.
SSC Periods	Students complete 1 SSC in the first year. This is done after the exams and runs over a two-week period. It consists of an essay and poster presentation that is done in a small group. In the second year, students take two SSCs. One is a taught module with classes/practicals, and the other is a library project which is an essay of 6-8,000 words. One day per week is set aside for SSC work in the second year and students complete one SSC in the first term and another in the second term. A wide range of projects are on offer, including scientific literature reviews, foreign language lessons and history of medicine modules.
Exams	***Year 1:*** Numeracy exam in term 1. Mid sessional exam in January. Three end of year exams in May/June. These are MCQs and SBAs. ***Year 2:*** Two mid sessional exams in January, one of which is a statistics exam based on a piece of clinical research. In April there is an ethics exam and a short essay exam. There are four end of year summer exams in May, three of which are MCQs and SBAs. The fourth exam is a 20-station OSCE. All examinations have a 50% pass mark and none are negatively marked.

Clinical/Years 3–5	
Topics	***Year 3:*** Cardiology, Respiratory, Neurology, Ophthalmology, Psychiatry, Renal Medicine, Endocrinology, General Medicine (abdomen), Public Health, Ethics and Law ***Year 4:*** Obstetrics and Gynaecology, Genitourinary Medicine, Paediatrics and Elderly Care, Dermatology, Emergency Medicine, Anaesthetics, Orthopaedics ***Year 5:*** General Medicine, General Surgery and General Practice Throughout the clinical years, there is community health teaching and various ethics and law teaching integrated into the clinical specialities.

SSC Periods	You have to do three SSCs in years 3, 4 and 5. They usually occur one per term unless you do a modern language where in one term you might be doing two SSCs. There is an extensive range of SSCs on offer and also the opportunity to self-design your own SSCs in an interest you want to expand on, a research opportunity or even an audit. Students also have the opportunity to do a SSC in a foreign language which are offered by the Modern Language Centre at King's College. It is very comprehensive and useful for those who have panache for languages.
Exams	All exams are MCQs (true or false), Single Best Answers (SBAs), where one correct answer out of a choice of five is chosen, and Extending Matching Questions (EMQs) – where you have to match each clinical answer to a scenario or a clinical presentation. In the final year there are no MCQs but only SBAs and EMQs. In years 3 and 5, exams are done at the end of the year. However in year 4, there is an exam at the end of each clinical speciality rotation, ie at the end of every term. How difficult the exams are, is a very subjective view – some find them easy and some incredibly hard. It really all depends on how well prepared you are and how good your grasp of clinical Medicine is. Failure rates are usually in the region of around 10%.

Hospital placements/academies

District General Hospital (DGH) placements are really good fun. These are the hospitals that are outside of the city. Usually the accommodation at the DGHs is very good, clean and convenient. However there are some horror stories with some of them (you can find these out when you come to King's).

In any of the three clinical years, you can be sent to a DGH for either a three-week period or for an entire term. Allocation is usually random but in the final year you do have the opportunity to rank your choices and hopefully get allocated the ones you have ranked highly – this does not always happen though. In each placement there are usually around 20-30 students. The well liked ones are King's, Canterbury, Woolwich and Ashford. Getting to the majority of the DGHs can take a bit of time but usually you can share a lift with friends, get coaches or even trains.

Hospitals and Travel Time from University	
Guy's Hospital	2 minutes
St Thomas' Hospital	10 minutes
King's College Hospital	20 minutes
Canterbury	90 minutes

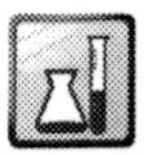

The medical school

Work	Reasonable work life balance
Facilities	24-hour library and IT facilities, restaurant and café, bar, pathology museum, Clinical Skills Centre, medical bookshop, ATM
Support	Support is provided via a tutor and clinical adviser. 'Papa and mama' scheme – older years providing support
Feedback	There is continuous feedback to the medical school. This allows for constant upgrade and improvements

Facilities

There is one main library at the Guy's campus. This library contains many computers and IT suites. During the exam period, it is open for 24 hours. There is also another small 24-hour library on campus too which does not house many books but provides desks, chairs and an IT suite. Students are also able to use any of the libraries at the Waterloo or Strand campus, or even the library at St Thomas' Hospital and King's College Hospital. In addition to this are various computer rooms including one that is open for 24 hours.

The Clinical Skills Centre is one of the largest of its kind in the UK. It provides a huge range of resources for medical students. Students are able to practise their clinical skills on anatomical models.

Student support

In the first two years, each student is provided with a tutor, who is then replaced by a clinical adviser for the clinical years. The Student Medical Council (SMEC) at King's College has also recently started the parent system and are hoping for this to take off. Otherwise if there is a problem students can contact head of the year. SMEC also offer a consular service.

A chaplaincy can be found on Guy's campus too and the chaplain is very friendly and approachable. In addition to this, the university itself has support services through the student union and welfare associations.

In terms of a healthcentre, there is the main one at the Strand where the students can be registered. The centre holds open clinics where you do not need to book appointments. For clinical years, medical students need to be cleared by occupational health which is situated at St Thomas' hospital.

Medical societies

There are many medical societies so highlighting the main ones would be difficult. Most of the main clinical specialties have a society and then there is Medsin, which is the global health society. Societies generally hold lectures and workshops for students so that they can improve their knowledge and additionally show their interest in a particular field. In addition to this, there are opportunities to get involved with committee roles and making decisions on how the societies are run.

Medics' sports again are very successful. There are a large number of teams in every sport and the quality tends to be much higher than King's College itself (probably an overestimate and a biased view).

Medic nights are varied but there is the annual Christmas Show which is always entertaining and also the notorious Fashion Show.

On top of this there is the well known Rag Week which raises thousands of pounds for various charities. During Rag Week there are lots of themed nights making it a very enjoyable, fun and drunken week!

Finance

Further info: www.kcl.ac.uk/funding

Student opinion

'Medical school truly is a wonderful experience. You make some amazing friends, gain an abundance of knowledge, realise what your true drinking limits are and become an expert in sitting MCQ type exams. There is so much to get involved in; catering for students from all backgrounds – sorry about this spiel – but it is so true. You are never bored unless you are a truly boring person!

During the clinical years you are able to experience hospital life and meet more and more new people, which is great fun. There is so much to do that you never realise how fast time passes and are suddenly faced with the prospect of revising for finals. Trust me, this happens to us all!'

The university

Accommodation	Non-campus halls of residence
Further Info	www.kcl.ac.uk/accomm www.kclsu.org/

Accommodation

Most first years live in Great Dover Street apartments, though a fair number of students live in other residences such as Stamford Street apartments and King's College Hall. Great Dover Street apartments are the most popular due to the close proximity to Guy's campus (10-minute walk) and the large number of medical students living there. King's College London has lots of student residences to its name, including intercollegiate halls as well as catered residences such as King's College Hall. These are all further from campus than Great Dover Street and necessitate the use of public transport.

After the first year most students rent properties in South London to stay fairly close to campus. Popular areas include Borough and Bermondsey.

Study facilities

Most medics use the libraries on Guy's campus. New Hunts House is the biggest and most popular, boasting a multi-level library with full IT facilities. It is open until 9.00pm but becomes a 24 hour library during exam periods. There is a 24-hour library in the Hodgkin building at Guy's campus called the Will's Library, though it is smaller and does not have comparable IT facilities. There is also a large library at the Waterloo campus which medics who live nearby tend to use. King's College Hospital in Denmark Hill also has a sizeable library in the Western Education Centre, which is predominantly used by clinical students placed at King's College Hospital and first years living in King's College Halls.

University sports & students' union

There is a small but well-equipped gym on Guy's campus, which costs around £150 for eight months' membership. There is also a pool at Guy's campus and gym membership including use of the pool costs around £160 for eight months.

The Waterloo campus also has a gym, which is larger, costing around £200 per year.

Wednesday afternoons are kept free for sport, and King's is host to a wide range of sports teams. Training for sports such as hockey, cricket, football and rugby takes place at facilities/fields spread over south London, with certain societies such as squash training on campus courts.

King's has two student unions, Boland House on Guy's campus is mainly used by medical and dental students, whereas the Macadam Building on the Strand is frequented by students from other schools within the university. Boland House contains bookable rooms for society meetings as well as Guy's Bar, which is the centre of many social events. Though host to Guy's Bar, the union at Guy's campus is not the social centre for medical students at King's, though many societies do make use of the rooms as well as the bar.

Student opinion

'Living in London has its advantages and disadvantages. Being in one of the most expensive and vibrant cities in the world is a challenge in itself. However this is what makes living in London as a student such a wonderful experience. There are so many things on offer and, even better, most of time it is free for students or offered at a discounted price. These 'things' include theatre shows, festivals, exhibitions and events. The beauty of being at King's is its proximity to all the major attractions of London. Most notable are Borough Market with its wide range of cuisine and coffee and Southbank which hosts some of the more enjoyable moments of London with the British Film Institute and the Royal Festival Hall. Living in London has certainly been an incredible experience but is expensive. However I would still rather pay more and have the luxury of living in one of the finest cities on the planet.'

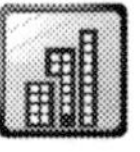

The city

Safety	🛡	🛡	🛡	🛡		Generally safe for students
Nightlife	☾	☾	☾	☾	☾	Excellent; London nightlife is among the best in the world
Transport	🚌	🚌	🚌	🚌		Cars are not recommended for pre-clinical medicine but can be useful for peripheral hospital placements in clinical years. London has excellent transport links with buses, tubes and rail
Cost of Living	🐖	🐖	🐖	🐖	🐖	Expect to pay £400-500 per month for rent. A night out can cost anything between £10 for a student night and £40 for a Friday night. The privilege of London study does come at a cost

Things to do

As the nation's capital, London caters for everybody. It has the well known art of the Tate and National galleries, the theatres of London's famous West End, as well as more bars, pubs and clubs than you could possibly ever visit (even if you intercalate!).

Although London is a big city, the tube and bus systems mean it is easy to get around, and attractions have a tendency to be within walking distance from one another.

In the summer months, you can take a stroll along London's famous Southbank, visit the zoo at Regent's Park, or just relax in one of London's many beautiful parks, Hyde Park being among the most popular.

For shopping, it doesn't get better than London's Oxford Street and Bond Street which together come to roughly a mile of shops interspersed with restaurants and cafés.

The IMAX cinema at Waterloo shows all the top new releases in 3D, and is an experience not to be missed by film lovers.

Places to go		
Place	**Brief Description**	**Entry Fee/Opening Time**
Waterfront Bar	Student bar at Strand campus with beautiful views of city and Thames	£Free, Open all day everyday until 11.30pm.
Tutu's	King's College night-club on the Strand doing student nights on Tuesday and Saturday	£4 Open 10.00pm – 3.00am. Tues, Fri and Sat.
Ministry of Sound	World-renowned club in Elephant and Castle – student night on Tuesday called 'Milkshake'	£5/£20 (depending if student night or not), Open 10.30pm – 5.00am Mon–Sat.
Guy's Bar	Basement student bar on Guy's campus	£Free, open until 11.30pm.

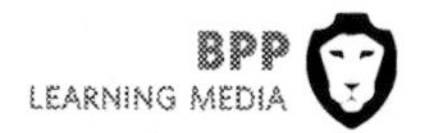

Student opinion

'London is one of the most exciting and cosmopolitan cities in the world. It has a lively student life, a vibrant nightlife, and is world renowned for its history and art. I wouldn't spend my six years as a student anywhere else.'

Student's view

Pre-clinical

'The day begins with a journey to Guy's campus (walkable from Great Dover Street but requires public transport from other residences) along with other students based at Guy's. Lectures usually start the day at 9.00 or 10.00am and take place in the Greenwood lecture theatre infamous for its bright orange walls and capacity for well over 400 students. They typically last an hour, but can vary depending on the amount of information to be covered as well as the lecturer's style. Histology and dissection room sessions also often take place in the morning and last two hours.

At about 1.00pm students have a lunch break lasting about an hour. A lot of students go to nearby cafés and shops around Borough High Street and Borough Market to buy lunch, though many use the on-campus restaurant in Henriette-Raphael House and others bring a packed lunch to enjoy on the grass in the centre of the campus.

Afternoons are normally a mix of lectures, small group tutorials, lab-practicals and dissection, though as I have mentioned, it varies between days, weeks and tutorial groups.

Lectures are for the whole year to attend, but for practicals, tutorials and dissections, students are split into their tutor groups of eight to ten students.

In the second year Tuesdays are free for SSCs, though taught modules often require students to attend classes/practicals on campus. Wednesday afternoons are kept free for sports and society activities.

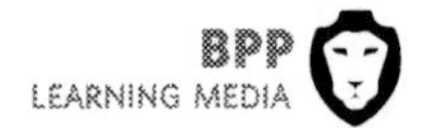

Highlights of my pre-clinical years were the well known KCL medical school Christmas shows and after-parties, which never fail to amaze both the students and medical school staff, packed with their own brand of crude humour, guilty laughs and bare-faced nudity.

Though located in one of the biggest and busiest cities in the world, King's College medical school has a very friendly and relaxed atmosphere.'

Clinical

'Clinical years at medical school are truly remarkable. A typical day includes ward rounds in the morning where they will be some bed-side teaching. After the ward round, coffee break and breakfast, there is organised teaching with either the registrars or junior doctors. If not this, then there is an opportunity to clerk patients and present patients to the senior doctors. Afternoons are spent either in outpatient clinics, clerking patients or organised teaching. Sometimes if luck is on your side then the afternoon is free and a chance to self directed learning or read up on diseases or just going home to "chill".

Teaching in later years tends to be in firms which are usually organised on the wards. It is a time for senior doctors to teach clinical skills, history taking and use patients for case-based scenario teaching.

The major plus point of clinical teaching is the wide range of exposure you get. In addition to this is the chance to meet new people who you never knew existed in your year (if you have a large year group). This makes it very exciting and enjoyable.

Clinical years allow you to put all the knowledge you have learnt into practice and get involved with everything and anything on the ward especially if you are at a good teaching hospital. It allows you to get involved with clinical procedures and diagnoses and also the chance to get scrubbed up in theatres – definitely the highlight of clinical years.'

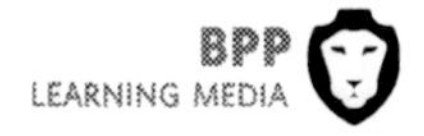

Once you get in...

Along with your offer of a place, you should expect to receive a pack containing several pieces of important information. Details regarding accommodation come in the form of a booklet, and students are required to submit their accommodation choices in order of preference through an online application form.

You will also receive occupational health forms, informing you of the specific health clearances and vaccinations required before starting the course in September.

Information regarding freshers' week such as timetables and fair information is obtainable online.

Information about sports teams and societies is available at the freshers' fair and many sports teams and societies have their own websites.

The Best Thing	Three of the best and most famous teaching hospitals in the world
The Worst Thing	Large class sizes

Student top tips

- Sort out your student Oyster card early on!
- Go to Borough Market for lunch after lectures on Fridays.
- Venture out and experience London and all its student deals – don't just stay south of the river.
- Join a sports team, even if just for fun, it's a great way to make lots of friends.
- Work hard, but also play hard. Well-rounded individuals will progress well in a medical environment.

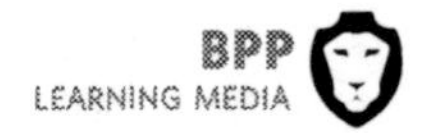

Summary Table

Positives	Negatives
Great location close to the centre of London	London living can be expensive unless you are careful with your money
Enthusiastic teaching from experienced staff	Large year group means difficulties getting to know everybody
World-renowned teaching hospitals	Distance of some residences from campus
Lots of research, publication, and BSc opportunities.	Little clinical exposure and teaching in first two years
Wide range of sports teams, societies and social events	Exam feedback can be vague

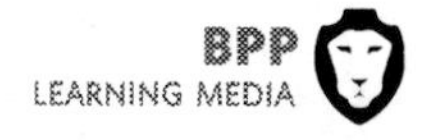

London: University College London

UCL Medical School
University College London
Gower Street
London
WC1E 6BT

www.ucl.ac.uk/medicalschool

UCL Medical School is a vibrant medical school in the centre of London. UCL is committed both to excellence in education and research, indeed UCL has recently come fourth in *The Times* Higher Education league table of world universities (behind only Harvard, Cambridge and Yale). It is one of the largest in the country and has the widest range of intercalated BSc courses of all UK medical schools. Clinical training is based at three main sites in central and north London, University College Hospital near Warren Street, the Royal Free Hospital in Hampstead and the Whittington Hospital in Archway.

The medical course

Key facts

Course Type	Traditional 6 years including an intercalated BSc year	Degree Awarded	BSc, MBBS
Basic Entry Requirements	AAA	Entrance Exams	BMAT
Year Size	330	Open Days	April – see medical school website for further details
Admissions Website	www.ucl.ac.uk/medicalschool/mbbs-admissions/entry-requirements/		

Getting in – student tips

There is no simple relationship between academic performance and making a good doctor. However evidence exists that those with low grades and those who need to resit modules and examinations are more likely to have academic problems. GCSEs are used as a general indicator of the candidate's academic background.

Strong determinants include previous experience (both personal and through work experience/volunteering) in healthcare/laboratory work. Or if the candidate has been involved among the sick, disabled, very young/elderly, being able to reflect on their experiences. Demonstration of motivation to study Medicine and an appropriate attitude is essential. Strong determinants include previous experience (both personal and through work experience/volunteering) in healthcare/laboratory work.

Course details

Foundation / Pre-Med	No	Graduate	Yes
Student Population	Male: female ratio: 40:60	Term Length	Pre-clinical: 12 weeks Clinical: Variable
Erasmus / Foreign Exchange	UCL Medical School has an Erasmus exchange agreement with: La Salpetriere, Paris, France. The agreement allows one student per academic session to join either year 3 or year 4 of the MBBS degree programme	Elective Period	Year 5 – 8 weeks

Intercalation

Stage	Post pre-clinical years (ie years 2, 3, 4)	**Degree Awarded**	BSc
Requirements	Compulsory	**Subjects**	Anatomy and Developmental Biology, Biochemistry and Molecular Biology, Clinical Sciences, History of Medicine, Human Genetics/Genetics, Immunology and Cell Pathology, Infection, International Health, Medical Anthropology, Medical Physics and Bioengineering, Molecular Medicine, Neuroscience, Orthopaedic Science, Pharmacology, Physiology, Physiology and Pharmacology, Philosophy, Medicine and Society, Primary Health Care, Psychology, Speech Science and Communication, Surgical Sciences

Anatomy teaching

Anatomy is taught with lectures and in the dissection laboratory with traditional robust dissections, prosections and modern imaging. This occurs all in the pre-clinical years. The quality of the anatomy teaching is superb with close supervision by helpful teaching staff.

Pre-clinical/Years 1–2	
Topics	***Year 1:*** Foundations of Health and Disease, Infection and Defence, Circulation and Breathing, Fluids, Nutrition and Metabolism. ***Year 2:*** Movement and Musculo-skeletal Biology, Neuroscience and Behaviour, Endocrine Systems Regulation, Reproduction, Genetics and Development, Cancer Biology.
Teaching	Lecture based. Coupled to small group tutorials and extensive laboratory work as assessed through continuous assessments and essays.
SSC Periods	Two are required per year to broaden a student's educational experience. These include a science SSC for in-depth study of a chosen topic in the sciences; a non-science SSC, for example, short courses in modern languages, art, ethics and law; research skills; community voluntary activities, peer mentoring and tutoring.
Exams	Formative assessments at the end of each module and summative end of year exams. Failure rates are variable though most students progress through each year.

Clinical/Years 3–5	
Topics	***Year 3:*** General Medicine General Medical Specialites, Surgery and Anaesthetics, Care of the Older Person, Trauma and Orthopaedics with Rheumatology. Also included in the third year curriculum is a two-week SSC block during which either a clinical subject or a language can be studied. ***Year 4:*** Child and Family Health with Dermatology, Women's health and Communicable Diseases, Psychiatry, Neurology and Opthalmology. ***Year 5:*** Preparation for Practice; Medicine and Surgery, Accident and Emergency, General Practice, Oncology, eight week Elective period, Student Selected Component.
SSC Periods	Two Student Selected Components, each four weeks in the length in final year. There are many on offer and it is possible to arrange to be involved in research and audits. It is possible to arrange an SSC in a topic of the students' choice, following discussion with the medical school. A limited number of students are able to undertake their SSC abroad.

Exams	There are assessments mid way through the third year and at the end of the year. There are assessments at the end of each module in the fourth year and final summative exams at the end of the fifth year. Once again the failure rate is variable and there are opportunities to resit. In addition there are in-course assessments in clinical Medicine that are undertaken in hospital and written a projects such as reflective practice. These are required to progress through the course.
Elective Period	Students can travel to almost anywhere in the world, with restrictions dependant on current political situations. There are a large number of prizes available and students travelling long-haul are entitled to a small amount of funding to help with the cost. A project must be written and this a compulsory part of the final year assessment.

Hospital placements/academies

During third year all placements are at one of the three main sites listed above.

In fourth year students also get sent to centres of excellence eg The National Hospital for Neurology and Neuroscience.

In fourth and fifth year all students will spend some time at District General Hospitals and be expected to live on-site. These are all within approximately an hour of London and include hospitals such as Basildon General Hospital, The Lister in Stevenage, Luton Hospital amongst others.

Hospitals and Travel Time from University	
University College Hospital	5 minutes
Royal Free Hospital	20–30 minutes
Whittington Hospital	20–30 minutes

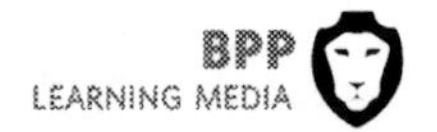

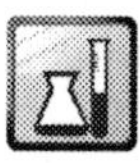

The medical school

Work	🞤	🞤	🞤			Well balanced though exams can be tough
Facilities	☕	☕	☕	☕	☕	Excellent library and computer services available
Support	👥	👥	👥			Walk-in welfare services are available on a daily basis
Feedback	📋	📋	📋	📋		Examination results are communicated via email. In course hospital assessments are more individual and provide the possibility for individual feedback and constructive criticism

Facilities

Dissection laboratory, many excellent libraries, clinical skills centres at all sites. There are multiple computer rooms and student union buildings, which act as common areas.

Student support

This has dramatically improved in recent years. Faculty tutors are assigned to the pre-clinical/clinical years and are contactable during normal hours. A medical chaplaincy service does exist at the medical school as well as those at each hospital. Numerous systems exist to catch students struggling due to the workload, external factors or for those who simply need a chat.

Medical societies

There is a huge range of sports and societies available. Students can choose to represent either the medical school or the main university teams.

Finance

Further info: www.ucl.ac.uk/current-students/money/2012_2013_fees

See scholarships: www.ucl.ac.uk/current-students/money/scholarships/scholarships

Student opinion

'UCL Medical School is an incredible place to study Medicine, bringing with it all the advantages of a world-class institute along with everything that London has to offer. Students are not lost in the big city but also belong to the community of the medical school and university, along with its social areas, sports and societies and bars and restaurants. The social life offers something for everybody from every walk of life.'

The university

Accommodation	Halls of residence are available: www.ucl.ac.uk/prospective-students/accommodation/residences/halls-of-residence
Further Info	www.ucl.ac.uk/ucl-union/

Accommodation

There are many halls of residence in central London (walking distance from the medical school) and some in Camden, north London (a short bus or tube ride away). They are of a good standard and are competitively priced. After the first year most students live in privately rented flats in central London or north London. Many graduates do not live in halls in the first year and do not find that this hinders the social aspect of the course.

Study facilities

There is a medical library as well as many other UCL libraries that the students can use. IT facilities are available in all libraries and hospitals have study areas and IT suites for students to use.

University sports & students' union

There is a main UCL student union with bars and restaurants which medical students use. There is also the University of London Union

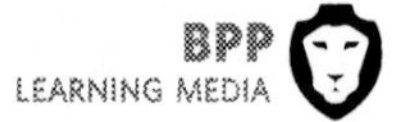

with more restaurants, bars and a gym and swimming pool, which medical students have access to. In addition there are the medical school bars on Huntley Street, at the Royal Free Hospital and all the sites have student common rooms and cafes.

University of London Union has a gym, which is competitively priced, and there is also a swimming pool. Most of the sports and societies have a small joining fee and then students have access to training areas and equipment.

Student opinion

'There is a tremendous amount for you to do and see and participate in around UCL Medical School. Medical school has been a ridiculous experience encompassing some tremendous highs and some rollercoaster lows. No matter your background and experience, Medicine has a habit of flattening the playing field where all things are equal on entry. One startling fact is how the often perceived immaturity of first year medical students transforms into efficient professionalism, not just in Medicine but in life by the time finals examinations approaches. My experience is more expansive than most, courtesy of me being a previous RUMS Pre-clinical President, RUMS Clinical President, ULU Medical Students Officer and editor of The Bell Magazine, collecting every student award in the process. My point is that you can do anything and do almost everything in medical school.'

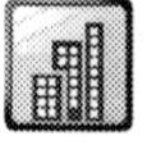

The city

Safety	🛡	🛡	🛡	🛡		Good transport links between most of the social areas and the halls of residence make UCL a safe university to attend, although being a large city, London has its dangers like any other
Nightlife	☾	☾	☾	☾	☾	Unmatched – the capital city has everything on offer!

Transport	🚌	🚌	🚌	🚌	🚌	Excellent transport links. Having a car would be of no benefit due to parking restrictions and the congestion charge
Cost of Living	🐷	🐷	🐷	🐷	🐷	Rent – between £100 and 150/week. Transport – £60/month Pint of beer – £3.10 – £3.60

Things to do

London is one of the world's greatest cities and boasts a host of things to see and do from bars and restaurants, to museums and parks. There really is fun to be had every day and night. Students from UCL tend to congregate around the university where there are cheap pubs. Another area that is densely populated by UCL medical students is Camden, which is full of bars and restaurants and has a world famous market. It has some of the liveliest nightlife in the city. As you get to know the city you begin to spread your wings and venture far and wide. The city is not geared up for students in the way that some smaller university towns are, but there are students' nights across London offering reasonably priced fun.

Places to Go		
Place	**Brief Description**	**Entry Fee/Opening Time**
The Roxy	One of the many haunts of medical students on a Wednesday night. This is a small club just off Tottenham Court Road. There are just too many other places to mention.	£3 on a Wednesday night
Clubs	Oxford Street and surround areas abound	£5-25. Open 10.00pm-4.00am
Museums	The list is monumental but something for everyone	£0-15
Concert Halls	Some of the world's best are featured in London	£4-250

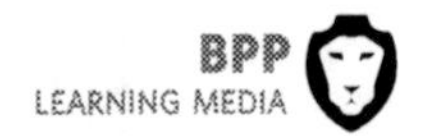

Student opinion

'The old maxim, study hard, play harder is apt to medical school life here at UCL. The beautiful thing about studying in London is the connectivity to the other four London medical schools and the opportunity to gain a greater understanding into their own culture as demonstrated through our sports teams competing vigorously against each other and through our Rag Weeks.'

Student's view

Pre-clinical

'The first two years are intense and you learn quickly to work hard and play hard. The typical day in pre-clinical years starts at 9.00am and finishes around 5.00pm, with gaps in between. This is when you really make your friends over a coffee and lunch at the medical school bar or in one of the many cafés nearby. I chose to study at UCL because of its reputation as a world-class university and also because of its location.

If you like London UCL really is the place to study. I got involved with playing rugby from the first year and made many friends through that, friends that I believe I will stay in touch with for life. Exam periods were stressful but ultimately rewarding and you really do feel yourself progressing. The exams are based on a number of formats with both practical and 'written' papers. In reality the written papers are mainly based on a number of formats of multiple-choice questions. If I were to give any advice to a new first year student at UCL Medical School I would tell them to throw themselves into both the work and social life. You definitely get out what you put in.'

Clinical

'Your life and experience of university changes totally when you begin Clinics at UCL. You start off in small groups attached to a clinical team and are taught by that team while you are with them. Late nights mid-week are harder to manage but when you are not at the hospital or in teaching you have all that London has to offer

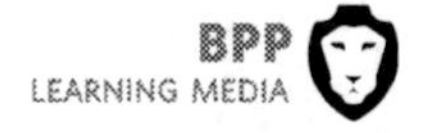

at your fingertips. Before each module you are taught in a lecture theatre for a week on the pathology and basics of the module you are about to enter. Following that week it is straight onto the wards to learn from the experts. Students are given the chance to present cases and be supervised while examining patients.

Feedback is given throughout and I feel that this facilitates learning and guides you on areas that you need to read up on. Again the exams are in two formats with practical and written papers The exams are tough but they teach you to work under a bit of pressure and I have felt that they are fair. My personal highlight was my elective period. The medical school was very supportive in helping me to organise going to America for this time. My advice to someone starting in the clinical years would be to turn up on the wards as often as possible because it really is there that you learn Medicine rather than in your room with a book.'

Postgraduate

'UCL is an excellent medical school to attend as a graduate. Being a traditional five-year long course the material is covered at the typical pace through conventional didactic teaching, and although small group tutorials do occur, it does not follow the problem-based learning system that many graduate entry programmes offer.

I found the mix of undergraduate and graduate students interesting, as graduates are fully encompassed into the main teaching programme and welcome at all of the social events so it does not feel at all segregated. Being a traditional course, there are also long holidays giving the opportunity to travel or earn money, which may be particularly desirable to a graduate. I feel that UCL suits younger graduates who are keen to get involved in the university and everything it has to offer.'

Once you get in…

The medical school send you the crucial lists to enable you to get to the first inaugural lecture where you will be reminded that you are, irrespective whether you are a school leaver or not, the top two per cent of all schools leavers anyway, and the first person you sit next to you may never speak to again throughout medical school as the year is that big. The first week flies by so do not take anything too seriously, but be as open minded as you can be and meet and greet anyone. One interesting thing is that any student representative who does a lecture announcement always gets a round of applause in the first week. This, of course, transforms into boos and hisses by the end of the term, depending on the announcement. Never, and people say 'never say never' but I tell you, never buy a book in the first couple weeks. Get them from the library. The only exception is D&P anatomy books, which you must purchase. The entire lists of things to do and sign up to is long but remember to read everything before you sign.

The Best Thing	Huntley Street, the medical school bar
The Worst Thing	Price of living (and drinking) in London

Student top tips

Jeremy Bentham's embalmed body is on display in the main UCL quad building!

Summary Table

Positives	**Negatives**
Excellent teaching	Cost!
First class hospitals	UCL can be an impersonal place
Good facilities	World renowned centres often forget students exist
Living and socialising in central London	It would be nice once in a while to have much smaller group tutorial teaching in the pre-clinical years

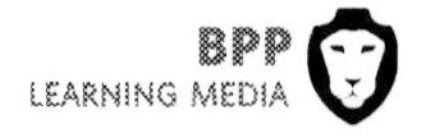

London: St George's

St. George's University of London
Cranmer Terrace
London
SW17 0RE

www.sgul.ac.uk/

Being part of the University of London and boasting such great names as Edward Jenner and John Hunter as part of its alumni, St George's Hospital is a name rich in heritage.

In 1733, St George's Hospital first opened its doors in Lanesborough House at Hyde Park Corner, and has been training medical students ever since.

Now residing in the suburb of Tooting, St George's still has all the enjoyment and excitement that London has to offer, as well as a friendly student atmosphere. The medical school offers a well-balanced course with particular emphasis on clinical and communication skills early on.

St George's offers an exciting, experience-centred course with a supportive student atmosphere in the stunning backdrop setting of the nation's capital.

The medical course

Key facts

Course Type	Integrated	**Degree Awarded**	MBBS
Basic Entry Requirements	AAA	**Entrance Exams**	UKCAT GAMSAT
Year Size	150	**Open Days**	Last Wednesday afternoon of every month except August
Admissions Website	www.sgul.ac.uk/undergraduate/		

Getting in – student tips

St George's looks for a personal statement demonstrating a genuine interest in Medicine, a compassion and commitment to helping others, a wide range of personal interests, examples of extra-curricular achievement, and at least one to two weeks of patient-related work experience (either directly with patients, or people in need of care).

All students will be interviewed for a place at St George's. St George's uses Multi Mini Interviews (MMI), which consists of a series of small interviews and simple tasks.

Questions asked at interview revolve around your interest in Medicine, your ability to work in a team, work experience, empathy, extra-curricular skills and interests, your ability to make decisions, as well as what you would bring to St George's. 'What role do other professionals play in a clinical setting?', 'Why do you want to study Medicine?', 'Why St George's?', as well as any questions on trips/expeditions.

St George's offers no preference between people who have or have not had gap years, although gap years do offer invaluable time to widen your extra-curricular interests, travel and gain work experience, which can give you the edge in your personal statement and more to talk about in your interview.

Course details

Foundation / Pre-Med	No	**Graduate**	Yes
Student Population	Male: female ratio: 40:60	**Term Length**	Pre-clinical: 12 weeks Clinical: 15 weeks
Erasmus / Foreign Exchange	Exchange with Flanders in Australia for one term in year 2	**Elective Period**	Mini Elective in year 2 – year 3 Elective in final year – 10 weeks

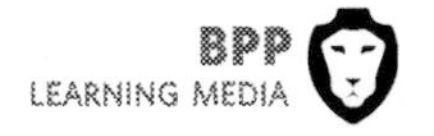

Intercalation

Stage	Year 2 to 3 and year 3 to 4	Degree Awarded	BSc in Basic Medical Sciences
Requirements	All that is generally required is to have passed years 1 and 2 of the medicine course	Subjects	The intercalated BSc year at St George's shares its modules with the final year of the Biomedical Sciences course. There are a wide variety of modules on offer including anatomy and physiology; psychology and neurosciences; genetics and cancer biology

Anatomy teaching

Anatomy is taught in the Dissection Room, in the basement floor of Jenner Wing in the Hospital. Anatomy sessions are once a week in the first and second year, usually lasting about one and half hours and are taught in groups of five to eight around a prosected cadaver, following instructions given before the session, with the assistance of an anatomist supervisor.

Pre-clinical/Years 1–2	
Topics	***Year 1:*** Inter-professional Foundation Programme (IFP, Semester 1): Principles of Pharmacology, Introduction to Human Biology, Physiology and Anatomy, Introduction to Cellular and Molecular Biology and the Biology of Systems. (Semester 2): Musculoskeletal, Cardiovascular, and Respiratory System, Epidemiology and Evidence Based Practice, Sociology. ***Year 2:*** (Semester 3): Dermatology, Human Molecular Biology, Genetics, Skeletal System, and Neurology. (Semester 3): Endocrine & Reproductive System, Child Development and Aging, Immunology and Cancer, Further Sociology, Epidemiology and Evidence Based Practice and Pharmacology. Throughout both pre-clinical years clinical skills, anatomy and communication skills are taught throughout (usually on a weekly session basis).

Teaching	Lectures, small group tutorials, GP visits, two-week clinical attachment, on-line study resources (moodle).
SSC Periods	During the first year, there is one, short formative SSC essay, with a small choice of subject areas. On completing the first year, you are given a choice for your two SSC projects in the second year (one for each semester). During the second year, afternoons are set aside each week in order for you to work on your project. There is a wide choice of subjects on offer for the second year, examples include: Hypnosis and Medicine, Alcohol and Sexual Health and History of Medicine. Assessment is carried out by your SSC tutor and an outside marker, and varies depending on the type of project chosen. If the work is promising, there is a good chance of an opportunity to get it published.
Exams	One set of exams each Semester, four in total in pre-clinical years: three-hour written paper (Single Best Answers, Multiple Choice Questions (negatively marked) and Short Answer Questions), Observed Structured Practical Examination (OSPE, 1 hour 20 min anatomy examination, Single Best Answer), Observed Structured Clinical Examination (OSCE, 1 hour clinical skills exam). Pass mark for written ~50%.

Clinical/Years 3–5	
Topics	***Year 3***: Firms include Junior medicine and surgery; Specialties (ENT, Opthalmology, Dermatology); Rheumatology and Orthopaedics. Systematic teaching covers Respiratory Medicine, Renal Medicine; Musculoskeletal Medicine; Alimentary; Pharmacology and Endocrinology. ***Year 4***: Fourth year firms cover Obstetrics and Gynaecology; Paediatrics; Neurology and Psychiatry; Care of the Elderly; Cardiology; General Practice; Senior Medicine and surgery; Investigations of Disease. ***Year 5***: Assistant House Officer posts in Medicine and Surgery; A General Practice placement; Anaesthetics and Emergency Medicine; Public Health and an Interprofessional practice placement.

SSC Periods	There are two SSC periods in the third and fourth year, each five weeks in length. There is a handbook listing a broad choice of SSCs for the third year SSC programme. These include library projects; clinical skills teaching; mini lab research projects and the opportunity to do audit work.
Exams	There are written exams at the end of the third year and the written final exams at the end of the fourth year. Somewhat confusingly both these written exams also include an OSCE (practical clinical) component which also has to be passed. Written papers consist mainly of Single Best Answer and Extended Matching Item questions with a few Short Answer Questions to cover ethics and statistics. Speaking from recent experience the written final exams are difficult but do-able – if you put the work in. Relatively few people (around 10%) fail the written final exams, though this varies from year to year.
Elective period	Electives take place in the final year following the final exams. The choice of where you go on elective is entirely up to you – as long as it involves a moderate amount of Medicine! Currently the elective period is ten weeks long and six of these are to be spent on a placement somewhere in the world, giving you plenty of extra time for travelling. Registry keeps a list of previous host institutions if you are in need of some inspiration.

Hospital placements/academies

St George's Hospital is one of the biggest hospitals in Europe and has a rich history going back over 250 years with many famous alumni, including Henry Gray (of the anatomy textbook fame not from the TV series!); Edward Jenner (discover of the smallpox vaccine) and John Hunter (the father of modern surgery). The hospital attracts a varied clientele from a range of social backgrounds and is a tertiary referral centre for many specialties ensuring a great number of interesting cases.

Generally, placements are five weeks' long, with the exception of the obstetrics and gynaecology, paediatrics and assistant house office placements which are all six weeks' long. Most of the time there will be no more than three students attached to a particular firm which means you get plenty of opportunity to see patients and get involved with the workings of the junior staff. The majority of consultants are more than willing to give plenty of teaching – as long as you get your face seen. Placements at George's can be very busy so you sometimes find Consultants more willing to teach at hospitals further afield.

Accommodation is somewhat variable in its quality and availability. Nearly all of the third year placements take place in hospitals, which don't require accommodation and are within a commutable distance. One of the third year specialties attachments is out at Guildford, which is a bit of a trek, but there is the bonus of getting free lunches every day for five weeks!

Hospitals and Travel Time from University	
St George's Hospital	0 minutes
St Helier Hospital	1 minute
Kingston Hospital	15 minutes
Mayday Hospital, Croydon	20 minutes
Tolworth Hospital	20 minutes
St Peter's Hospital Chertsey	25 minutes
Frimley Park Hospital	40 minutes
Redhill and Crawley Hospitals	30 minutes
Springfield University Hospital	5 minutes

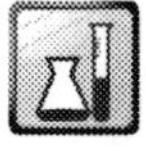

The medical school

Facilities						St George's has undergone massive investment over the years and now can boast facilities to be proud of. Almost all of the medical school and students' union have undergone multi-million pound refurbishment
Support						The family system is still really strong and there is also good support on offer from the personal tutor system and the students' union

Feedback	🩺	🩺	🩺			Exam and coursework feedback has improved but could still be better

Facilities

The medical school library stocks pretty much every book that you could ever need to get you through the course. There are plenty of copies of all the major textbooks. There are three well-stocked computer rooms but getting a computer around hand-in time for SSCs can be a challenge. Most people now have their own laptops and there is a wireless network, which can be accessed throughout the medical school. One of the computer rooms is open overnight to provide 24-hour study space.

There has been major investment in the clinical skills department. There are plenty of skills labs including a self-directed learning room with all of the necessary models and other equipment for honing your practical skills.

St George's still boasts the only bookshop in Tooting which is always competitive in its pricing. The school shop stocks everything from sandwiches to stationery and is run by a lovely bunch of ladies who are always willing to offer a hug around exam time! There are plenty of other places to get food including the students' union café – Eddie Wilson's (named after the doctor on Captain Scott's ill-fated expedition to the Antarctic and who is another George's alumni).

Student support

Student support at St George's is very good. Our relatively small size leads to an excellent sense of community. The family system ensures that you have a social network from day one and there are notes and other wisdom passed down from generation to generation! Every student has a personal tutor who you tend to see once a term for the first couple of years and then as needed from the third year onwards. There is also a multi-faith chaplaincy service available as well as an excellent team of counsellors. The students' union also has a sabbatical officer in charge of student education and welfare and they are always on hand to give advice and support. He or she is the first port of call if you ever have an issue. The students' union is also affiliated to London Nightline, which provides a listening service out of hours.

There is a hospital staff and student occupational health department. Students are encouraged to register with a local GP and there are plenty to choose from in the Tooting area.

Medical societies

There are loads of different societies and sports clubs at St. George's. If there's anything that's not available you can always start up your own or head up to ULU!

A quick glance at the students' union website will give you an insight into the abundance of societies that George's has to offer. The Revue society performs at the Edinburgh Fringe Festival every year and there is also an active Play society and Musical society.

Sports on offer range from rugby to rowing and include our newest sports club – Ultimate Frisbee! Sports teams compete in United Hospitals events with other medical schools from within the University of London, as well as on a national scale in BUCS and NAMS (National Association of Medical Schools) tournaments. George's teams consistently punch above our weight on a local and national level, with the netball and hockey teams being particularly strong.

Finance

Further info: www.sgul.ac.uk/studying-at-st-georges/student-finance/

See scholarships : www.sgul.ac.uk/studying-at-st-georges/student-finance/undergraduate-students-2012/grants-and-bursaries

Student opinion

'I can honestly say that I have loved the five years I have spent at St George's. The small size of our medical school benefits us as students in many ways. For a start our firms tend to be smaller than those at other larger medical schools so the clinical teaching is great. St George's is an incredibly friendly place to study and it is hard to imagine anywhere where it is so easy to get involved with so many aspects of student life. You get out what you put in and I would encourage people to take full advantage of the opportunities that being a student gives you wherever you end up.'

The university

Accommodation	Non-campus halls of residence
Further Info	www.sgul.ac.uk/studying-at-st-georges/accommodation/accommodation

Accommodation

Most first year students at St George's live in halls of residence at Horton Halls, a brief 15–20 minute walk from the university. Built in 2007, each room in these new halls has an en-suite and internet access, with four to six rooms in a flat, sharing one kitchen/living space. Blocks A to E have its own common room with TV and seating area. Horton Halls also has 24-hour security and on-site laundry facilities.

Most upper years choose to rent around Tooting near to the university.

Study facilities

The St George's University Library can be found on the first floor of Hunter Wing. Re-developed over 2009, the library offers a wide selection of medical textbooks and journals for reference, as well as areas just outside for discussion and socialising.

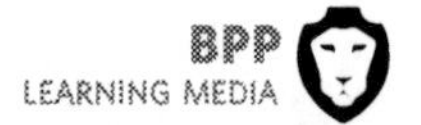

University sports & students' union

St George's student union can be found on the second floor of Hunter Wing of the medical school. In many respects it can be regarded as the heart of St George's. Recently re-developed, the SU bar usually hosts St George's events and discos. During the day, it also offers a place to relax, socialise, and play table tennis and pool.

On-site at the university is the Rob-Lowe Sports Centre. Annual membership cost £40 for students and while being small, it offers a good selection of equipment and workout classes. There is also a sports hall and four squash courts that can be reserved. St George's also has a wide selection of sports teams, the more popular being rugby, hockey, netball, football and rowing.

> **Student opinion**
>
> *'Being in Horton Halls when they were newly built in my first year could only be described as a joy. Not only did you have the luxury of an en-suite room, but you were never more than a couple of doors away from new friends, in the comfortable setting of a greener area of Tooting!'*

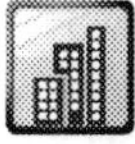

The city

Safety						Tooting is relatively safe and is certainly lively into the small wee hours of the morning
Nightlife						Central London, Wimbledon, Clapham are all close by. Plenty of curry houses in Tooting offering food from all corners of the Indian subcontinent. Some lively, trendy pubs

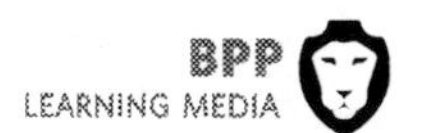

Transport						(Tooting, Earlsfield) are 5–10 minutes away by bus. Plenty of bus routes going to Tooting Broadway. Bike racks requiring security access available on campus
Cost of Living						London taxis are not so abundant here. Minicabs are available at reasonable process; confirm a price before travelling! Standard beer/lager: £2.75–£3.50

Things to do

There is a huge variety of curry houses in Tooting offering some of the best and cheapest Indian (south or north), Sri Lankan, Tamil, etc food you will find anywhere in London. Two different covered markets are open daily for fresh produce, cooked food, and all sorts of weird and wonderful things. Other large stores in Tooting include Sainbury's, Primark, TK Max, Boots; most of the major high street banks are represented.

Lively pubs in the area generally have a discounts for St George's students.

London is right on your doorstep. In just 20 minutes you can be in Oxford Circus.

The medical school sport centre does not have a swimming pool. Fortunately, Tooting Leisure Centre is right next-door and the famous Tooting Bec lido, the UK's largest open air swimming pool, is a short distance away. Wimbledon is just around the corner, within easy walking distance to get those valuable tickets to watch the championship in June.

Places to Go	
Place	**Brief Description**
London Clubs	Take your pick from the whole of London!
London Theatres	The West End

Student opinion

'Throughout the course I have lived about 10 minutes' walk from St George's. Rent is certainly affordable in this part of London and it is easy to find a large house to share with three or four students. Often, student houses get passed down from year to year to new students and many St George's students live in the area so it is easy to meet up in one of the local pubs after class.

I have joined many of the clubs and societies at SGUL. These organise evening events or weekends away so I have definitely kept myself busy. There are also plenty of opportunities for competitive or recreational sports and Tooting Bec Common, Wandsworth Common and Wimbledon Common are all popular local places to got for a run or cycle. With central London on the doorstep, there is always something exciting to do. I often hop on the Northern Line and take advantage of Student Standby tickets at the London theatres or concert venues. Being in London also means that I have been able to take advantage of the library, facilities and events (free drinks reception) at the royal Society of Medicine. I have been very lucky to avoid the hustle and bustle of central London but have access to it while living in the cheaper and vibrant outskirts.'

Student's view

Pre-clinical

'In the first year at St George's, a lot of emphasis is put onto introducing the different areas of Medicine first, including new topics such as pharmacology, sociology, epidemiology, clinical and communicating skills. Work-life balance at the university is usually very easy, with Wednesday afternoons being reserved for sport activities, even until the clinical years!

A typical day usually starts with lectures at around 9.30am. It takes about 20 minutes at a leisurely pace to get to the university from halls, so leave around 9.00am. The day usually lasts until about 4.00pm, at the latest (rarely) 5.30pm. Anatomy, Clinical and/or communication skills are usually on a Tuesday, with case base learning groups (CBL) on a Thursday morning.

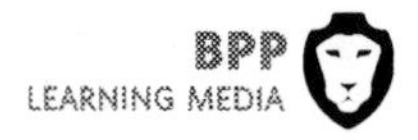

Lectures last about 45 minutes, with 15-minute breaks between them. Lunch can last anywhere from two and half hours to 30 minutes, but almost always last more than an hour. Food can be bought either from the Eddie Wilson's café on the second floor of Hunter Wing, M & S Simply food on ground floor, or the school shop and Peabody's.

In the second year, Monday afternoons are set aside to allow you to work on your SSC project.

For exams, I have found that generally, as long as you study what is in the lectures and sessions, they pose little difficultly. Even being a committed member of the St George's Hospital Boat Club, I have found easily enough spare time to stay on top of my work as well as having time to train and socialise when the time calls! What St George's gives is not a course to teach you to be a doctor, but the opportunity to learn to become one, as well as the chance to learn more about yourself as a person, in what I can only describe as an atmosphere so friendly, it's close to family.

Personal highlights for me in my pre-clinical years include: freshers' fortnight (all of it!), The Boat Club 'Cheesetastic' Tour to Cardiff, The RAG (raising and giving) Ball at the Barbican, The Summer Ball at Cobham, as well as countless fancy-dress themed discos in the SU bar!'

Clinical

'A typical day might involve heading in for an early morning tutorial, followed by a morning sitting in clinic. After lunch there may be another tutorial, and then clerking a patient for the next morning's ward round, before heading down to Chiswick or the gym for some rowing training.

I've spent the majority of my time in the third and fourth year on clinical placements. There is one morning each week given over to lectures in the third year. In the fourth year the year is divided into three separate groups, which rotate through the different terms' placements and lectures. Many of the lecturers for the later years are also your Consultants and are always very approachable.

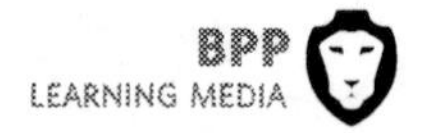

I really like the close-knit community that exists within George's. Another benefit of our relatively small institution is the small firms, which go with it, and excellent teaching this brings. Unfortunately the George's grapevine is still going strong so everyone knows everyone else's gossip!

Regarding exams, it was initially quite a shock to go from having exams each semester back to having them just once a year. They were definitely a step up in terms of difficulty, purely from the point of view of the massive quantity of information you are required to retain. The OSCEs become trickier too, with much more thinking on your feet required!

There have been many highlights over the past five years, in terms of my Medicine course; the first time I got to suture for real was pretty cool. Outside of medicine, reaching the BUSA rowing final was awesome, as was the feeling when we raised over £60,000 for charity in my year as RAG officer.

Make sure you go in and make the most of your clinical placements, five weeks is precious little time to learn the ins and outs of each specialty. Take advantage of any teaching that anyone offers you – it is always useful and you will thank yourself come exam time!'

Postgraduate

'Teaching in the first two years of the course is by PBL (problem based learning). I was surprised how structured this was! I had thought that it was pretty much teaching yourself, however, while this is somewhat true (you have fewer lectures and the onus is on you to do the reading) we were quite carefully guided to what to go away and study. During these two years there are many opportunities to gain clinical experience: regular visits to community care centres. I found this was good preparation for my first clinical year (year 3), which I am just about to finish.

At the start of my third year, I had a 12-week placement at a local hospital during which time I spent eight weeks attached to a general medicine firm and four weeks attached to a surgical firm. Much of this time was spent on ward rounds, helping in the wards (phlebotomy, inserting cannulae /catheters etc) clerking and presenting patients in A&E as well as attending numerous clinics.

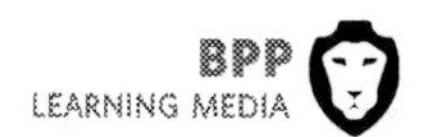

This is the advantage of the graduate course: you can decide for yourself what you want to do or not do. If you want the experience you are encouraged to go for it yourself.

After this, I had three-week mini-elective. I could choose to do whatever I wanted to do (within the medical realm) and wherever I wanted to do it. I went to Africa.

In the second term, I had Obstetrics and Gynaecology, Paediatrics and Psychiatry (each a five-week placement) at other local hospitals giving an opportunity to experience different NHS Trusts and how different medical teams function. St George's is lucky to be close to a large mental hospital. Plus we even had a fabulous day trip to Broadmoor!

The final placement was for another 12 weeks, this time at St George's. As a tertiary referral centre, there are so many opportunities to see rarer conditions / diseases. In the final term our minds are much more focused on the end of year exams and again, the flexibility of the graduate course enabled me to plan which clinics, ward rounds or operations, as I wanted to attend. I also appreciated that the staff realised our anxiety about the exams and were happy to give impromptu teaching or point out patients with interesting signs to examine.'

Once you get in...

Once you get in you will receive a fresher's pack, containing essential information about halls of residence, the course itself, as well as information about Sports, Societies and freshers' fortnight!

You will also be given the option of purchasing a 'Fresher's Pass'. This pass allows you to enter all the discos at freshers' fortnight for a hugely reduced price.

Closer to the start of term, another letter will be sent containing instructions on moving to halls, as well as a timetable for the first week.

As far as books are concerned, on the first Monday evening when you are introduced to your St George's 'family', it is best to ask

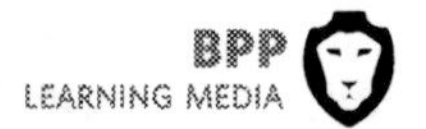

them what books they recommend for study (ie which ones to borrow from the library or buy).

The Best Thing	Small class sizes. Making it very friendly
The Worst Thing	The difference of experience depending on your hospital placement

Student top tips

- Don't be afraid to turn up to A&E to try to clerk and present patients.
- Take advantage of situations as they present themselves.
- Most of the staff, no matter which hospital, and provided it isn't crazy busy, are happy to help students and guide them in their learning.

Summary Table

Positives	Negatives
PBL	PBL not suited to everyone
Flexibility in learning	Not central London
Friendly	Some may find large city daunting
Cheap area of London to live in	

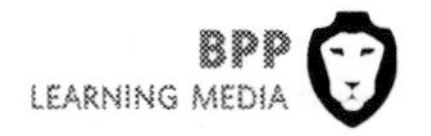

Manchester

School of Medicine
The University of Manchester
Oxford Road
Manchester
M13 9PT

www.manchester.ac.uk/medicine

Manchester, the city where Rolls met Royce, has something for everyone, including first class education. Among its staff and alumni the university boasts more than 20 Nobel Prize winners and no doubt has plenty more to come. As part of the prestigious Russell Group, Manchester has always been a strong contender in the academic world, particularly in the sciences, and is consistently ranked very highly not only in European, but also in world league tables. As such, the university receives approximately 65,000 applications annually from would-be undergraduates. Those lucky enough to gain admission can look forward to years of...anything and everything they want, the diverse city really does cater for all tastes. The medical school's innovative PBL curriculum teaches medicine to 'tomorrow's doctors' in a fun and interesting way while still holding onto the best part of the more traditional courses of days gone by, dissection!

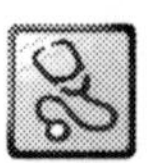

The medical course

Key facts

Course Type	PBL	Degree Awarded	MBChB
Basic Entry Requirements	AAA	Entrance Exams	UKCAT
Year Size	Approx 350	Open Days	June
Admissions Website	www.medicine.manchester.ac.uk/		

Getting in – student tips

Manchester requires all prospective candidates to have some experience in medical or community care. They like to see how a student can show humility, commitment to an activity (sports, music, charity, etc), leadership skills, and teamwork skills. On top of this, Manchester really want to know a good reason why you'd be right to study Medicine there. The interview panel usually consists of three tutors from the School of Medicine or the Faculty of Life Sciences. The interview process has changed recently and now consists of a group discussion for 30 minutes on an ethical situation, followed by two one-on-one interviews lasting around 15 minutes each. Outside of the ethical discussion, the interviewers want to know about why you want to do Medicine and outside interests.

Course details

Foundation / Pre-Med	Yes	**Graduate**	No
Student Population	Male: female ratio: 40:60	**Term Length**	Pre-clinical: 10 weeks Clinical: 13-15 weeks
Erasmus / Foreign Exchange	N/A	**Elective Period**	Year 5 – 8 weeks

Intercalation

Stage	End of year 2 or year 4	**Degree Awarded**	BSc (Hons)
Requirements	Passed all exams at first attempt.	**Subjects**	Medical Sciences

Anatomy teaching

Two hours of anatomy teaching takes place each week for the first and second year, with an additional two hours each fortnight scheduled for teaching neuroanatomy in the second year. Classes take place within PBL groups of about 12 students taught usually by a house officer. Each session typically involves the use of various learning resources including cadaveric dissection, prosections, pathology pots, skeletons and prosthetic models. Where it is appropriate, surface anatomy is also taught. It's Manchester's policy that all

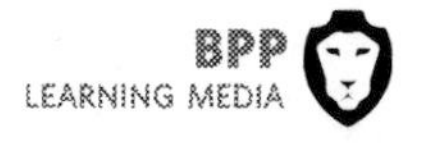

students must participate in cadaveric dissection. Manchester students tend to make the most out of anatomy classes, as it is one of the few opportunities in which formal teaching takes place.

Pre-clinical/Years 1–2	
Topics	***Year 1:*** Introduction to PBL learning, reproductive system, genetics, immunology, physical and psychosocial development, ageing, cardiovascular system and respiratory system. ***Year 2:*** Nervous, musculoskeletal, digestive, renal and hepatic systems, and metabolism. Throughout years 1 and 2, psychology, sociology, epidemiology, healthcare ethics and law are covered when relevant in a PBL case.
Teaching	A PBL approach to learning means that contact hours are kept to a minimum. Three hours a week of PBL take place over two sessions, in which a clinical case is read out, the salient points are then discussed within a group and learning objectives are derived from discussion. It is then up to students to go away from the group and learn about different learning objectives. The PBL group will then reconvene and discuss the learning objectives and talk about the case in more detail in the second session.
SSC Periods	There is one SSC in each academic year pre-clinically. In year 1, this takes the format of an individual literature review on a wide variety of topics (there is an element of choice in that students put down a list of topic preferences, and these are accommodated for as best as possible). In year 2, the SSC is a group poster presentation on any topic covered in the second year that the group can agree on.
Exams	At the end of each semester there is a knowledge test on topics covered in that semester with the format being MCQ and EMQ. Along with this, there is an MCQ progress test sat universally by all Manchester medical students with the rationale behind it showing that students have more medical knowledge as each year progresses. There is also an OSCE in year 1 and 2 which tests students' ability of basic clinical skills. For written examinations, grade boundaries are normal-referenced, and usually few people fail them; while OSCEs are standard-referenced and while there's the possibility that many can fail, only the minority do. There are opportunities to resit examinations in the summer. For the high achievers, there are prizes for the top two students in year 1 and for the top five students in year 2.

Clinical/Years 3–5	
Topics	*Manchester runs the course through PBL which continues through the clinical years and adopts a holistic approach to the modules covering diverse areas at the same time, getting you to look at clinical practice from multiple directions simultaneously. By the end of the fourth year you have spent time in all the major specialities.* ***Year 3:*** Heart and Lung and Nutrition, Metabolism and Endocrine ***Year 4:*** Mind and Movement, Families and Children ***Year 5:*** Consolidation and Preparation for practice
SSC Periods	There are four SSC periods through the third and fourth year, each roughly four weeks long, in many areas. If you think ahead then it is possible to use these as audit or research projects. They are assessed with reference to your performance and a report. There is a project option at the end of the fourth year, for three months, allowing you to undertake some serious research in any field you choose.
Exams	Assessment is through OSCEs at the end of modules and twice a year there is a progress test which is a multiple choice. Overall those that work, pass. If the clinicians think there is a problem you will be told and helped to fill the gaps in knowledge or performance.

Hospital placements/academies

There are placements at various District General Hospitals around the north west which last a semester. Accommodation is usually provided and, although not luxurious, is clean and warm. In the fifth year most get to spend a semester at Christies, the world famous cancer hospital.

In all placements those that show an interest can get involved in research which is going on in their allocated hospital.

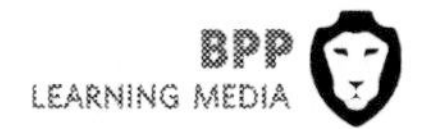

Hospitals and Travel Time from University	
Manchester Royal Infirmary	2 minutes
Royal Preston Hospital	55 minutes
Hope Hospital	20 minutes
Manchester South	15 minutes

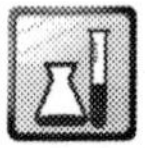

The medical school

Work	Good work life balance
Facilities	Good facilities. All the hospitals have well stocked libraries and internet access
Support	Lots of peer support and some tutor support. Being able to choose a clinical partner for years 3 and 4 is invaluable!
Feedback	Feedback from exams is adequate but could be better

Facilities

The course is run through a website which provides times, announcements and other helpful resources. Each base hospital has a good library, with helpful staff who can get any books/articles you desire. At each base hospital there are good well-equipped clinical labs to help your practise and at some, ie Preston, a full simulation suite with computerised patient dummy who bleeds and dies without the need for a death certificate!

Student support

During the first and third years (which is the first year of clinical placement), the students organise a group system that allocates a student to a group supervised by students from the year above, to help with anything. Through the clinical years you are allocated a tutor who is extremely useful if there are problems or you need careers advice. There are all the usual student helplines through the university but the medical school operates an unofficial open door policy so if there is a problem there are many to ask for help.

For the third and fourth year, you arrange between yourselves to find a clinical partner, who accompanies you on all your placements, apart from the SSC, which really helps, particularly when you are adjusting to the clinical environment.

Medical societies

The medsoc runs loads of events throughout the year, the Scrubs bar crawls, with all five years stopping at bars through the city is legendary. There is a strong surgical society, Scalpel, which hosts lectures and practical training in surgical skills and the Medical Acorn Foundation hosts the annual National Medical Student Research Conference each year.

There are strong teams in football, rugby, basketball, golf, hockey with a marathon and diving club, all who do not take it too seriously.

Finance

There are various university wide scholarships and bursaries worth up to £5,000 per year. Need based access to learning fund.

Further info: www.manchester.ac.uk/undergraduate/studentfinance/

Student opinion

'Despite being home to Coronation Street, and tending to be damp more than other parts of the world, Manchester is a vibrant place with more to do than you'll have time for. There are great parts of the city which are hubs for bars and clubs. Manchester remains a real clubbing capital with loads of festivals. There are lots of places to hang out around the university, but take a short walk and you're into a large city centre. There is of course always a certain football Mecca if you follow the religion that is United.'

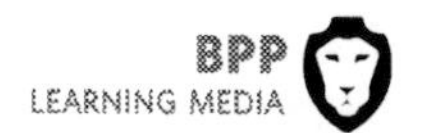

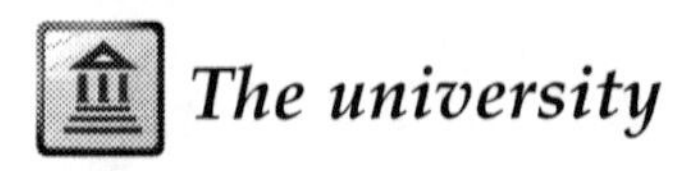

The university

Accommodation	Accommodation is spread around the main campus on Oxford Road and down to the student village called Fallowfield
Further Info	www.accommodation.manchester.ac.uk

Accommodation

The proximity of accommodation to the medical school varies. A popular hall with medical students is Whitworth Park, a two-minute walk away from the medical school. Many other students tend to favour living in Fallowfield where there is a large student population and many halls of residence. The types of hall can vary significantly, from en-suite self-catered flats for those who wish to be more self-sufficient, to traditional catered halls offering a more communal environment. The university also provides single-sex halls. University accommodation is guaranteed to most first year students.

Study facilities

The John Rylands University Library is one of the largest academic libraries in the whole of the UK and spans over ten sites. The Main Library has recently been piloting 24-hour opening times with very positive feedback. The library in the Medical School has a large collection of all the texts and journals necessary for medical students to use, with dozens of copies of core textbooks available to borrow.

IT resources are plentiful at the university. Computer clusters exist in halls of residence, libraries and all over each faculty. Each student has an individual Webmail account, and medical students have their own intranet called MedLea which has lectures and other resources uploaded. Halls of residence have their own internet network (Hornet) which provides a very fast Ethernet connection to users.

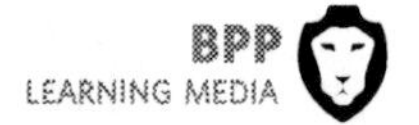

University sports & students' union

Sports facilities are plentiful at the University of Manchester, but are generally not free. The Armitage and Sugden Centres both have well-equipped gyms available for a reasonable price for students. Discounts are also available for students to use the Manchester Aquatics Centre built for the 2002 Commonwealth Games which has two 50m pools and fitness suites. The Armitage and Sugden Centres have indoor sports halls, all-weather pitches and grass pitches which are used by many of the sports teams.

Two students' union buildings exist; one on the North Campus near the city centre, and one on the South Campus, opposite the medical school. The students' union is where the elected sabbatical officers can be found and is also home to the gig venue, Manchester Academy. It boasts many facilities including a bar, cafeteria, shop and a hairdresser. This is the venue of the Freshers' Ball, as well as other popular events such as the end of year party called Pangaea. Because of the gig venues, many bands and artists can be found playing there such as Mika and Nickelback to name but a few. While there are events for medics here, it is popular for pre-clinical students to go here to get lunch or go to the bar.

Student opinion

'Being a large university may make it seem intimidating and impersonal, but on the contrary: halls of residence, small seminar groups, sports teams and societies provide everyone with a very sociable time. On top of this, the high academic standard and teaching styles employed gives students the chance to become independent learners and develops a wide range of transferrable skills. With a good nightlife and regular events out, Manchester is a very fun and social place to study.'

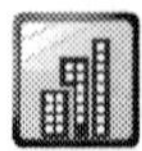

The city

Safety	🛡	🛡				Despite a good partnership between the university and police, and security patrols, students can often be seen as easy targets with many expensive goods such as laptops and phones
Nightlife	☾	☾	☾	☾		From comedy clubs, to theatres, to nightclubs, there is something to cater for all tastes on a night out
Transport	🚌	🚌	🚌	🚌		With one of the busiest bus routes in Europe, student travel from the city centre to Fallowfield is very frequent and affordable. A car is not really necessary for pre-clinical years and there is very limited parking on the university site around the medical school
Cost of Living	🐷	🐷				Living in Manchester is relatively cheap, with weekly rent in houses not usually exceeding £80

Things to do

Home to the Curry Mile, Old Trafford, the MEN Arena and where bands such as Chemical Brothers and Oasis started, Manchester is a hub of culture. With a street full of curry houses, the Curry Mile makes the perfect start to a night out or for student groups to get together. With many mid-week student nights, many students can be found out on a Wednesday night in clubs around the city centre. Nights out are often very enjoyable, but drunken students can often be targeted walking back so it is important not to go back alone.

Places to Go		
Place	**Brief Description**	**Entry Fee/Opening Time**
5th Ave	A popular venue for indie music-loving students.	£3-4, Mon; Wed-Sat 10.00pm-2.00/3.00am
Tiger Tiger	Bar, club, restaurant, Tiger Tiger is an experience over four floors with varied music.	£4.50-7, Mon-Sun 12.00pm-12.00/2.00/3.00am
42nd Street	A rock and indie venue, very popular with students.	£3/4, 10.00pm-2.00/3.00am
Baa Bar, Sackville Street	Two floors full of disco and pop with £1 shooters.	£Free, 9.00pm-2.00/3.00am

Student opinion

'My time at Manchester Medical School has been awesome and a lot of fun. I start to feel ready as a junior doctor and I am off to Aspen and South Africa for my elective.'

Student's view

Pre-clinical

'I first chose Manchester because of the course, I thought PBL would suit my learning style and I thought that being an independent learner would make me a better clinician. After pre-clinical years, I still feel I've made the right decision. With not many scheduled contact hours, I've been able to take control of my learning, and deciding how much detail to go into and how many hours I work has been a learning curve in itself. Typically there are two PBL sessions, six lectures and dissection taking place each week. Sometimes there will be clinical experience or physiology practicals. Occasionally we also have portfolio sessions where we learn about reflective writing and developing our professionalism. After two years, I feel that I've got the dynamics right between working and social activities, although it has taken time to get used to this. I

can now go to hockey practice, choir rehearsals and go out socially when I want to and not compromise on work.

Early patient contact has meant that I have been able to apply what I have learnt real situations and has been a real highlight. To actually know what biological actions are going on and see how it affects people gives what I have learnt a real purpose and acts as an incentive to do better.

Examinations every semester appear intimidating at first, but you soon learn that everyone else is in the same boat and after the first winter examinations you learn how to revise for examinations and develop your learning skills. Coming straight from school, the MCQ and OSCE styles are fairly new concepts, but appropriate guidance from staff and practice OSCE sessions help, and you adapt to knowing how to answer MCQs very quickly'

Clinical

'The last couple of years in hospital as a medical student has been hard work, a bit scary at times, exciting and a lot of fun. I got to undertake lots of procedures and assisted in theatre, delivered a baby and got some research papers/presentations under my belt. There has been a continual round of exams and hours studying but the rewards of patient contact and exam success have made it worthwhile. There have been many highlights, for example, when I got to suture in theatre was amazing and then, on seeing the results of my work a couple of weeks later, experienced both a relief and a real sense of achievement.

The wards start out as foreign environments where you are not sure even where to stand but within a short period of time they become familiar and places where not only are you able to learn but also where you can start to make a difference in helping patients, even if only with a cup of tea. I have yet to spend some time with a patient which, with the benefit of hindsight, I consider a waste.

Within the base hospital there are so many opportunities at first it is difficult to know where to start, but everyone has welcomed and encouraged me to exploit this time. There has been a lot to get to grips with quickly but the satisfaction of being able to be a baby clinician at the moment is very satisfying.

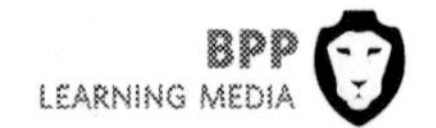

The more time you spend on the wards the easier it will be in exams and in the future. I would advise you to grab the opportunities with both hands. Be willing to do extra projects or stay late and the dividends will pay off now and in the future.'

Once you get in...

The moment the offer becomes unconditional, Manchester send information about what accommodation you've been offered, your timetable for the first week, information on the social activities for freshers' week (including selling tickets for the Freshers' Ball) and information on the MedSoc. It's important to confirm your accommodation offer as soon as possible. While Manchester has a reading list available, they prefer that students read different texts before buying key core texts and do not advise you to do any reading in advance. The first week which coincides with freshers' week consists of introductory lectures, student registration and explaining about how PBL works. This light timetable allows for students to bond in social events organised for freshers' week. It's a good idea to gel with your PBL group as soon as possible and to attend social events with them where possible.

The Best Thing	Variety! Variety of teaching methods, variety of things to do in the city, variety of people you meet
The Worst Thing	No real personal tutor system. Your PBL tutor is meant to act as a personal tutor to some extent but they change every semester

Student top tips

- Don't get your library card in the first few days, you will be waiting for hours!
- Don't forget your swipecard! If you don't have it you aren't getting into the Stopford building no matter how nicely you ask.
- Don't believe all the rumours about the fourth floor!
- Be careful walking up the steps of the Stopford building, they are oddly spaced and even have their own facebook group because of it!
- Be on the lookout if you like Hollyoaks, lots of the actors are spotted in and around Manchester.

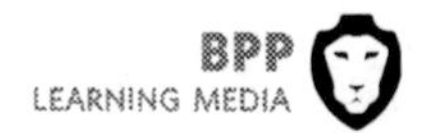

Summary Table

Positives	Negatives
Dissection	No real personal tutor system
Medics socials	Long gaps between exams and results
The city	Not enough practice exam questions
Develops independent learning	Few contact hours may impact on the quality of teaching for some
Early clinical experience	Lots of rain

Newcastle

Medical School
Newcastle University
Framlington Place
Newcastle upon Tyne
NE2 4HH

https://mbbs.ncl.ac.uk/

Land of the Geordies, Brown Ale, the Magpies and Ant and Dec. The university was built around one of the oldest medical schools in the country and continues a long tradition of producing excellent doctors. Newcastle is an electric, vibrant city that welcomes any student with open arms. From being one of the most densely packed cities in the country for nightlife haunts, to famous cultural hotspots such as the Baltic and the Sage, the city definitely caters for everyone's needs. Newcastle's medical school is famous for its early clinical involvement and 'hit the ground running' approach, the benefits become apparent as you quickly become immersed in the medical world in the north east. With a work hard play hard ethos the medical students of Newcastle enjoy a life packed with excitement and rewards.

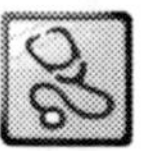

The medical course

Key facts

Course Type	Traditional	Degree Awarded	MBBS
Basic Entry Requirements	AAA	Entrance Exams	UKCAT
Year Size	Approx 300	Open Days	August
Admissions Website	http://mbbs.ncl.ac.uk/public/index/		

Getting in – student tips

At Newcastle, in relation to the standard five-year programme (A100) and the four-year programme (A101), applications fulfilling the academic threshold will be assessed on their UKCAT scores. This score is now used to identify applicants for interview.

All students will be interviewed for a place at Newcastle. The interview will be conducted by two selectors. There will be the standard questions eg 'Why Newcastle?' A large focus will be on your personal statement and being able to draw and expand on examples. Another tip is that Newcastle like candidates who can reflect, ie why you have done something, what you have learnt from it and how you can improve.

From my experience, it was a relaxed setting, the interviewers were friendly and overall far from the daunting experience I anticipated. The interviews process at Newcastle ends in late March, so don't worry if you have not heard anything for a while!

Course details

Foundation / Pre-Med	No	**Graduate**	Yes
Student Population	Male: female ratio: 40:60	**Term Length**	Pre-clinical: 10 weeks Clinical: 15 weeks
Erasmus / Foreign Exchange	N/A	**Elective Period**	End of year 4 – 8 weeks

Intercalation

Stage	Between years 2 to 3 and years 4 to 5	**Degree Awarded**	BScMedSci (Hons)
Requirements	Pass all exams first time around	**Subjects**	Medical Sciences

Anatomy teaching

Anatomy is taught in the first and second year using cadaveric prosections (parts of the human body that have already been dissected prior to the session), and is an important focus for the first two years. The setup involves the year being split into two and each half of the year is further split into smaller groups, so there is enough personal guidance. The facilities are excellent – the

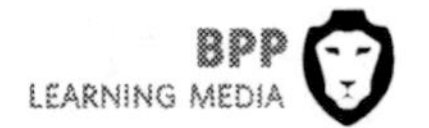

anatomy and clinical skills centre is modern and now provides students instructional video screens to aid teaching. Handouts are also given before the sessions which mean you can prepare if you like and they also help in guiding each of the sessions, so you always know what is going on. Individual or small group sessions may be arranged with prior notice – excellent for last minute revision before exams!

The anatomy sessions are taught by surgical trainees, the 'dems'– they are really friendly, willing to help and make it a relaxed and fun atmosphere. You can also get to know them better at their notorious 'dems night out' in December – an annual event not to be missed!

Pre-clinical/Years 1–2	
Topics	***Year 1:*** Molecules to Community, Cardiovascular, Respiratory & Renal Medicine, Life Cycle, Nutrition, Metabolism & Endocrinology, Clinical Sciences & Investigative Medicine Unit, Personal & Professional Development, Medicine in Community. The topics are taught through a series of twenty case studies, for example, 'A Young Man with Cystic Fibrosis', 'Sophie and Paul – Having a Baby' and 'A Woman with Weight Loss and Tiredness'. ***Year 2:*** Thought Senses & Movement, Life Cycle, Clinical Sciences & Investigative Medicine, Personal & Professional Development, Medicine in Community. Examples case studies in the second year include 'A young boy who stopped breathing', 'A young woman from Africa', 'A man who couldn't finish lunch'.
Teaching	Lectures, small group seminars, Computer assisted learning (CAL), Clinical Demonstration', Case Presentations, Clinical Skills Training, GP visits, Hospital visits.

SSC Periods	There is no SSC period in the first year. In the second year, the SSC is a written 3,000 word assignment – it is where you look at research articles on a topic of your choice. The Family Study – This is not an SSC, but is the main project you do in first year. It involves following a pregnant patient and family through their experiences of pregnancy and childbirth. This is done in pairs and involves a variety of visits to see the family – a good first step to patient contact. The Patient Study – This is a similar project undertaken in second year following a patient and their experience of living with a chronic illness.
Exams	Multiple choice questions (NOT negatively marked), Extended matching items, OSCEs based on clinical skills.

Clinical/Years 3–5	
Topics	***Year 3:*** The first clinical year is mostly split into your essential junior rotations, which consist of foundations of clinical practice, obstetrics and gynaecology, child health, infectious diseases, psychiatry, public health and then a large rotation covering what is essentially hospital medicine and some surgery. You are also attached to a primary care placement for the year. ***Year 4****:* Clinical and Investigative medicine. This is all group and lecture based at the medical school. SSCs and elective occur after Christmas. ***Year 5****:* Essential senior rotations which consists of primary care, mental health, obstetrics and gynaecology, hospital based practice, which includes your major surgical rotations and preparation for practice which among others helps familiarise you with administrative duties of the wards.
SSC Periods	There are three SSC periods lasting six weeks which all occur after the first term of the fourth year. At least two must be clinical selections. The medical school offers an assortment of SSCs, which can be battled for in a fastest fingers first arena via an online selection page or many students organise a private option which is agreed between you, your supervisor and the medical school before hand. The non-clinical options include medical photography and medical Spanish. The first SSC must include an audit or research topic.

Exams	During the third year there are OSCE examinations and written papers. These happen both before Christmas (one OSCE and one written paper) and during summer term (one OSCE and two written papers). In fourth year there are only two written papers before Christmas. Finals occur in the Summer of fifth year and consist of two written papers an OSCE and a MOSLER (which is a multiple long case examination). Fourth year exams have got a reputation for being the most difficult. The failure rate is always low throughout.

Hospital placements/academies

In Newcastle, hospital placements are controlled by the base unit allocated to you in the third and fifth year. The clinical placement area is one of the largest of any medical school in the country. The base units are Tyne, Northumbria, Wear and Tees. You will be allocated to one of these regions for the entire year during the third or fifth year. The hospital placements last roughly four to eight weeks. The majority of hospitals can be reached from Newcastle but some require you to be housed there. All hospitals that fall into this category offer adequate accommodation. Unless your hospital placement falls within the Tees base unit in either the third or fifth year the majority of students will stay in Newcastle. On each rotation there are approximately 20-30 students but this is broken down into smaller tutor groups for teaching and ward work so you should never feel any pressure for finding patients to examine or take histories from. There are no good or bad placements but the majority of students prefer their base unit hospitals to be accessible from their student house in Newcastle (unless they were in the Stockton campus during the first two years). A Teeside placement generally implies a move away from Newcastle for one year. All the hospitals are fantastic teaching hospitals and many such as the Freeman cardiothoracics department are national leaders in their discipline. Many of the consultants and teaching fellows from the hospitals are very amiable to embark on a research topic with you if you show enough interest; the fourth year is an excellent opportunity to complete some if you are well motivated.

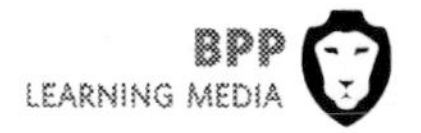

Hospitals and Travel Time from University	
Royal Victoria Infirmary	1 minute
Newcastle General Hospital	10 minutes
University Hospital Durham	30 minutes
Sunderland Royal Hospital	40 minutes

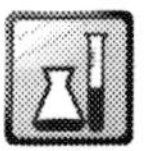

The medical school

Work	✚	✚	✚			Good work life balance
Facilities	☕	☕	☕	☕	☕	Very good learning environments. Library packed with resources and helpful staff
Support	👥	👥	👥	👥		The parenting system and personal tutor work well if used. The undergraduate office is an excellent base of support
Feedback	📋	📋				Poor in course assessment feedback. On a positive note there is a critical appraisal at the end of each year for every student

Facilities

Newcastle medical school has always scored highly for its facilities. The medical sciences faculty building houses a large medically orientated library and five large computer clusters. The medical students have there own common room complete with pool and football tables. Most of the teaching during your first two years will be in the David Shaw lecture theatre, a large, modern and comfortable place to learn. The clinical and dissection rooms are also there for your benefit and can be booked when not in use for revision purposes. The university is very fortunate to be linked with the Centre for Life, which is a large hub for genetics (stem cell research) in the UK. The benefit of this is medical students are taught by some of the country's leading academics in their field.

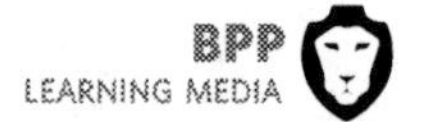

Student support

Generally the support receives consistently high feedback from the students. There is a parenting system for first years with an annual cheese and wine greetings night to meet your parent. You are also assigned a personal tutor for academic and pastoral support, however it may be the case you see them only once in your whole time during university. The undergraduate office team is a constant source of advice and support and are extremely helpful in redirecting your query if they can't help. The students' union is another helpful contact and offers a range of services including health and financial advice if it is required.

Medical societies

The Medical Society of Newcastle dominates many medical students' social calendars, and from the Metroline pub crawl to the winter ball, there is plenty to keep you entertained. The MedSoc usually meets every Friday in the union. The surgical society has also become more prolific recently and is open to all years. It's an excellent way to try some surgical techniques and hear from eminent speakers when formal opportunities are lacking in the first two years. Med Sex is another well managed society that organises sexual education in local primary schools. The medics' sports teams have been a dominating force in both university intra mural and local leagues in the past years. A strong rugby and football team, with also good hockey and netball teams, many non-medic students also compete for places in these squads due to the high standard. There are also second teams in some of the bigger sports to allow a wide participation. For the last two years there has also been an intra year football competition, which always produces fierce rivalry.

Finance

Newcastle offers an undergraduate bursary of £1,340 for those from low-income households (<£25,000), with a smaller bursary of £670 available for income between £25,001 and £32,284. Achievement bursaries, excellence scholarships and NCL+ bursaries are also available. For students on the four-year accelerated programme, NHS bursaries are available throughout the course. The NHS pays the fees for years 2, 3 and 4 for these students.

Further info: www.ncl.ac.uk/undergraduate/finance

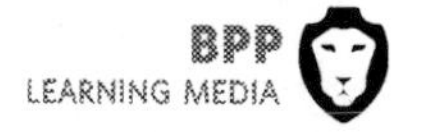

Student opinion

'The amazing teaching and fantastic facilities at Newcastle have completely prepared me for the rigorous academic and emotional challenges medicine will offer. Not only has Newcastle given me a good medical education its also offered many opportunities outside Medicine that have let me develop my life outside the clinical environment and will make me a better doctor.'

The university

Accommodation	Non-campus
Further Info	www.unionsociety.co.uk www.ncl.ac.uk/undergraduate/accommodation/university.htm

Accommodation

The two main catered halls of residence are Castle Leazes and Henderson Hall. Most medical students stay at Castle Leazes as it is just a five-minute walk from the medical school – perfect for first year late nights and 9.00am starts! Richardson ('Ricky') Road is a popular self-catered accommodation which is a two-minute walk to the medical school. Both Castle Leazes and Ricky Road are near the university gym and less than a ten-minute walk to the city centre. There other self-catered halls located even nearer the city centre, eg Windsor Terrace – it just depends on what you want but there's plenty of choice to suit everyone's taste! In later years, the main student areas are Jesmond, Sandyford and Heaton, all less than 20 minutes' walk from the medical school.

Study facilities

Walton Library is the main library for medics, with plenty of computer clusters and located conveniently on the fifth floor of the medical school, which makes it useful for your time between lectures. There is also the main student library, Robinson Library, located a five minute walk from the Walton Library, where all other Newcastle students study. Many medics use this library during

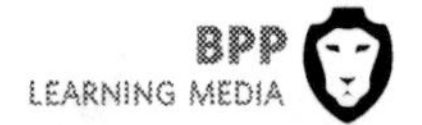

revision time – when the Walton gets quite busy. There is also a 24 hour cluster available for those last minute deadlines.

University sports & students' union

The university gym is located literally a minute's walk from the medical school, ideal for a quick workout between lectures. It cost £55 for just a recreational pass – this is a pass that allows you to join the sports societies and it is an extra £155 (one year's membership) for using the gym and £180 for the gym and pool. It is a small gym, and can get busy. The gym also hosts a really fun Intra Mural programme, including five-a-side football and mixed hockey. They also have classes for dance, yoga and aerobics as well as some squash courts for racquet sports. The university has strong rowing and rugby teams.

The Newcastle student union is the social hub of the university. It has a lot to offer during your time as a student. It has five cafés for a quick bite to eat between your lectures, six bars for a quick drink or two and is the venue for many gigs and events. It also has JOB shop if you are looking to find work as a student, a post office and a student advice centre. As a medical student, it is a good place to chill and go for lunch especially in your first two years when you are more based in the medical school.

Student opinion

'The fast pace of the city will make sure there is always something new to do. It has a reputation for being one the best nights out in the UK and once you start being a student here it's easy to see why. Living in Newcastle for me has been a truly remarkable experience. It was easy to settle in and the opportunities the city and surrounding countryside boast made the transition of moving away a very trouble free experience.'

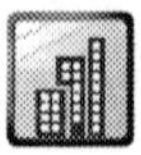

The city

Safety	⛨	⛨	⛨	⛨		Newcastle is generally a safe city
Nightlife	☾	☾	☾	☾		The city centre has a variety of cheap and trendy clubs and bars to suit all tastes. Many popular bars are also located in the student living areas in particular around the Jesmond area
Transport	🚌	🚌	🚌	🚌		Car is useful for clinical years but there is an excellent metro system that links many areas in Tyne, Wear and Northumberland. Parking is difficult around the medical school and the city centre
Cost of Living	🐖	🐖				Expect to pay £300/month for accommodation in Jesmond, more reasonable in Heaton and Sandyford, £4 for a taxi into the centre and £15-25 for a good night out

Things to do

Newcastle offers a nice blend of culture, relaxation and fun. There are beautiful sights and attractions to see – the Baltic, the Sage and Angel of the North to name but a few. Tynemouth and Whitley Bay are the local beaches – popular with students in the summer for barbecues.

In terms of nightlife, there is something for everyone, from a classy night on the beautiful quayside to a cheaper night out on the infamous Bigg Market. The quayside itself boasts some of the nicest restaurants, pubs and bars including the Baha Beach club (a good student night out) as well the gorgeous views from Millennium Bridge.

Shopping isn't the best in Newcastle, but the city centre does have numerous shops and boutiques including a Primark. There is also the Metro Centre which has a bit more choice. It is a 20-minute car or train journey from the student areas, but well worth the trip!

Metro Radio Arena and Carling Academy hosts gigs from various bands and artists. The Theatre Royal is a gorgeous theatre located right in the city centre that hosts popular plays and musicals. St James Park hosts the home games for Newcastle United – I don't know whether that's a positive or negative for coming to Newcastle!

Places to go		
Place	**Brief Description**	**Entry Fee/Opening Time**
Liquid & Envy	Cheap popular cheesy student night	£5;Mon,Thur–Sat 10.30pm–3.00am
WHQ	Smaller cool alternative club	£5; Fri and Sat 10.30pm–3.00am
Digital	Attracts great DJs, David Guetta, Pete Tong and Axwell – great house music.	£8-15; Mon, Thur–Sat 10.30pm–2.00/3.30am
Tiger Tiger	Located in the GATE	£5; Mon–Sat 12.00pm–2.00/3.00am

Student opinion

'Newcastle's first two years really allows you to have a balance of doing medicine and time to be a normal student. Good teaching along with a busy a social calendar makes it a perfect choice for university.'

Student's view

Pre-clinical

'I found first year quite difficult to adjust to from sixth form – lectures are useful, but there is a lot of self-learning involved to achieve the "learning outcomes". However, you soon get used

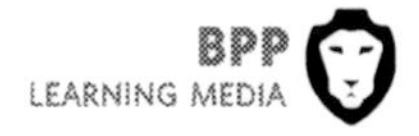

to the system, and I found the anatomy and case-based teaching really good.

A typical day is a 9.00–10.00am lecture; 10.00am–12.00pm break for going to gym, library or a well deserved break after waking up so early; 12.00–1.00pm another lecture; then head off for lunch to the dental café (great sandwiches) or the union.

Afternoons usually entail a couple of hours of seminars or lectures. They are not necessarily till 5.00pm, some days you can be home by 3.00pm – it depends on what group you are in! These groups are assigned at the beginning of the year – they can be really fun, especially if you have a good social secretary that can organise fun group socials!

Second year structure is the same. The first term is based mainly on the "thought, senses and movements" module – the teaching for this module is excellent. In the second year, you also get a lot of "self study time" for your SSC. The second term of the second year is probably my hardest term of the pre-clinical years. You have to juggle doing your patient study, SSC and end of year exams. Students get through it, even with some fun in between, especially around Medsoc campaigning – which many students in the second year will get involved with!

I feel that Newcastle really allows you to have the notorious medic 'work hard, play hard' mentality! There is lots of time to get involved with sports and societies, and you can really live life as a student. The exams are do-able if you have revised – a brilliant thing is that they are not negatively marked! The medic nights are amazing, especially the Christmas and Summer Medic balls. Highlights for me, were Metroline pub-crawl, Teddy Bear Hospital and Medsoc.'

Clinical

'The clinical years certainly make you feel more like you are training to be a doctor. For me the day usually started with a small lecture outlining the learning objectives of the week. It would be followed by ward work either in pairs or by yourself, your history and examination would then usually be discussed with a doctor on the ward. The afternoon would then consist of teaching or

more focused based clinical work. This may involve the use of out patients to practise histories and examinations of specific medical conditions. I felt this was an exceptional way to learn, you began to appreciate how diseases impact on a person's life and it really cemented your pre-clinical learning. Even though there's structure I felt the onus was on me to make what I could of it, the freedom of the clinical years encouraged my curiosity and helped me to learn more effectively. I did find that I had less time to socialise with other friends and some sports commitments became harder. It definitely helped me become more successful at managing my time! I also found that the teaching was very variable but as a rule I found that the smaller hospitals were better for teaching. What I enjoyed most about my clinical years was having an active role in managing a patient, even though small, it gave you a sweet taste of what was yet to come. My SSCs were also a highlight, I organised and tailored my SSCs to do what I wanted to do. It was also the longest attachment to any ward I've ever had and so I could really value how a ward functions. The clinical OSCEs are always a nervous experience for any student as it's usually the first time you've been marked by an examiner sitting in the room. The only way I knew I was going to pass was with lots of practice and that's the best guidance I can give. As for other advice it is always useful to talk to the older students who were in your placement previously, they are usually a wealth of knowledge and know which members of staff you should become acquainted with.

Finally, there is no substitute for experience and that is what your clinical years are all about so use your time wisely and dive in head first.'

Once you get in...

Once you get the 'conditional offer', you will be sent a lot of information. This includes Criminal Records Bureau Form, CRB Identity Check List, BMA information, term dates, smartcard letter, MEDSIN leaflet, Learning Agreement, first week timetable (subject to change), ATC note, biology book, Student Conduct Letter, list of GP surgeries, Blackwell leaflet, Peacocks flier, Newcastle Wilderness Medics, Newcastle University campus map.

First, you need to send your application for your halls of residence. Get this done early to be assured your first choice.

You also need to sort out getting your fresher's wristband, to be entitled to all the freshers' events. Make sure you make the deadline for this – this date is after you get your A level results.

To sign up for societies and sports, there is a freshers' fair in the university gym. This is really worth a trip – there is all sorts, from Irish dancing to rock climbing clubs!

You can sign up for the university gym before freshers' week as well, but most students do this once they are settled.

The Best Thing	Well-structured, highly reputed course with good student support
The Worst Thing	Having to potentially change geographical locations for clinical placements in the third and fifth years

Student top tips

- It's worth spending a day walking around the city with a map – once you've found the shortcuts, you can get around the place in no time.
- Home of Ant and Dec, Cheryl Cole and Alan Shearer to name but a few – it's definitely worth investing in an autograph book!
- Bring warm clothes. Newcastle's on the same latitude as Moscow.
- Make sure you get to see a match at St James' Park – it's quite something to see 52,000 Geordies cheering (or shouting!).
- Register with the gym early to avoid the queues.

Summary Table

Positives	Negatives
Early clinical contact	Very little in course assessment feedback
Excellent student support	Lack of formalised surgical training in early years
Campus and student areas in close proximity to city	Subjective marking at the end of rotations
Good transport systems	Difficult access to surrounding countryside
Incredible nightlife	Base unit allocation can move you away from where you want to be

Nottingham

Faculty of Medicine and Health Sciences
University of Nottingham
Medical School
Queen's Medical Centre
Nottingham
NG7 2UH

www.nottingham.ac.uk/mhs/index.aspx

The Nottingham Medical School, situated in one of Britain's busiest teaching hospitals, (The Queen's Medical Centre), was opened in 1970. The medical school is rich in tradition and presents a whole host of opportunities to its students! Those studying in Nottingham are spoilt for choice for places to go as a break from their hard work. Whether it's the trendy Lace Market or the historical parts of the city that suit you best, an enjoyable and interesting time is guaranteed!

The medical school currently spans two campuses, (at Nottingham and Derby) with top quality facilities and a friendly attitude at both. The course is refreshingly detailed with a mixture of traditional lectures and small group work. Nottingham remains original in the sense that its students are awarded a degree at the end of year 3 (while only a five-year course); an encouraging reward after the hard working clinical years.

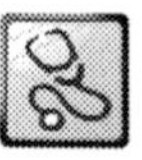

The medical course

Key facts

Course Type	Traditional	Degree Awarded	BMBS
Basic Entry Requirements	AAA	Entrance Exams	UKCAT GAMSAT for Grad entry
Year Size	Approx 240	Open Days	All year
Admissions Website	www.nottingham.ac.uk/mhs/index.aspx		

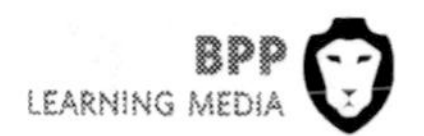

Getting in – student tips

The Nottingham admissions department considers each applicant carefully, from a variety of different sources. The UCAS personal statement and predicted grades are assessed in addition to the candidate's UKCAT (UK Clinical Aptitude Test) score, and special online questionnaire submission. The questionnaire is offered to every applicant, giving them the opportunity to provide evidence that they have the attitude and integrity to meet GMC approval.

There is a large emphasis at interview on empathy and ability to reason in an honest and appropriate manner. A good knowledge of the structure of the course and surrounding location is additionally of benefit.

The interview will often explore the candidate's opinion on current ethical issues, in addition to looking for a general interest in Medicine, academic achievement and involvement in extra-curricular activities. The panel normally comprises two members of staff. The Nottingham interview is not intimidating, and a good experience if a reasonable amount of preparation has been done!

Course details

Foundation / Pre-Med	Yes	**Graduate**	Yes
Student Population	Male: female ratio: 40:60	**Term Length**	Pre-clinical: 11 weeks Clinical: 14 weeks
Erasmus / Foreign Exchange	N/A	**Elective Period**	End of year 5 – 8 weeks

Intercalation

Stage	Between years 2 and 3	**Degree Awarded**	BScMedSci (Hons)
Requirements	Passing the first two years. Everyone does it	**Subjects**	Medical Sciences

Anatomy teaching

First and second years at Nottingham are fortunate enough to be able to participate in full student led dissection, typically with one cadaver between six at a time. Students have one three-hour session every week which is broken down into three one-hour sections: 1) Student briefing and teaching, 2) Supervised dissection, 3) Verbal assessment of dissection task. Examination each week counts towards the final module grade and is particularly helpful in reinforcing anatomy knowledge in preparation for the end of year written assessments. Prosections are used in addition to dissection, to aid teaching. There is lecture based anatomy teaching to supplement time in the dissection room.

Pre-clinical/Years 1–3	
Topics	***Year 1:*** Molecular basis of Medicine, excitable tissues and cell signalling, Histology (with microscope teaching), anatomy of the thorax and limbs, cardiovascular, respiratory and haematology physiology, clinical laboratory sciences, behavioural sciences, public health and communication skills, Clinical skills. ***Year 2:*** Alimentary system and nutrition, renal and endocrine physiology, General and biochemical pharmacology, clinical laboratory sciences II, anatomy of abdomen, pelvis, head and neck, functional and behavioural neuroscience, epidemiology in practice, early clinical and professional development and communication skills II, clinical skills. Community follow up project commences, (students follow and record the progress of a patient in the community for 18 months). ***Year 3, (honours year pre-clinical):*** At Nottingham, the first half of the third year is dedicated to completing a research project to complete the pre-clinical course and to attain a separate BmedSci honours degree. Students are allowed to specify a field of interest from an available choice, and then are allocated a project randomly within their chosen homebase.
Teaching	Lectures, seminars, practical sessions – clinical skills lab, DR, microscope lab and voice recording suite for communication skills. GP visits and hospital visits.

SSC Periods	No SSCs are offered in the first year of study, however there is a choice of a module in the second year, and of two courses to complement the research project in the pre-clinical third year. Instead of intercalation, an honours degree is compulsory and is completed during the first half of the third year. All three years of the course actually count towards the grade of the BmedSci achieved at the end of year 3.
Exams	***Years 1 and 2*** – multiple choice, (negatively marked), multiple choice, (marked with a random adjustment), short answer questions and longer extended essay questions. Anatomy is examined twice yearly with an MCQ paper and spotter exam. ***Year 3*** – MCQ and essay papers, VIVA in front of a panel in order to pass the research project. Pass mark 40% for most examinations and typically, one resit is permitted.

Clinical/Years 3–5	
Topics	***Year 3:*** General Medicine and Surgery attachments, pathology, therapeutics, community follow up project completed. ***Year 4:*** Obs and gynae, Paediatrics, Psychiatry, Healthcare of the elderly, ENT, opthalmology, dermatology, SSM, (student selected module). ***Year 5:*** Advanced general medicine and surgery, GP placement, rheumatology, orthopaedics, emergency medicine, clinical chemistry, rehabilitation medicine, elective, SSM, anaesthesia and preparation for F1 year.
SSC Periods	A student selected module, (four weeks) is chosen in the fourth and fifth year. This is typically selected by ranking preference from an organised list, but occasionally self arranged choices are arranged after approval. Publications are usually in the form of the third year dissertation, but additional audits can be arranged in a self-directed manner in all clinical years.
Exams	Clinical exams take the form of OSCEs, OSLERs, MACCS and MCQ papers. Some are negatively marked and others are marked with a random adjustment.

Exams continued	MACCS, (mandatory assessments of clinical skills) are examined during the attachments, and can be retaken once at the end of the attachment if not satisfied. Clinical OSCEs and OSLERs are assessed usually at the end of an attachment and typically count towards the module grade. Resitting of a module usually follows failure of both a practical and written exam. Nottingham is unusual in allowing one resit of finals without the need to repeat the year. Pass marks range 40–50% for clinical modules.

Hospital placements/academies

Placement length varies depending on clinical year, but usually rotations range from 7–14 weeks. In the third year, firm size is tailored to the hospital that the student is attached to, but most clinical teaching groups consist of no more than ten students. Occasionally firms are subdivided to give Consultant led teaching in groups of two or three and this is beneficial.

Accommodation is provided for all years placed in Mansfield, Lincoln and Boston – although this does currently not extend to psychiatric placements in Mansfield where accommodation must be self-funded. Students in the third year are allowed to rank their preferences between hospitals, but there is no choice in the fourth and fifth year. Car sharing is encouraged by the university to Derby, as they currently they provide no free means of transport for those who do not drive.

The Derby Royal Hospital is new, with excellent facilities and a student's mess where free tea and coffee can be found. There is also an excellent undergraduate education centre.

Hospitals and Travel Time from University	
Queens Medical Centre	10 minutes
Nottingham City Hospital	20 minutes
Derby Royal Hospital	45 minutes
Boston Hospital	90 minutes

The medical school

Work						Hard first two years
Facilities						Excellent facilities
Support						Good tutorial system throughout, slightly less time with tutor in years 4 and 5
Feedback						Very helpful 'insight' area of the medics NLE. Shows place in the year for some exams and question areas answered incorrectly

Facilities

The Medical School at QMC, has a useful and well organised library. There is no common room, but plenty of cafés for students to catch up during well-earned breaks! Derby Royal Hospital has a student's mess for those on clinical attachment where free drinks are available. The QMC has several lecture theatres, a series of tutorial rooms and an excellent drop-in clinical skills centre.

Student support

There are many sources of support available for Nottingham medics. Within the medical school, all students are assigned a tutor who is seen regularly throughout the first two years to deal with any problems or queries. In the clinical years, students are additionally assigned a tutor who is usually a clinician/physician on placement. Regular meetings are again ensured and student self-appraisal is encouraged. All students in the medical school are provided with a 'pastoral care in the medical school' booklet which contains the contact details of other trained individuals, appointed to provide advice to students with problems. Outside the medical school, Nottingham University offers a free, confidential counselling service run by students, for students. All advisers are trained to deal with the problems they may encounter, more information may be found at www.nottingham.ac.uk/counselling. Within the main university, chaplaincy service is available and the Portland Building houses a multi-faith quiet room, Muslim prayer rooms and a chapel.

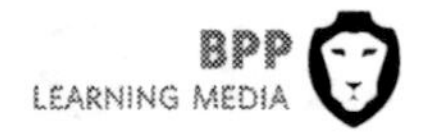

Medical societies

There are some excellent medics' sports teams at Nottingham, and joining one of the many clubs is a lively and fulfilling experience. In particular the medics' rugby team is very successful; having recently work the NAMS sevens, a national competition. Medics also get involved in tennis, football, hockey and swimming and regularly compete and go on tour with their teams. During the summer of the fourth year and fifth year, the medics' 'Summer series' is organised in the absence of the pre-clinical students! This is an entertaining and more relaxed inter-school competition, followed by an exciting night out to celebrate / commiserate in the local bars of Nottingham.

The third years annually put on the 'Medic's Musical' – a highlight of the social calendar which hopes to display the large amount of musical talent within the medical school, while raising money for a good cause. In addition medics take part in their own choir, orchestra, and societies such as sexpression, (teaching younger teenagers sex education), and open art surgery, (offering art opportunities on the paediatrics ward).

Finance

Further financial support, such as hardship loans can be applied for through the university Student Services centre in Nottingham.

www.nottingham.ac.uk/studentservices/financialsupport/studentfunding/index.aspx

There are three scholarships available to GEM students. For more information visit:

www.nottingham.ac.uk/studentservices/financialsupport/bursariesandscholarships.aspx

Student opinion

'There are countless exciting opportunities from being a medical student at Nottingham. The homely feeling of being on campus is contrasted brilliantly by a vibrant and cosmopolitan city, with plenty to see and do when you need a break from a busy day!'.

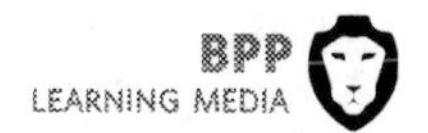

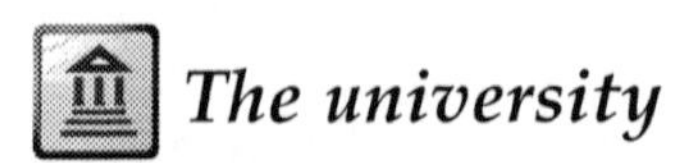

The university

Accommodation	Campus halls of residence
Further Info	(students' union) www.su.nottingham.ac.uk/ (accommodation) www.nottingham.ac.uk/acc/

Accommodation

Most first year students will live in halls of residence on the main campus, Jubilee campus or Raleigh Park. Off campus accommodation is also available with good bus links to the QMC hospital, where the medical school is located. The 14 halls available on the main campus are no more than 30 minutes' walk away and there is around 10–15 medical students on average in each. Second years mainly choose to rent properties in Lenton, about 20 minutes' walk from the hospital. Those that don't want to rent private property are welcomed back onto campus should they wish.

Study facilities

The main library on university campus, (Hallward) is available to all students and is convenient particularly for first years living on University Park. For those living off campus or medics in higher years, Greenfield Library at the QMC is tailored more specifically for the medical student. In reality, most spend time at both locations for a bit of variety! IT services at both libraries offer internet, printing/scanning and photocopying on presentation of a valid student card.

University sports & students' union

The university gym and fitness centre are located next to the Cavendish and Ancaster halls of residence on the main campus. The sports centre additionally offers a nice swimming pool, squash and badminton facilities and two decent sized sports halls. The hockey team, among other clubs, have access to an astroturf pitch. The gym is medium sized with two floors, but can get busy, particularly on a Wednesday afternoon. Students can obtain a gold, silver or bronze membership.

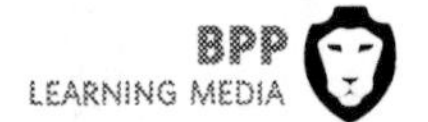

Nottingham medics, along with other students, have access to a vibrant and recently refurbished students' union. The SU is located conveniently on the main campus at Portland building, surrounded by the greenery of the university downs. Although the union bar is a quieter spot for socialising, the Portland building cafe, SU shop, Boots and Natwest Bank are all really useful resources for campus based first years! The SU is the hub of the Nottingham uni run charity organisation, 'Karni.' The medics nominate separate Karni reps who organise weekly rag raids for first years, to collect money for a good cause in some of the country's major cities! Rag raids are well known for their return journey, when there is plenty of Karni cocktail at hand for those that wish!

Student opinion

'As a student from Cavendish Hall, I would absolutely recommend living on the main campus if you can. The hospital is not too far to walk and the social experience is fantastic with plenty of medics and non-medics alike to get to know. Enjoy the first year as much as possible – take advantage of all the social and sporting events on offer!'

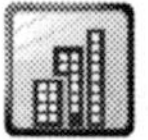

The city

Safety	⛨	⛨	⛨			The Nottingham student areas are generally safe places. As with all major cities, Nottingham has some less desirable areas and these are better avoided!
Nightlife	☾	☾	☾	☾		Nottingham boasts an incredible choice of bars and nightclubs. Only problem is deciding where to go!

Transport						Student cars are not allowed on campus which can be a problem. It is rarely possible to apply for extenuating circumstances. Parking in Lenton as a second year is much easier
Cost of Living						Due to bar and nightclub competition drinks are fairly cheap! Average night out costs between £10–30. The price of accommodation ranges from £55–100 a week

Things to do

Nottingham, (infamously the home of Robin Hood) boasts many tourist attractions, places to eat, and shopping! The city is extremely student orientated with many restaurants and bars offering a variety of discounts on presentation of a student card. While full of authentic architecture and surroundings, (the running tram system being one of them) the city is undergoing many new developments to add to its rich culture. Top places to visit include the Lace Market, (plenty of swanky shops and bars), the Nottingham Playhouse, (housing some top quality theatre and international drama productions), the National Ice Centre and Sherwood Forest, to name but a few. Students at Nottingham are rarely short of ideas for places to go or things to do and access to the city centre is particularly easy with ample buses and trams running frequently.

Places to Go		
Place	**Brief Description**	**Entry Fee/Opening Time**
Ocean	Students only nightclub, a MUST	£5. Every Friday 9.30pm–4.30am
Isis	Houses the weekly AU night, out of city centre	£4 standard tickets, £6.50 VIP. Every wed 10.00pm–3.00am
EQ	£1 drinks party. Wide variety of music	£4 entry
Stealth	Lots of live music!	£4–7 every Saturday

Student opinion

'The clinical years at Nottingham Medical School are interesting and varied. Aside from academic opportunities, there are many clubs and activities to immerse yourself in during the summer holidays when the other students are away!'

Student's view

Pre-clinical

'Having heard prior to the start of uni that Medicine at Nottingham was fairly intense, I had some apprehensions on arrival. There was in fact no need to worry. The course is well organised and varied with enough social events on offer to balance out all the hard work!

The first year began by extending knowledge gained at A level, with modules in molecular biology and biochemistry. After Christmas we were introduced to some new topics such as dissection and microscopy. Basic clinical skills are integrated within the course so it never felt like this side of Medicine was ever too far away! I enjoyed my time spent in smaller groups in both the first and second year; it was nice to see familiar faces regularly in a year of 250 students!

Lectures in the second year were more physiology based. The course was organised so that dissection could tie in with the body system taught at the time which was helpful when trying to remember what had been learnt. I felt there was more free time in the second year to catch up on lectures. The medical school understands that being able to plan some of your own time is an important part of learning, in addition to time spent at lectures.

The structure of the working day is very much the same for the first two years. The day begins bright and early at 9.00am, with a walk across the scenic campus to the QMC and the LT1 lecture theatre. Lunch is typically scheduled between lectures around 12.00–1.00pm and then an afternoons teaching may finish around 4.00pm. In both first and second year, Wednesday mornings are reserved for clinical placement eg GP visit or skills centre teaching and afternoons are left free for sport. Many early Wednesday mornings were spent waiting for the bus to take us to another hospital or GP surgery and it was always fun to catch up with friends along the way! I had dissection for three hours on a Thursday morning and group based workshops on Friday around lecture topics.

The pre-clinical part of the third year is tailored slightly differently. I was allocated a research project in the laboratory, (library was also available) and spent September to January, planning, carrying out, and recording an experiment for my dissertation. This was hard work but very satisfying on completion. Lab time was usually Mon–Fri 9.00am–5.00pm, but this will vary depending on your project. Gaining the compulsory BmedSci has felt like a great achievement, and it is taken into consideration when Nottingham students apply for junior doctor jobs. By today's competitive standards this can only be a good thing!'

Clinical

'The clinical course at Nottingham begins with CP1 in March of the third year, and ends 14 weeks later with three exams at the end of June. Throughout this time, students typically spend time in general Medicine and Surgery while gaining experience in theatre, clinic and on the ward.

The teaching Clinicians at Nottingham City were helpful and keen to teach, and there was a mixture of ward based bedside teaching, outpatients shadowing and small tutorial group teaching. Students at City are taught a separate pharmacology module by a visiting senior Pharmacist. CP1 is examined with a written MCQ paper, written therapeutics MCQ paper, (marked negatively) and a practical OSLER.

CP1 is an enjoyable introduction to clinical work, but there is some difference to the course depending on your allocated hospital. In general for clinical work, City Hospital operates a more self directed timetable than Derby, which produces a heavily timetabled program. Lunchtimes at Derby, are spent in the Doctor's mess where free drinks and common room facilities are available. At the other hospitals, there is more of a canteen environment with plenty of cafés and restaurants to choose from.

Throughout the three clinical years, practical skills are examined on attachment by MACCS, (mandatory assessments of clinical skills) – these are good to monitor progress along the course of the rotation. These are continued through to the more specialised year, CP2, and the advanced clinical year, (ACE or CP3). Students are encouraged to take histories, and meet patients on the ward throughout all the clinical placements. Most F1s at Nottingham are happy to teach, and from experience will very kindly find you a teaching slot in their busy schedule. Students learn to cannulate, take bloods and put in catheters in their third year.'

Once you get in...

On acceptance to Nottingham Medical School, a large brown envelope is sent in the post containing all that is needed to confirm a place on the course, sort out living arrangements for the coming year and plan what is and is not needed to take to uni! Students are allowed to select not only whether they would like to be catered / self-catered but also which hall of residence they would like to be on campus. The information pack also contains some forms about immunisations which are ideally in place for the beginning of the course – it is worthwhile to check with the medical school if these are offered at Nottingham at the beginning of the academic year.

The students' union and MedSoc send out several newsletters and brochures to provide a taster of what is to come. During the weeks leading up to freshers' week, the week one microsite at www.su.nottingham.ac.uk goes live and the line up for the events of fresher's week is released! Most events are hall specific so its a good idea to take note of what theme the hall parties are so you can be prepared ready with some fancy dress ideas!

The Best Thing	Well organised course with extra degree at the end of year 3!
The Worst Thing	A high revision load at times, but it will be worth it...

Student top tips

- Don't go rushing out to by all the books on the reading list until you've spoken to older students to find out what was helpful and what wasn't.
- Sometimes additional textbooks are not necessary as the lecture notes are very thorough.
- Attend the Medics Celebrity Cocktail Party with an original costume!
- Try to be familiar with lectures as you go along – it's tempting to leave them till the end of term, but it's less stressful to revise them during the course.
- Do get involved with hall events as well as medics' ones. During the first two years there is enough time to get to know as many people as possible!
- Try to work hard but relax and have fun too!

Summary Table

Positives	Negatives
If course passed, guaranteed BmedSci at end year 3 with no intercalation needed	Cars on campus are disallowed
Small amount of problem based learning to meet requirements but otherwise traditional lecture based teaching	Information to learn overwhelming at times
Fantastic, vibrant city to explore	Extra science work integrated into lecture program for BmedSci degree
Great medics social scene	Some lectures during freshers' week
Work in small groups with access to many resources. Full dissection available	Getting to placements at Derby/Mansfield is a struggle if you do not drive

Oxford

Medical Sciences Office
John Radcliffe Hospital
Oxford
OX3 9DU

www.medsci.ox.ac.uk/

As the oldest university in the English-speaking world, Oxford is commonly known for its history, academic excellence and tradition. However, that is only one side of a city which at one time or another has housed the national parliament, played a pivotal role in the development of antibiotics, been the location where Roger Bannister first broke the four-minute mile and provided the set for productions including Inspector Morse and Harry Potter! The historic buildings and stunning architecture make Oxford a beautiful place to live. Recent investments, including in the medical students' club, Osler House, have provided outstanding facilities to learn, relax, play sport and socialise. Furthermore, the collegiate system means you are based in a small, friendly environment, but still have access to the facilities and opportunities of a large university.

Overall, the combination of world-renowned research, the tutorial system, colleges, vast recent investment in facilities and stunning surroundings, make Oxford a fantastic place to be as a medical student.

The medical course

Key facts

Course Type	Traditional	Degree Awarded	BM Bch
Basic Entry Requirements	AAA	Entrance Exams	Pre-clinical: BMAT Graduate: UKCAT
Year Size	150	Open Days	July
Admissions Website	www.medsci.ox.ac.uk/study/medicine		

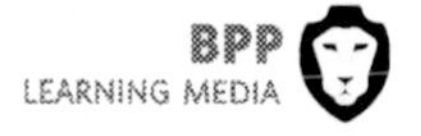

Getting in – student tips

The standard offer for Oxford is AAA (or equivalent) at A2. The personal statement is generally considered less important for Oxford than some other medical schools. The decision over which candidates to interview is based primarily on the BMAT (bio-medical admissions test) score and GCSE results. This seems to provide a very fair method of selection to interview. The best preparation for the BMAT can be found at www.admissionstests.cambridgeassessment.org.uk, where there are specimen papers and an excellent BMAT guide written by the examiners.

Candidates are normally interviewed twice in each college and in at least two colleges; expect plenty of science based/problem solving problems, and be prepared to build arguments and criticise opinions. Do not expect many typical questions such as 'why do you want to be a doctor.' Interview candidates will stay overnight in Oxford. More information can be found on the medical school websites and sometimes mock interviews can be seen at open days. Gap years are rare but seem to be acceptable if you are doing something useful – ask your college at the open day.

Course details

Foundation / Pre-Med	No	**Graduate**	Yes
Student Population	Male: female ratio: 44:56	**Term Length**	Pre-clinical: 10 weeks Clinical: 15 weeks
Erasmus / Foreign Exchange	N/A	**Elective Period**	February of final year – 10 weeks

Intercalation

Stage	Year 3	**Degree Awarded**	BA in Medical Sciences
Requirements	Compulsory part of pre-clinical course. Passing first two years	**Subjects**	Medical Sciences

Anatomy teaching

The anatomy teaching at Oxford is excellent and taught in detail. In the first year general concepts in anatomy are taught during the 'Organisation of the body' module. There is focus on embryological origins and patterning of the body, which makes understanding both anatomy and medical problems involving anatomy easier and more logical. At the end of the third year there is an intensive three week 'principles of clinical anatomy course' where the fine details required for clinical school are taught and examined on a weekly basis. There is a focus throughout both courses on living anatomy. All anatomy is taught with lectures, seminars, prosection in a state of the art laboratory and excellent Oxford specific web resources.

Pre-clinical/Years 1–3	
Topics	***Year 1:*** Organization of the Body, Physiology and Pharmacology, Biochemistry and Medical Genetics, Medical Sociology (minor module), Patient and Doctor Course (minor module). ***Year 2:*** Systems of the Body: Integrative Aspects, The Nervous System, General Pathology and Microbiology, Psychology for Medicine (minor module), Patient and Doctor Course (minor module). ***Year 3:*** Intercalation as mentioned above.
Teaching	For the first two years the teaching consists of lectures, practical classes, seminars and tutorials. There is a strong focus on practical classes and much of your time will be devoted to these. The tutorial system is really the jewel in the crown, focusing less or not at all, on learning facts or exams, but rather on developing thought processes, analytical and problem-solving skills. The timetabled content is very light compared to other medical schools with self-directed learning filling much of the time, this allows you to schedule it around your own extra-curricular timetables.

SSC Periods	There are no special study components during the first two pre-clinical years, however the third year is obviously very student directed. However throughout the pre-clinical years the essay based nature of the tutorial system means there are ample opportunities to explore personal areas of interests then discuss them with tutors. Excitingly you can have your views in those areas challenged and perhaps challenge the views of your tutor, who is an expert in his or her chosen field!
Exams	Exams come at the end of first year and after term 2 in the second year (term 3 being dedicated to starting work for the intercalated degree. The exams are in two parts, part a) is multiple choice conducted on the computer, part b) is essay based and hand-written. The exams are challenging and much revision is needed, the pass mark for part a) is 70%. If you fail either part a) or b) by a small amount you are given a 'viva' (oral examination) to redeem yourself. The average resit rate for the first year exams over the last three years has been 18%.

Clinical/Years 4–6	
Topics	***Year 4:*** Laboratory Medicine (Pathology Course); General Medicine; General Surgery; Ethics and Law. ***Year 5:*** Obstetrics and Gynaecology; General Practice; Public Health; Dermatology; Geratology; Palliative Care and Oncology; Paediatrics; Psychiatry; Neurology; Ear, Nose and Throat; Opthalmology; Orthopaedics and Musculo-Skeletal Medicine; Emergency Medicine. ***Year 6:*** General Medicine; General Surgery; Elective; Preparing for Practice.
SSC Periods	There is a four-week Special Study Module in the fourth year, and a further eight-week period after finals in the sixth year. In both occasions, you can choose from a wide selection of topics suggested by various clinical and basic science departments. There selection is very large, ranging from Anaesthetics to Pre-natal diagnostics to lab based research. Alternatively, you can organise your own module in an area which interests you.

Exams	***Year 4:*** Pathology Course (December): MCQ and EMQ; May/June OSCE and formative written assessment. ***Year 5:*** Written assessment (MCQ, EMQ, short notes) and OSCEs after each of the six, eight-week rotations during the year. ***Year 6:*** Finals are held in late January/early February. They consist of a written short answer paper; an MCQ/EMQ paper; computerised data OSCE; and a clinical OSCE. The exams are aimed to assess clinical competency and the majority of people pass. If you fall just below the overall pass mark, or fail one section (eg one OSCE station), you can retake only the section you failed, often very shortly after the first sitting (eg there is a rescue OSCE a few days after the first attempt OSCE for those that fail one station first time round). At the other end of the spectrum, merits and prizes are awarded.

Hospital placements/academies

Placements in hospitals outside of Oxford typically last between four to six weeks. The number of students at each placement varies according to the hospital and the placement you are on. For example, six students are assigned to Northampton for the general medicine/surgery district general hospital rotation in the fourth year, while there are three students assigned to High Wycombe for Obs and Gynae in fifth year. Teaching is usually very good, and some hospitals have areas of special interest eg Stoke Mandeville incorporates the National Spinal Injuries Centre.

Accommodation is provided free of charge at all sites, although its quality varies. At some (eg Stoke Mandeville, Swindon) there are en-suite rooms, while at others (eg Banbury, Northampton) accommodation is a little more basic, but still pretty good. There is access to a kitchen in all accommodation.

All hospitals have a post graduate centre, where there is a student co-ordinator who organises student attachments and timetables while on placement and is there to help with any problems. The post grad centres also provide access to library and IT facilities and most have a common room and teaching rooms.

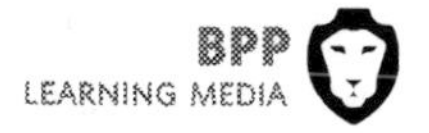

Hospitals and Travel Time from University	
John Radcliffe, Oxford	5 minutes
Churchill, Oxford	5 minutes
Banbury	35 minutes
Reading	60 minutes

The medical school

Work						OK work-life balance. Tough first year exams
Facilities						Excellent academic facilities provided by the medical school, university and college. State of the art medical student common room
Support						Very good support throughout. Provided by the medical school, college and peers
Feedback						Clinical school feedback generally good, feedback on pre-clinical exams is limited

Facilities

Academic facilities are excellent. The Bodleian Library has the right to claim a copy of every book published in the UK, and the university libraries stock many copies of the most popular textbooks for loan. In addition, each college has a library, and there is a well-stocked medical school library in the John Radcliffe Hospital, and library facilities are provided at all district general hospitals. IT facilities are available in colleges, including network/internet access in rooms; at the pre-clinical school and at all hospitals. The pre-clinical school is based in a state of the art new building in the university science area. There is a large lecture theatre, including a histology suite and computer-aided learning suite and a dissection room.

The clinical medical student's society, the Osler House Club, is based in a fantastic, refurbished building at the John Radcliffe. The building has undergone a multi-million pound extension and

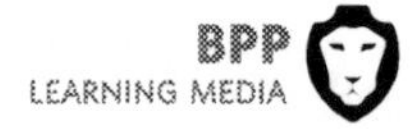

renovation which boasts a large common room, complete with plasma TVs, game consuls, big sofas, a café, bar, IT facilities, office space, kitchen, seminar room, showers and a beautiful garden. In addition, each college has a common room.

Student support

The structure of the collegiate system at Oxford means provision of support is extensive. Students have access to support from peers, colleges, the medical school and the university. Each college has at least one pre-clinical and clinical tutor who, along with providing teaching, are available for support. In addition there are senior tutors at each college who can provide support and guidance in academic and personal matters.

Student run support is very good. Colleges tend to run 'parenting' schemes for pre-clinical students, where a second year becomes your 'parent' and can help with practical things, such as where the best place to go out is, as well as academic and pastoral problems. A parenting scheme is also run for fourth years when you join clinical school. In addition, you are taught history taking and examination skills at the start of the fourth year by sixth years. This 'med-ed' course runs for two weeks and is a fantastic scheme, where you learn a huge amount about clinical skills and life in the hospital from people really keen to teach and can dedicate a large amount of time to make sure you have a strong grounding in basic clinical skills.

Medical societies

A feature that makes Oxford different to the majority of other universities is the set-up of sports and societies. Unlike many universities, the collegiate system means competition is between colleges rather than between faculties. This means that teams/clubs have a mix of people from many different subject areas so you don't spend all your time only socialising with medics (although there is still plenty of time for that!). All levels are provided for, with teams ranging from those who have never played before, to high achievers.

Sport and societies are also an integral part of the university, with competition ranging from the boat race, to the annual Oxford v

London Wasps rugby match. This means that all levels of ability are provided for, from more 'social' college teams, to high achieving university teams.

Clinical students are also well taken care of. During pre-clinical, most students take part in sport and societies with their college, while in clinical school, the majority of students choose to take part in sport/societies with Osler House Club. These teams/clubs work in a similar way to colleges, and compete in the same leagues/competitions. In addition, each year, there is a weekend competition against Cambridge Medical School, finishing with a big party. There is a huge variety of different activities on offer, including sports, orchestra, bands etc. One highlight is the annual Christmas medics' pantomime called Tingewick. The whole of the fourth year take part, either acting, playing music, or behind the scenes. It is written, produced and directed by a group of fifth years, who also put on several events throughout the year to raise money for charity.

Finance

Tuition fee and college fee loans may be available from your local authority.

NHS Bursaries for the clinical years are non-repayable and in the order of £3,000–£4,000, to cover the tuition fees.

Further info: www.medsci.ox.ac.uk/study/medicine/pre-clinical/fees

Student opinion

'The combination of the outstanding one-to-one teaching, great facilities and world-renowned research taking place in stunning surroundings bound in tradition and history makes your years at Oxford truly some of the very best of your life.'

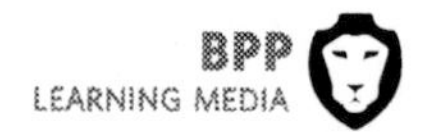

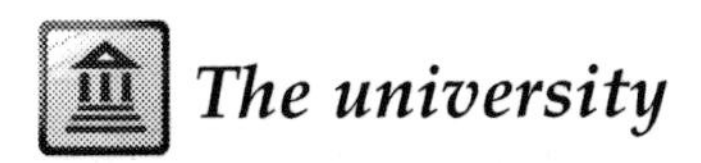

The university

Accommodation	College accommodation
Further Info	Visit individual college websites from: www.ox.ac.uk/colleges

Accommodation

Some colleges offer accommodation for all three or even all six years, the quality and cost of the rooms does vary by college, some may be beautiful old rooms, with en-suites overlooking traditional Oxford quads (though usually these are reserved for second and third years!) others are more typical student rooms but all reach a reasonable standard. Generally all first year accommodation is located on or near the main college sites meaning resources such as catered hall, college libraries, bars, common rooms and chapels are on site for the first years. Generally college accommodation for second years is in annexes, but many third years return to the main college site.

Study facilities

Library facilities in Oxford are exceptional, every college has a library which will stock at least the core medical text books on a reference-only basis and some are open 24 hours a day. The main university science library – the Radcliffe Science Library (RSL) is part of the Bodleian copyright library and thus claims a copy of every book published in the UK which can be ordered by students from the stacks and normally arrive within a couple of hours. The RSL also has an excellent selection of non-UK books and all the core medical text books are available on loan in reasonable numbers. The library is fully equipped with computers, copiers, scanners, a café area and ample desk space. Students are free to visit any other library including the main Bodleian library and Radcliffe Camera, which can provide much needed variation when studying! Medical students also enjoy online access to an inordinate number of scientific and medical journals.

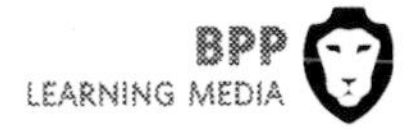

University sports & students' union

All colleges provide sports facilities which may include football, rugby, cricket, tennis squash, or onsite gyms. The university also has the Iffley Road sports centre, where Sir Roger Banister famously ran the first four minute mile. The facilities provided here are extensive including a recently built pool. There are extra costs to the pool and gym area; however colleges or JCRs may provide bursaries to university sports people.

The student union at Oxford is termed 'OUSU' and is rather unlike many other university unions as many of the typical functions of a union are taken by college JCR (junior common room committees). They do not therefore have a central venue, mainly because it would probably only see limited use. OUSU do however have an organisational role, sorting freshers' week, student campaigning and helping with student complaints. They also produce the *Oxford Student*, one of two award winning student newspapers in Oxford.

> **Student opinion**
>
> *'I have had such a great time over the last three years that I cannot recommend Oxford strongly enough, though I could never get across a true sense of its appeal in a few short words, therefore my recommendation to you is to go and see the university, colleges and medical faculty on an open day – you won't be disappointed!'*

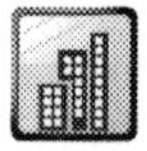

The city

Safety	🛡	🛡	🛡	🛡	🛡	Generally a very safe city and certainly feels this way. Some theft, particularly of bikes
Nightlife	☾	☾	☾	☾		Limited number of clubs but college bops (parties), college bars, pubs, student theatre and comedy make up for it!

Transport						Limited parking in the centre but then you don't need a car there, almost everyone rides a bike and its a quick convenient way to get around. Excellent links to London – 24 hour bus plus fast train
Cost of Living						Not London prices, but price of living is above average, room rents variable, pint £1+, £4 club entry

Things to do

You'll never be short of things to do in and around Oxford, after dining in college be it at a grand formal hall or a quick canteen meal, there's always something going on, down the bar or in the common room. While not renowned for its clubbing scene there's a variety of decent, good value clubs. During term time you'll always find students in one of the many outstanding Oxford pubs, be it the White Horse; Oxford's smallest and oldest pub popular with Winston Churchill, Bill Clinton, Tolkein and Morse, or the King's Arms which reportedly has the highest IQ per square foot of any pub in the world! The Arts have a proud place in Oxford be it productions at the New Theatre or Oxford Playhouse, student productions in colleges are a must see, with an outstanding quality that usually draws crowds of both students or locals. Become a life member of the Oxford Union and there'll be debates, famous speakers, cheap drinks and termly balls a plenty. On the topic of balls, Oxford does them very well, from a grand all-night college quincentenary ball with champagne, fairground rides, fireworks and headline acts, to one of the smaller quainter and cheaper college balls. Both are a must-do at least once during your time in Oxford! It's easy enough to escape Oxford for a lazy afternoon, be it for retail therapy at Bicester shopping village, exploring the grandeur of Blenheim Palace or simply punting down the river to a pub.

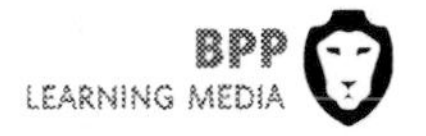

Places to Go		
Place	**Brief Description**	**Entry Fee/Opening Time**
The Bridge	Club, multiple floors, varied music	£4; Mon–Sat open to 3.00am
Purple Turtle	Underground club, student feel	£Free union members/2.00am
Union Bar	Cheap drinks, plush furniture	£Free Mon–Sun till late
Living Room	Gorgeous cocktail bar and restaurant	£Free Mon–Sun till 2.00am

Student opinion

'There is always so much going on within college, the med school and around the city that it is always a challenge to fit everything you want to do in, especially in the summer when your free time is quickly taken up relaxing on a punt on the Cherwell with a cold glass of Pimms!'

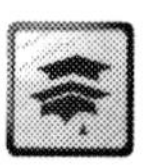

Student's view

Pre-clinical

'Oxford is a great place to live, work and play; it really is a privilege to study here. I have access to some of the best 'medical minds' in the country during lectures, seminars and tutorials and they have a genuine interest and desire for me to succeed. It is a strange situation whereby I live among the grandeur of Oxford's centuries-old sandstone architecture, yet am taught cutting edge science in state of the art facilities. Yes the workload is sometimes heavy, and yes it can be stressful around exam time, but the skills and expertise I have gained and fun I have had in and around Oxford by far outweigh this. The strict science focus has given me the confidence that I can understand any medical condition, and the intercalated year has given me powerful abilities to read, understand and criticise the research literature.

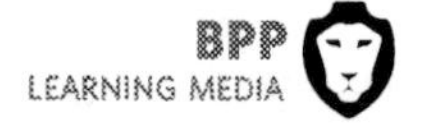

Certainly do not let any stereotypes associated with Oxford put you off applying, in terms of the people there is such a diverse mix you will always find someone on your wavelength, and probably make friends with those you thought you had nothing in common with. The university is traditional, be it wearing "sub-fusc," gowns to formal hall, or waking up at 6.00am on May Day morning to listen to choristers sing from Magdalen Tower, but it's all part of the experience and fun, and being in a college environment means there are always people around to experience it with. Don't be put off either by the amount of work that needs to be done, you'll certainly find time to go out, continue your hobbies and probably take up some more, plus your tutors will expect/demand this of you!'

Clinical

'After having done three years of pre-clinical medicine, where you have experienced very little clinical medicine, starting clinical school is a particularly exciting and enjoyable experience. You very quickly get used to using knowledge which you have picked up during the first three years to apply to the large variety of clinical scenarios which you come across in clinical medicine. As you progress through clinical school, you experience a wide range of different specialities and ways of practising medicine. During rotations in Oxford you have the opportunity to work in teams, which often include eminent consultants and professors and come across interesting, more complex cases, which have been referred to Oxford for specialist care. In contrast, at District General Hospital you typically experience a more common caseload, but have more freedom to go to the clinics and surgery lists that you want to.

During a typical day, you join the morning ward round and help out the F1 with writing in the notes, taking blood and putting in cannulas, while trying to answer the questions the Consultant asks you! During surgery rotations, on the days when your Consultant has surgical list, you join them in theatre. This is a particular highlight as you sometimes will be asked to scrub in and can assist in the operation. After lunch in Osler House, where the café sells delicious made-to-order gourmet sandwiches, you can go to clinic, help out the junior doctors with jobs, or go and practise taking histories and examining patients.

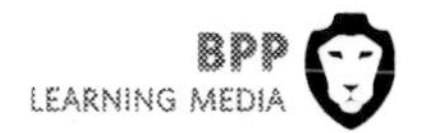

Teaching at clinical school is, on the whole, very good. A particular highlight is small group practical sessions with Dr Lancaster who is an excellent teacher and very enthusiastic.

Of course, for all the highlights of clinical medicine, there are times when you wonder why you chose such a hard career! Ward rounds can sometimes last for hours and sometimes you will turn up for teaching, which then is cancelled at the last minute, which can be frustrating at the time. But in the end, I would never think again about choosing Medicine, and would struggle to think of somewhere where I would rather study it than Oxford.'

Once you get in...

Offer letters are generally received before Christmas Day. You may get a reading list from college or the medical faculty – read them as they may be useful, they are all general interest medical books – no text books or learning to do! You'll get a lovely letter from your college parents, at least one of whom will be a medic and they will hopefully look after you for three years and perhaps beyond! The course starts at a gentle pace and ensures everyone is at the same place.

The Best Thing	One of the world's best universities with fantastic clinical teaching and a great college atmosphere
The Worst Thing	Tourists

Student top tips

- Get a cheap bike. You'll use it for everything but they're liable to get stolen.
- Do the student pantomime (Tingewick) as a way to meet everyone in the clinical school.
- Do as many activities as you can outside Medicine.

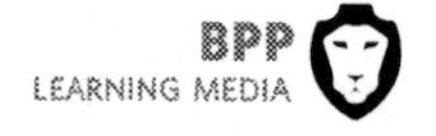

Summary Table

Positives	**Negatives**
Outstanding facilities and teaching	Little integration between pre-clinical and clinical schools
World-renowned research	Limited clinical experience in first three years
Beautiful, historic city	Limited anatomy teaching
Collegiate system	Academically pretty demanding
Loads to do outside medicine	Fairly high living costs

Peninsula

Peninsula Medical School
The John Bull Building
Tamar Science Park
Research Way
Plymouth
PL6 8BU

www.pcmd.ac.uk/

Set in a variety of locations throughout the south-west, from the beaches of Cornwall to the busy streets of Plymouth, Peninsula Medical School (PMS) offers students a diverse range of settings in which to study for their medical degree.

PMS is one of the newest medical schools in the UK. Founded in 2002 by Professor John Tooke, the school uses innovative teaching techniques and early clinical exposure to equip students with the knowledge and skills needed to work in the ever-changing world of the modern NHS.

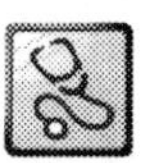

The medical course

Key facts

Course Type	PBL	Degree Awarded	BMBS
Basic Entry Requirements	AAA	Entrance Exams	UKCAT, GAMSAT (if A levels sat more than two years ago)
Year Size	215	Open Days	Plymouth: June Exeter: April
Admissions Website	www.pcmd.ac.uk/		

Getting in – student tips

The medical school, like many, would like your personal statement to show that you have a good understanding of what it means to

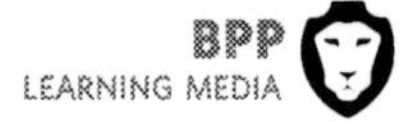

be a doctor, and a high level of motivation towards what can be a long, challenging career.

The PMS interview is very different from the standard medical school interview. For starters the interview panel will not have seen your personal statement so it will be up to you to demonstrate your experience and qualities all over again in the flesh. The same set of questions are posed to all candidates. The questions 'why Medicine?' or even 'why PMS?' will **not** be asked as the school believe that your reasons for studying Medicine will change throughout your career. The interview will start with a questionnaire to fill out (this can be used to select candidates in a tie-break situation). Candidates then pick one of three ethical scenarios, which will form the basis of the first interview question. There then follows a series of questions that should last around 20 minutes. Interviewers mark your answers using a relatively strict mark scheme and those with the highest marks will be offered a place.

While this might sound pretty daunting, the interview is actually a very relaxed affair. On the day there is also a tour of the campus and a chance to chat to some current students.

Course details

Foundation / Pre-Med	N/A	**Graduate**	N/A
Student Population	Male: female ratio: approx 45:55	**Term Length**	Pre-clinical: 12–14 Clinical: 12–15
Erasmus / Foreign Exchange	PMS takes part in a student exchange programme facilitated by the International Federation of Medical Students' Association (IFMSA). These exchanges allow a student in year 3 or 4 to exchange with another medical student from a variety of countries worldwide as part of a four week placement	**Elective Period**	9 weeks from mid-August to mid-October. The start of year 5 is immediately after

Intercalation

Stage	Between year 4 and year 5	**Degree Awarded**	BSc (unless otherwise stated)
Requirements	Maximum 15% of cohort can intercalate. Offered first to students ranking highest in exams and SSCs	**Subjects**	Biosciences, Human Biosciences, Emergency Care, History of Medicine, Animal Science, Exercise and Sports Sciences, Environmental Sciences, Wildlife Conservation, Sport and Exercise Medicine (MSc), Paediatric Exercise Physiology (MSc). Sport and Health Sciences(MSc), History (BA), Education Studies (BA), Childhood and Youth Studies (BA), Psychology (optionally as a BA),English, Media (BA)

Anatomy teaching

Anatomy teaching is integrated with the rest of the course material rather than in distinct anatomy classes or lectures. For example, lectures on the digestive system will normally include parts on the anatomy and embryology of the digestive system as well as the physiology and pathology. Peninsula also put a big emphasis on learning clinically relevant anatomy and applying what you learn to clinical situations. This means that students spend a lot of time interpreting medical imaging such as X-rays and CT scans. 'Living' anatomy is also taught for around an hour per week. During living anatomy students learn to identify anatomical landmarks on each other and on volunteer models so that they are comfortable and competent in the art of physical examination.

Pre-clinical/Years 1–2	
Topics	The course is broken up into Case Units, each centred on a different clinical scenario. There are 16 Case Units that cover the major bodily systems throughout all stages of the human life cycle. Year 1 looks mainly at basic anatomy and physiology whereas in year 2 there is a much bigger focus on disease. Throughout the two years student are also taught the basics of EBP and Clinical Skills.
Teaching	PBL, lectures, small group tutorials, community placements.
SSC Periods	In years 1 and 2 students will undertake five SSCs each lasting three weeks. The topics are wide ranging and all come from three core themes (Biomedical Science, Healthcare Environments, Medical Humanities). In general, Healthcare Environments SSCs are heavily clinical topics involving numerous hospital placements whereas Biomedical Sciences tend to require a much more library based approach. Medical Humanities give students the chance to think of Medicine in a wider context and in relation to other topics like law, art and religion. During each SSC, students will meet an SSC 'provider' a minimum of three times to discuss their progress. Most projects will take the form of a review article which some students do manage to get published.
Exams	Students sit the Applied Medical Knowledge (AMK) test four times per year. The exam is a negatively marked multiple choice exam based on all areas of Medicine. All students from year 1 to 5 sit the same AMK paper. As students progress through the year they will be expected to show clear improvements in their exam marks. Pass marks vary according to how well the year as a whole has performed with the top 10% gaining an 'excellent' and the bottom 5% being deemed 'unsatisfactory'. As the topic base is so broad it's extremely difficult to revise for so the pass marks in the first and second years are very low. There are also various clinical competencies to pass which build up to the end of year 2 ISCEs (Integrated Structured Clinical Examination) where students are assessed on their history taking and physical examination skills. While not an exam as such, professionalism judgments are given in many of the small group sessions which are taken into account when deciding which students pass and fail the year.

Clinical/Years 3–5	
Topics	In the third and fourth years the programme is divided into six, 'Pathways of Care' (with roughly one occurring each term). Each pathway itself is divided into nine weeks with each week corresponding to differing specialties or varying aspects of one specialty. Students rotate through the different weeks, which consist mostly of hospital placements with some community and GP placements as well. Although these are essentially, 'the clinical years', one day a week is also dedicated to lectures, small group sessions, and clinical skills sessions, aimed at supplementing your learning. In the fifth year the emphasis is on the practical implementation of what has been learnt during the previous years. The year is divided into five week blocks in various specialties and students work as part of the healthcare team.
SSC Periods	In the third year there are four SSCs, two of which are similar to the ones undertaken in the first two years, one called, 'working together' – which focuses on multidisciplinary team working, and one called 'management' – which focuses on managerial structures in the NHS. In the fourth year, there are also four SSCs, one of which is again similar to the ones undertaken in the first two years, with the three others focusing on 'Medicine as Art', 'Teaching', and 'Research'. The latter involves an attachment to one of the school's research teams.
Exams	The exam format is the same – the Applied Medical Knowledge (AMK) exam. At the end of the fourth year is a structured clinical exam.

Hospital placements/academies

In the third and fourth year, placements usually last one week and students rotate through the different specialities, whereas in the fifth placements are much longer, comprising five week blocks. There are usually two, occasionally three, students per placement, which is great in terms of access to clinical experience. Peninsula doesn't have large groups of students following consultants around.

Academically, Peninsula has an excellent research reputation in key areas including diabetes, obesity and vascular risk, neurosciences and mental health, and clinical education. As part of the 'research' SSC, students join research groups and are encouraged to develop links with the Medical School researchers.

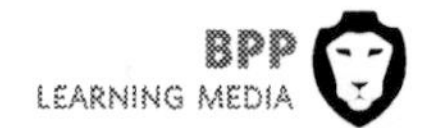

Hospitals and Travel Time from University	
Derriford Hospital	10 minutes
Royal Devon and Exeter	5 minutes
Truro	2 minutes
Exeter DGH	5 minutes
Torbay	10 minutes

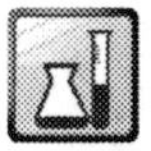

The medical school

Work						Not overworked
Facilities						All the books and clinical equipment you could need are provided and most places have decent opening hours
Support						Every student has an academic tutor and the staff are very approachable
Feedback						AMK results highlight key areas of strengths and weakness. Students get written feedback each term for most group sessions

Facilities

The Life Science Resource Centre has plenty of books, computers, and anatomical models. There is usually the odd member of staff if you get stuck. Due to the university being so new all of the equipment and buildings are modern. Rooms in the Clinical Skills Resource Centre can also be booked with all the equipment to practise a whole range of skills like blood taking and intubation. You can also watch back recordings of yourself taking histories from mock patients in previous clinical skills sessions.

Hospital affiliated libraries, often with rooms available for group study, are open for access 24/7 and have every book you will ever need.

Students also have access to the internet based 'Emily' website. Emily has a number of web resources including recordings of lectures, study guides for clinical skills and life sciences as well as many other computer based resources.

Student support

The two main forms of student support are your academic tutor and your second year 'parent'. Meetings with your parent happen in the first week when you all go out for dinner together. They are there to answer any questions and pass on some of their infinite wisdom as well as to generally to help you settle in throughout the first year and ask how your exams are going. Meetings with your academic tutor happen every term but you can always get in touch with them if you need to ask some questions or have a chat.

Any other problems or enquiries are best directed to the office team at either campus who will usually put you in touch with the right people.

The level of support is generally good as most members of staff are more than willing to help you out if you ask them.

Medical societies

As a Peninsula student you join either the students' guild at the University of Exeter or the students' union at the University of Plymouth giving you access to more than a hundred clubs and societies ranging from football, rugby and hockey through to archaeology, music theatre, surfing and sailing.

If that wasn't enough, there a large number of specific medical societies as well. These range from Medsoc (ie the par-tay society), which organises social events, activities and drinks discounts, to MedSin Peninsula which, arguably, has a slightly more altruistic purpose in that it aims to promote awareness and action concerning humanitarian and health issues across the world. Examples of others include Peninsula Undergraduate Surgeons, Peninsula Marrow, MedCinema, and the Peninsula Undergraduate Newsletter.

Medic sports are well represented and include football, netball and rugby teams (amongst others).

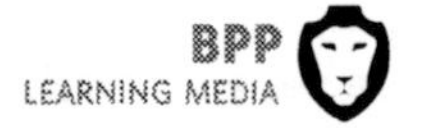

Finance

www.pcmd.ac.uk/finance_undergraduate.php

There is a means-tested national bursary of up to £1,500 pounds available from the college. Students whose household income is less than £35,000 are guaranteed to get something.

Students can also apply for a regional bursary if they have completed their A levels in Devon, Cornwall or Somerset. Bursaries are awarded based on a number of criteria including household income, number of parents, higher education etc.

Student opinion

'So far I've really enjoyed learning Medicine at Peninsula. In the prospectus they emphasised the patient-centred aspect of the course and I think, in fairness, that that has been borne out by my experiences so far. As a new medical school, the staff are determined to ensure that their students do as well as possible, resulting in an environment with a high level of support.'

The university

Accommodation	Campus
Further Info	www.plymouth.ac.uk/pages/view.asp?page=6777 www.exeter.ac.uk/accommodation/residences/selfcatered/rowancroftmews www.exeter.ac.uk/accommodation/residences/selfcatered/rowancroftcourt

Accommodation

Exeter students are all in the same halls based at Rowancroft. The halls are split into two main areas called Rowancroft Court and Rowancroft Mews. There are five people to a flat in Mews but the flats are grouped together in fours so it can feel like there are 20 people in there, so it definitely has a more social atmosphere. Mews also has a very large kitchen in each flat but the bedrooms are pretty tiny. Court however has nine people to a flat with much

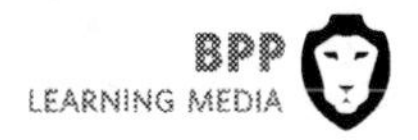

larger rooms but a rather cramped kitchen. Both are a 5- to 10-minute walk from the medical school but a 30-minute walk from the main university campus at Streatham. Both cost £84 per week with bills included.

Students allocated to Plymouth are free to apply for any of the university halls or cluster flats. All are self-catered and within five minutes of the main university campus. Prices range from £76 for a basic single to £121 for large en-suites.

Students at PMS are expected to change locality twice throughout the five years. Students in phase 1 (years 1 and 2) are randomly allocated either Plymouth or Exeter campuses. In phase 2 (years 3 and 4) students could then be placed in either Plymouth, Exeter or Truro and are expected to move away from their phase 1 locality. Phase 3 (year 5) requires students to change locality once more with Torbay and Barnstable also possibilities.

Study facilities

Plymouth University library is open 8.30am–10.00pm on weekdays with a slightly shorter opening time at weekends. Streatham Library is also open. Medics tend to use LSRC rooms or hospital libraries but during SSC periods university libraries are popular as they are pretty quiet and a lot of the research doesn't need medical textbooks (just a heavy dose of pubmed).

University sports & students' union

Both Plymouth and Exeter have large student unions with a variety of eateries, bars and games rooms, doubling up as clubs on the weekends. Exeter union in particular has hosted a fair few well known bands in the past such as the Kooks, Radiohead and Keane. Medics in both localities use them, although arguably the Plymouth union is frequented more often as it is closer.

Sports facilities at Exeter have varying levels of membership ranging from pay as you go (although there is a £30 induction fee) to £235 per year. The sports centre at St Lukes is pretty basic with a swimming pool, a small gym and an indoor sports hall. There are free, non-university affiliated tennis and basketball courts very close to campus.

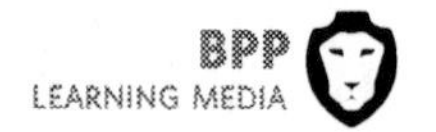

The main Streatham sports centre has a well equipped air conditioned gym, and a huge sports hall.

Freshers' week at Peninsula is incredible. Medsoc hosts events every night, often ending up in drunken fancy dress and late night flat parties. Students can look forward to pirate nights, toga nights, superhero nights and many, many more. Past events for those not keen on clubbing have included dodgeball tournaments, beach trips and paintballing so whatever you're into, freshers' week will definitely be one to remember.

During the daytime you will mainly sit/sleep/cough your way through a few introductory lectures, get yourself formally registered with the medical school and get shown around all the facilities. The medics' freshers' fair is also a great place to sign up to societies and pick up a couple of useful freebies. Popular societies to join are Medsoc, Medsin and PUS.

After the first week, medics then join in with the main university freshers' week which is a great chance to meet a whole new crowd of people. The main campus freshers' fair is also a must, with the chance to join a whole host of societies, ranging from the Rowing society to Beats and Bass society. During the day you will be settled into to all of your teaching groups and even run through a practice PBL case.

Student opinion

'It's unusual to be a member of two universities, but as you progress through the course you come to appreciate the sheer variety of options open to you. Exeter union has access to a great number of bands that pass through the region and concerts are frequent. Plymouth union is great for socialising and you invariably end up bumping (sometimes literally) into someone you know. As a Peninsula Medical School student you literally get two for the price of one!'

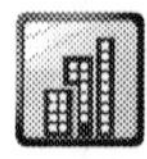

The city

Safety	🛡	🛡	🛡			Exeter is very safe, Plymouth is generally fine
Nightlife	☾	☾	☾			Plenty of cheap pubs and clubs at both campuses
Transport	🚌	🚌	🚌			Parking is very limited at both campuses. Traffic in Exeter can be terrible, Plymouth has pretty average traffic. You can happily get by without a car
Cost of Living	🐖	🐖				Average rent is around £70–80 (but can be as low as £55) in Plymouth a week. Pints range from £1.50–£2.20

Things to do

Exeter and Plymouth are both exciting cities, albeit in different ways. During the day in Plymouth you can relax down by the seaside on the famous Plymouth Hoe, wander around the theatres, galleries and restaurants of the Barbican, or head into the town centre. Exeter, in contrast has a huge amount to offer in terms of shops (both chains and kooky independent ones – you'll know what I mean), many of which are located around its beautiful cathedral.

The nightlife in both cities is pretty good as well. Students in Plymouth tend to head to the student union, smallish bars named 'Cuba' and 'Ride', and the bigger clubs called 'C103' and 'Oceana'. In Exeter, in addition to the student union, students have been known to frequent bars such as, 'The Old Firehouse' and clubs such as the infamous, 'Arena'. A lot of the clubs and bars boast either student discounts or nights dedicated to students. This is in addition to the fact that Medsoc negotiates with some bars to provide discounts during medic socials.

Both cities are safe for the most part, although Plymouth's Union Street is well known for being a bit rough, especially on Saturday nights.

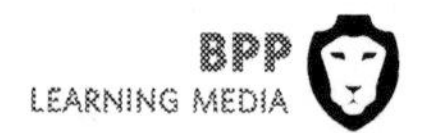

Places to Go		
Place	**Brief Description**	**Entry Fee/Opening Time**
C103 (Plymouth)	Club, student nights on Weds	£3
Cuba (Plymouth)	Bar	Open till 4.00 or 5.00am!
Firehouse (Exeter)	Bar/restaurant	£Free/£1
Arena (Exeter)	Club, student nights on Tues and Thurs	Student nights on Tues and Thurs

Student opinion

'Being a student in Plymouth and Exeter is great fun. Both cities are large enough to contain everything a student would want, but not so sprawling that you end up feeling lost within them. Being close to the sea is a huge bonus, and many medics enjoy the region so much that they end up applying for their Foundation jobs there too.'

Student's view

Pre-clinical

'The pre-clinical years can be frustrating for those who want to just get stuck in with seeing patients, but I remember quite enjoying being eased into Medicine. It helps that the first two years at Peninsula don't just consist of sitting in lecture halls while trying (sometimes unsuccessfully) to stay awake. Rather, the focus is more on learning in teams and small groups, which accurately reflects how doctors actually work in the NHS. It is appealing that Peninsula utilises a wide variety of teaching methods in the first two years – ranging from group tutorials, to sessions in the Life Sciences Resources Room (essentially the medical library for the first two years), to the more traditional lectures (or 'plenaries' as they're called here). Peninsula is one of the newest medical schools in the country – so it goes without saying that everything

is pretty much state of the art. In fact, that was one of the things that impressed me most when I attended the open day.

One of the interesting things about the medical school is that for the first two years the cohort is split in two, with half starting off in Plymouth and the other half in Exeter (in the latter years everyone gets mixed up). Although the actual curriculum is exactly the same and both localities have the same facilities, this ultimately means that the student experience is slightly different. In Plymouth I think it would be fair to say that the medics mix more with non-medics by virtue of the fact that everyone lives in the same halls, whereas in Exeter the medics form more of a community. Additionally, having two localities means there is a degree of (friendly) competitiveness.

Some first years about to start worry about which locality they've been assigned to; however both experiences are equally valid, both cities will provide awesome nights out, and as you progress through the course your closest friends will almost inevitably end up being medics anyway.'

Clinical

'The clinical years are when you make the transition from medical student to student doctor. The emphasis is much more on the clinical approach and symptom-sorting rather than pure science, although of course that's still important. At Peninsula, students are divided up between the three clinical localities (Plymouth, Exeter and Truro) so interestingly you meet some people in your year for the first time (ie those who started off in a different locality). This is unusual but ultimately keeps things fresh, not to mention that it reflects the shifting rotations of a junior doctor.

A typical day might involve joining the medical team on their ward round in the morning, where the Consultant will either teach you or quiz you on what you should know. These rounds provide a good time to get to know the patients on the ward and afterwards normally you would clerk (take a history and examine) some of them. Then, following some lunch, you might head back to the hospital for a fixed placement, (there are usually three or four per week), which vary, depending on the specialty you are attached to that week. For instance, if you were attached to the gastroenterology team, then you might be required to sit in with the Consultant during his outpatients' clinic. A timetable is provided each week, which is normally pretty clear in outlining where you need to be, when, and who with. At the end every week there is a fixed teaching session with the designated Consultant, during which you present an interesting case and are grilled / politely questioned about what you have learnt.

There is an understandable degree of trepidation prior to being let loose on the wards, but most students (myself included) prefer the clinical years. You feel much more like a doctor and I greatly enjoyed simply getting stuck in. This new freedom comes with a degree of responsibility – the onus is more on you in terms of learning and your spare time is curtailed to a greater degree – but most students manage to happily strike up a good balance between Medicine and having a social life. I'm loathe to use the old cliché of "working hard/playing hard", but that's precisely what the clinical years are about.'

Once you get in...

The medical school sends out all the information you need to get you started with things like vaccinations etc. The main thing they will want you to have done *before* you turn up is to have a Hepatitis B *surface antigen test*. Be very specific about the exact test you need as large number of GPs have been known to send the blood samples for the wrong test. In your first fortnight you will have a meeting with some occupational health people to get a plan of jabs in place.

There is also a brilliant leaflet from Medsoc telling you all about freshers' fortnight and the things you might need to bring. Later on you get sent all the details about applying for accommodation (which can all be done online) along with the reading list and a couple of student agreement forms to sign.

On the accommodation front, it is worth thinking hard about what accommodation would suit you best as even in Exeter, while there are only two options, the experiences in halls can be very different. In Plymouth, where the choice is much greater, you need to think carefully at the money side of things. While a big room with an en-suite may sound nice, come the end of term when money is tight, you might be wishing you had a bit more money to go out with.

The Best Thing	Hands-on teaching and beautiful locations
The Worst Thing	Finding motivation during a heavily self-directed course

Student top tips

- An interesting fact about Peninsula would be that the Dean, Professor Sir John Tooke, led the independent inquiry into 'Modernising Medical Careers', the post-graduate training structure for medical doctors in the UK. Given that this training programme affects pretty much every doctor in the country this is, like, a big deal.
- Whatever you do, do NOT buy everything on the reading list, even all the ones with a star next to them. You can do fine using library loans and the internet. Find out what ones you like before splashing out hundreds of pounds. By all means buy a few, if you wish but it is by no means essential. The only book that pretty much every student finds useful is Kumar and Clark.

Summary Table

Positives	Negatives
Regular feedback on all areas of the course	Moving location
Early clinical training placements and chances to practise history taking on actors	A bit isolated from main campus at Exeter
Strong focus on applying knowledge to clinical practice	Lack of dissection
Beautiful scenery and beaches close to all locations	As the campuses are split you don't get to see everyone in your year at first
Friendly, relaxed teaching	

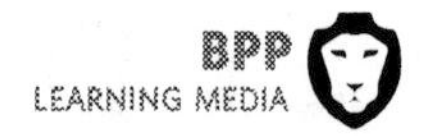

Sheffield

The Medical School
University of Sheffield
Beech Hill Road
Sheffield
S10 2RX

www.shef.ac.uk/medicine/

Sheffield, renowned for its steel working history, the Full Monty and the Snooker World Championship at the Crucible, is a vibrant and exciting city, which also has the delights of the Peak District on its doorstep.

The city, the university and the medical school are a mixture of tradition and new developments, with the students' union renowned as one of the best in the UK.

Sheffield offers quite a traditional approach to medical education in a well-organised and friendly manner, incorporating clinical teaching from early on.

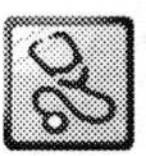 *The medical course*

Key facts

Course Type	Traditional	Degree Awarded	MBChB
Basic Entry Requirements	AAA	Entrance Exams	UKCAT
Year Size	Approx 250	Open Days	June/July/Sept
Admissions Website	www.shef.ac.uk/medicine		

Getting in – student tips

There is usually a member of the faculty, a senior student and a medical professional eg a GP on the interview panel. They will all have a copy of your personal statement, which will have been highlighted and scribbled on, so know it inside out, because the vast majority of question will come from it! Standard questions include 'Why Medicine?', 'Why Sheffield?', 'What recent medical news have you read about?'. They may ask about ethical issues eg euthanasia. You must know the structure of the course well before the interview. It is easy to find out about and a very easy way of slipping up in an interview.

Course details

Foundation / Pre-Med	Yes	**Graduate**	Yes
Student Population	Male: female ratio: 45:55	**Term Length**	Pre-clinical: 10 weeks Clinical: 15 weeks
Erasmus / Foreign Exchange	N/A	**Elective Period**	Year 4 – 7 weeks

Intercalation

Stage	At any stage after phase 1 (after finishing year 2)	**Degree Awarded**	BScMedSci
Requirements	Top half of the year	**Subjects**	A broad range of research subjects with associated funding is available each year including Cancer Studies, Physiology, Psychiatry, Immunology and Pathology

Anatomy teaching

Students at Sheffield are very lucky because anatomy is taught in the traditional way by cadaveric dissection. During the first and second year, two to three hours per week is dedicated to time in the dissection room. A group of eight shares a cadaver and throughout the first year the thorax, abdomen and parts of the head are dissected. During the second year the limbs, the brain and other organs not covered in first year are dissected (eg the kidneys and the thyroid gland). Both experienced anatomy teachers and F2 doctors, who provide very high quality teaching, supervise all of the dissection.

Pre-clinical/Years 1–2	
Topics	***Year 1:*** *I*ntroduction to medical sciences: eight weeks Cardiovascular system: four weeks Respiratory system: four weeks Introductory Clinical Experience (ICE): three weeks Gastro-intestinal system/liver/neoplasia: eight weeks. ***Year 2:*** Genitourinary, endocrine, skin, immunology, reproduction: eight weeks Neurosciences and musculoskeletal medicine: eight weeks Research SSC: six weeks.
Teaching	Lectures, small group teaching.
SSC Periods	There is one SSC in the second year. This is a six-week research attachment. Pairs of students are attached to a research team (varies from lab based research, to medical education research, to clinical research). Students are involved in collecting data, analysing it and presenting it. All students must write up what they have done and this is assessed. Some are asked to present to their supervisor or research team. There is a chance of achieving a publication as a result of this attachment.
Exams	Modified Essay Question (MEQ) paper. This consists of short answer questions based around cases. Often found to be the most challenging exam. Extended Matching Question (EMQ) paper. 90 multiple choice questions (not negatively marked). Multi-station exam. Takes place in the dissection room. Anatomy spotter questions, histology and a small number of clinically-based stations.

Clinical/Years 3–5	
Topics	***Phase 2 (first half of year 3):*** Introduction to clinical skills and clinical practice, two nine-week clinical attachments. ***Phase 3 (second half year 3, year 4, first half year 5):*** Obstetrics & gynaecology, paediatrics, psychiatry, GP, specialties (infectious diseases, haematology, oncology, etc), A&E, anaesthetics, general care (rheumatology, orthopoedics, etc). ***Phase 4 (second half year 5):*** Prescribing and preparation for foundation years.
SSC Periods	20% of the course is SSCs. There is a six-week period in phase 3a where there is an opportunity to do any non-medical topic, chance to do something abroad eg learn a language! There is a one-week SSC at the end of specialties to experience more of one of the specialties you enjoyed.
Exams	At the end of each phase: years 1 and 2 May / June, year 3 Dec, year 4 Dec, year 5 Jan and May / June. MEQs, EMQs, OSCE from year 3 +. Students failing have to resit all parts of the exam. Failing resits involves re-doing the whole year. Can only repeat a year once throughout the course.

Hospital placements/academies

Free accommodation is provided at all of the hospitals. The quality of accommodation varies in each hospital from quite dingy shared bathroom rooms in Grimsby to en-suite rooms with a TV in Scunthorpe. Placements are in blocks of eight weeks, however it does vary. During phase 3b there are eight specialty placements, which last one week, and four general care placements lasting two weeks. Phase 3b also has A&E and anaesthetic attachments that last four weeks each. The number of students on any one placement varies depending on the hospital you are placed in. In the central teaching hospitals there can be up to 10 students split into pairs, compared to the district teaching hospitals where there are usually two to four students.

Although the central teaching hospitals are more convenient, teaching on the whole is better in the district generals. Placements at Chesterfield and Rotherham are very enjoyable. Being placed in Scunthorpe or Grimsby can be a bit lonely, however you can only be there for phase 2 or 3b. Sheffield has a children's hospital to which many unusual cases get sent. Placements here are very interesting and provide a good opportunity to observe unusual cases.

Hospitals and Travel Time from University	
Northern General Hospital	20 minutes
Royal Hallamshire Hospital	2 minutes
Barnsley Hospital	30 minutes
Rotherham Hospital	20 minutes
Doncaster Hospital	30 minutes
Chesterfield Royal Hospital	45 minutes
Grimsby Hospital	1 hour
Scunthorpe Hospital	1 hour
Bassetlaw hospital	30 minutes
Pontefract Hospital	50 minutes

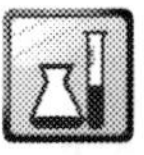

The medical school

Work						Good work life balance
Facilities						Plenty of IT facilities and small group rooms in the library
Support						Many opportunities for support and guidance throughout the course
Feedback						Currently starting to introduce more individual feedback on examinations

Facilities

Sheffield medical school is attached to the royal Hallamshire hospital itself. Within the hospital there is a medical library with plenty of computers available and small group rooms available for students to book. There are three main lecture theatres and numerous seminar rooms. There is a large histology lab and a clinical skills centre. There is a very good simulation suite in Mexborough available to medical students later on in the course.

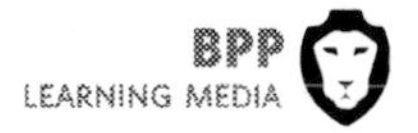

Student support

There is plenty of student support available at Sheffield. From the start of the course a 'parenting' system is in place. You are assigned to two third year students who will meet up with you when necessary. Each set of 'parents' differs in how they offer support. It can vary from emailing to meeting up regularly for a drink and a chat.

All halls of residence have tutors as well who are open to chat about any problems you may have, academically or socially. Medical students are also assigned a mentor, usually someone involved in the medical school such as a professor. You meet up with them each term to check there are no problems. If there are any problems with any of the mentors the medical school can assign you a more suited mentor. You can contact any of these people if there is a problem. The mentoring system is especially good if you think a problem may affect your work, as they will liaise with the medical school to make them aware of the problem.

University health offers a good general practice to all students. They also have an online booking appointment system so there are usually available slots when needed.

Medical societies

There are 250 different sports clubs and societies to get involved with at Sheffield. MedSoc is the largest society in the university. It is student-led and supports med students throughout the course organising social and academic events. Medsex and Stop AIDS are also good societies that educate schools and the public as well as organising fund raising events. Being a medic at Sheffield makes it very easy to meet new people as there is so much going on.

There are a wide variety of sports to get involved in with varying standards – football, rugby, running, bouldering, golf, hockey, tennis, badminton etc. Give-it-a-go sessions are available for beginners and more advanced players are welcomed to the teams. There are some high standards in the sports teams with the mixed hockey team reaching the final three times and semi-final once in recent years.

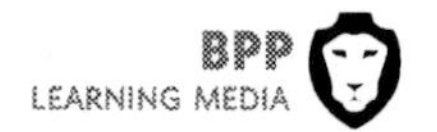

Sheffield medics are renowned for playing and partying hard and hosting the famous fancy dress four-legged bar crawl when 1,300 medics and some non-medics get involved.

Finance

There are a few hardship funds available to students. Full Maintenance Grant of £2,906 available to students whose household income is classed as low income (below £25,000). Partial grant available for those from a 'middle-income' (between £25,001 and £50,000). Scholarships and awards available for international students.

In the final year the NHS provide an income-assessed bursary.

www.shef.ac.uk/medicine/prospective_ug/applying/feesandbursaries.html

Student opinion

'I have thoroughly enjoyed all aspects of Sheffield Medical School. There is so much opportunity to be involved in both socially and academically from the start. The friendliness of the city also adds to the experience.'

The university

Accommodation	There are a number of different halls in different areas, all within a ten-minute walk from the university
Further Info	www.shef.ac.uk/union/

Accommodation

There are three main areas of university accommodation:

1. In the city centre – about ten minutes to the main university and 15 minutes to the medical school. Mainly self-catered accommodation.

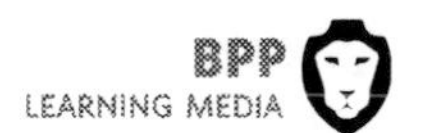

2. Endcliffe village – about ten minutes from the med school and 15 minutes to the main university. Catered and self-catered. Around the nice area of Broomhill. There is 'The Edge' in this area, which includes IT facilities, a bar and laundry area and the dining room for the catered areas.
3. Tapton Hall – one of the older halls. Ten minutes from the med school, 15 minutes from the main university. Catered accommodation, and there are two main blocks; the older fondly named 'prison block' and the newer more luxury block. You get the most authentic 'halls experience' at Tapton.

Study facilities

The medical school library is heavily used, as are the other university libraries. The Information Commons (IC) is very popular and includes a lot of computers, library books is open 24 hours per day. It even has a café which is open during the day. There is the much older 'western bank' library which is far more traditional, but very quiet and great for revision.

Medics often use the other libraries instead of the medical school library, especially during revision and exam time to get away from stressed medical students!

University sports & students' union

The main gym 'S10' and the attached Goodwin Sports Centre is about a five-minute walk from the medical school. The gym has very up-to-date machines and offers good student and also a special medics' membership. For peak yearly membership it usually costs about £250 at the start of the year when there is an offer or monthly peak membership costs around £30 per month. This gives access to the 33m swimming pool and all exercise classes as well. Goodwin Sports Centre includes a sports hall, four squash courts, the 'matrix' indoor climbing and bouldering wall and astroturf pitches which are used for sports matches and can be booked for personal use.

The students' union at Sheffield is one of the biggest, best and most well renowned in the UK. It is situated at the heart of the university and is about a five-minute walk from town and a five-minute walk from the medical school. It has many facilities including the 'Interval

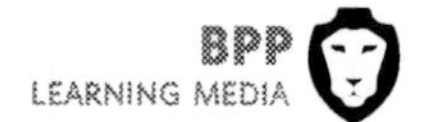

Café' which is very popular, Coffee Revolution, more places to eat and drink than you can imagine, the 'Fusion and Foundry' which is used for club nights and the Box Office. There are IT facilities, 'The Source' where you can find out everything that is going on with the union societies and even a cinema on the lower floor which is used for lectures during the day and cheap films in the evenings. Any student support needed can be found at the union.

Student opinion

'Sheffield is a fantastic place to live as a student and has got a lot to offer. The city and surrounding Peak District fulfils the interests of anyone. It is a cheap city to live in and isn't too big so it never takes too long to get anywhere around the university or the city. The nightlife is varied and great fun. The students' union offers a huge amount in terms of student support, activities and fun. The facilities for accommodation, study and revision are vast and these meet the needs of any student.'

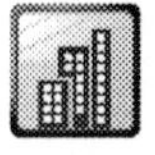

The city

Safety						Safety is about average for a British city. Just be sensible – don't walk through the common at night, or leave your new bike unlocked
Nightlife						There're some popular, sticky-floored student favourites in Portswood, a handful of bars and clubs in Bedford Place and more still further into town
Transport						Parking can be a bit tricky close to the uni and in town, and roads do get quite busy at rush hour

Cost of Living						Quite low, especially if you're not set on living in the middle of the student ghettos, such as Portswood. In the region of £275–£300 pcm. Taxis are fairly average – £10 back to campus or halls from the middle of town

Things to do

Sheffield is a fun place to be a student with great nightlife and lots of things to do in your spare time.

Places to Go		
Place	**Brief Description**	**Entry Fee/Opening Time**
Plug	Spacious range of music, indie, 80s, 90s, chart music	Different depending on event
Embrace	Massive club with five rooms	Around £5
DQ	Chilled night out with a variety of music	Depends on night

Student opinion

'It's fun being a student living in the city, as all the bars and pubs are close together. Everything is literally on your doorstep and you can walk anywhere. If you are an indie music lover, you are spoilt for choice!'

Student's view

Pre-clinical

'The first and second year (phases 1a and 1b) focus on medical science of the main body systems with some clinical teaching, but there is always a clinical slant to the lectures given. Lectures are performed by experts in their prospective fields with enthusiasm and a love for their subject. Anatomy classes are especially good.

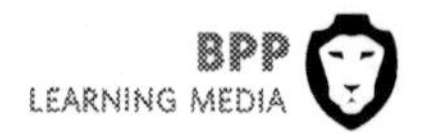

The timetable for the first two years isn't too heavy. A typical day has lectures in the morning and either a free afternoon or a practical session (anatomy is once a week in the afternoon and there is rarely more than one other afternoon practical during the week). This leaves plenty of time for both study and for people to live a 'normal student life' and get involved with sports and societies.

Exams aren't easy, but steady work throughout the year and learning lectures as you go will give you everything you need to pass. The MEQ paper usually proves tough in both the first and second year. Feedback from exams and feedback in general throughout the course has improved and more work is being done to improve this after student comments.

The reasons I chose Sheffield were because of the course, especially because of dissection and high quality anatomy teaching, the city itself because it really lends itself to a fantastic student life and the proximity of the Peak District.

Highlights of my pre-clinical years were the two-week attachment (ICE) in the first year, anatomy teaching, helping to set up the medics' running club and medics' big band and of course the medics' four-legged fancy dress bar crawl.

The advice I'd give to anyone starting at Sheffield is to get stuck in to every aspect of university life. Work hard and play hard and you will love life as a pre-clinical student in a fantastic city.'

Clinical

'I have enjoyed the clinical part of the course the most. It is brilliant to experience what the clinical setting is like and to view how life as a doctor might be. Teaching can literally take place anywhere; my favourite has to be over a take-away pizza lunch in the doctors' mess with a cup of tea!

A usual day of placement would start with teaching on a ward round. This can be a bit tedious but it is an important aspect of clinical placements and there are opportunities to be involved in the plan of the patients, making it a bit more interesting! Helping out the junior doctors with their jobs is always appreciated and can provide a good teaching opportunity as this will be you in a

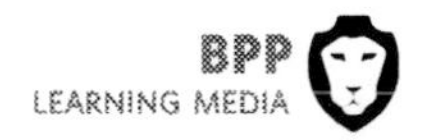

couple of years! In the afternoon there are usually clinics taking place that you can attend and receiving teaching from the more experienced doctors is really useful. In some clinics, seeing new patients is a great way to practise history taking and presenting to the doctors. I find this the most useful although it can be a bit daunting to start! The best way to take advantage of the clinical opportunities and increase your learning is to be proactive.'

Postgraduate

'I can remember many spent days spent as a first year medical student. The timetable for most days comprised a whole day of lectures with some practical classes. I found the lectures sometime tedious and boring even though they were well taught. The whole year would attend in a massive lecture theatre and one of the highlights was getting to meet new people everyday. Sometimes the lecturers were very good and I would listen and pay attention. However at other times you could not hear properly and they would be pointless.

Being a postgraduate, it was harder to mix with everyone but I soon found out there were other postgraduates on the course.'

Once you get in...

Once accepted and you have got your exam results you will be sent information on the university and the different halls of residence. You put your top choices of where you would like to live during your first year and whether you would like to be self-catered or catered and send this back to the university.

You will be sent information on the sports centre and the opportunity to join the gym at a discounted rate before you get to Sheffield. This is definitely advisable as during freshers' week the gym will be very busy with students trying to join. Also when you arrive it is worth booking your induction as soon as possible.

You will also be sent information about freshers' week, what events there are, maps of how to get around and the chance to buy your Freshers' Ball tickets to avoid disappointment. After you have been allocated a hall of residence, you will be sent more detailed information on where to go on your first day.

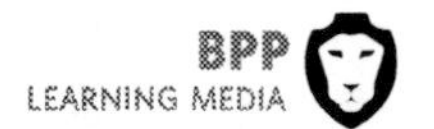

The Best Thing	The way the course is run
The Worst Thing	There's not much to show your mum when she comes to see the city

Student top tips

- One of the first UK med schools to embrace the idea of offering graduate medicine, I think they are getting better and better at it and offer a very good course for graduates.
- Expect to meet a diverse group of very driven people who all motivate each other to do well.

Summary Table

Positives	**Negatives**
Early clinical teaching	Excessive reflection
Fancy dress four-legged bar crawl	Steep hills
University / town / medical school all very close	Placements in Grimsby
Beautiful peak district 10 minutes away	No top flight rugby or football teams to watch
One of the best union's in the country	Traffic delays, one-way system in centre

Southampton

School of Medicine
Southampton General Hospital
Tremona Road
Southampton, Hampshire
SO16 6YD

www.som.soton.ac.uk

Southampton is the largest city on the south coast with a population of over 300,000. Despite it's size, Southampton has a small city feel and as a result may appeal to those wanting the best of both worlds: decent nightlife, varied leisure opportunities, fantastic shopping facilities and great places to eat and drink can all be found alongside beautiful parks (the city being one of the greenest in the UK), bustling marinas and fascinating heritage attractions. The university itself is based in lovely welcoming surroundings with an exciting campus culture. The city is also within close proximity of the New Forest and historic cities of Winchester and Salisbury. The cities of Bournemouth, Poole and Brighton are nearby, and traveling to London takes just over an hour by train. Southampton Airport connects Southampton with the rest of the world for those a little more ambitious!

The medical school is spread across three of the university's six state of the art campuses and is based at a top teaching hospital – Southampton General.

The medical course

Key facts

Course Type	Traditional	Degree Awarded	BM BMedSci
Basic Entry Requirements	AAA	Entrance Exams	UKCAT
Year Size	Approx 175	Open Days	Sept
Admissions Website	www.som.soton.ac.uk		

Getting in – student tips

Southampton is one of the few medical schools in the UK that does not normally interview students applying for the five-year undergraduate course. Students applying for the four-year graduate course and six-year widening access course are required to attend an interview as well as certain mature non-graduate and foreign students. As a result, applicants who meet the academic entry requirement are chosen primarily on the quality of their application and personal statement. The medical school looks for students who are 'self-motivated and have initiative', are 'literate and articulate', 'able to interact' well with others and 'have learnt from their experience of interacting with people in health or social care settings'.

Course details

Foundation / Pre-Med	Yes	**Graduate**	Yes
Student Population	Male: female ratio: 40:60	**Term Length**	Pre-clinical: 12 weeks Clinical: Variable
Erasmus / Foreign Exchange	N/A	**Elective Period**	Between year 3 and 4 lasting 8 weeks

Intercalation

Stage	Between year 3 and year 4	**Degree Awarded**	BSc
Requirements	Those achieving best marks in Intermediates at end of third year	**Subjects**	Medical Sciences

Anatomy teaching

Anatomy is taught by a combination of the study of prosected specimens in the dissecting room, lectures, and small group tutorials with one of the anatomy lecturers for troubleshooting. It amounts to about two or two and half hours per week. Arguably, you'd be likely to forget a lot of the intricate, in-depth anatomy knowledge which you simply don't draw much upon in the clinical context –

wait until you're sitting your exams to be a surgeon if that's your cup of tea; no need to fixate anatomy at this stage.

Pre-clinical/Years 1–2	
Topics	***Year 1:*** Foundation of Medicine Nervous and Locomotor Systems Respiratory, Cardiovascular and Renal Systems. ***Year 2*** *(builds on Year 1 knowledge and skills):* Nervous and Locomotor Systems Respiratory, Cardiovascular & Renal Systems Gastrointestinal System Endocrinology and the Life Cycle.
Teaching	The teaching in the first two years is made up mainly of lectures, symposia and tutorials with some practical sessions. Weekly or fortnightly an afternoon is spent with either a GP or hospital consultant as part of the Medicine in Practice Programme (MIP).
SSC Periods	One afternoon/morning a week students have the opportunity to work on a health-related topic of choice. There are two student selected units (SSU) units in each of the pre-clinical years. In the first unit of year one students choose a local community group and carry out an agreed project with them (eg producing literature or running a workshop). The second unit involved exploring areas of medicine through humanities (ie drama, creative writing, art etc).
Exams	The first two years are divided into four semesters. At the end of each semester there are exams on the material covered. These exams consist of a mixture of Short Note, Extended Short Notes, One Best Answer and Extended Matching Answer papers. Anatomy & Histology are assessed by a spotter exam (several specimens, slides and pictures in the dissection room which students are expected to identify and/or answer questions – one minute is given for each station). In addition there are practicals, presentations, coursework and assignments throughout the year.

Clinical/Years 3–5	
Topics	***Year 3:*** Medicine Block (12 weeks – Medicine and Elderly Care), Surgical Block (12 weeks – Surgery and Obs and gynae), Community Block (12 weeks – Child Health, Psych and Primary care). ***Year 4:*** Study in depth and short specialist attachments – Head and Neck, Ophthalmology, Neurology, Dermatology, Genito-Urinary Medicine, Orthopaedic Surgery and Rheumatology. Also 14 half days of Primary Care. ***Year 5:*** Six weeks Medicine in practice (four weeks acute and two weeks community) followed by attachments in Medicine, Surgery, Obstetrics and Gynaecology, Child Health, Psych, Primary care and a Clinical student selected unit.
SSC Periods	Four-week clinical SSU in the fifth year – options to spend more time in a speciality of your choosing. Possibilities to organise an SSU anywhere in the world.
Exams	Exams in each semester in the first two years. BM Intermediates at end of third year include OSCEs and writtens, must be passed to go on elective and are basis of quartiles used for Foundation Application. BM finals at end of final year consisting of OSCEs and writtens covering the whole course content.

Hospital placements/academies

Third year placements are based in Southampton, Winchester and Portsmouth and are non-residential. Travel expenses are reimbursed by the school of medicine for travel outside Southampton. Placements can be quite busy in Southampton due to large numbers of students.

Fourth year placements are all based out of Southampton and Portsmouth and are also non-residential.

Fifth year placements involve placements all across the south of England in hospitals in Hamsphire, Wiltshire, Dorset, Sussex and Surrey. Accommodation and atmosphere varies between hospitals however there are many opportunities for BBQs on the beaches and mess nights out with the junior doctors.

Hospitals and Travel Time from University	
Southampton General	15 minutes
Royal South Hants	10 minutes
Winchester	20 minutes
Portsmouth	30 minutes
Basingstoke	40 minutes
Chichester	45 minutes
Bournemouth	45 minutes
Salisbury	45 minutes
Poole	55 minutes
Frimley Park	1 hour
Dorchester	1 hour 20 minutes
Guildford	1 hour 20 minutes
Isle of Wight	1 hour 20 minutes
Wexham Park, Slough	1 hour 20 minutes

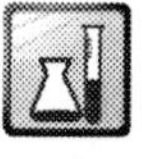

The medical school

Work	■	■				Good work life balance
Facilities	■	■	■			Facilities vary hugely between hospitals. Hospitals outside Southampton often have the most to offer
Support	■	■	■	■		The support at Southampton is renowned for being great and helping people whatever their problems
Feedback	■	■	■			Feedback is steadily improving however but feedback received for submitted essays remains limited

Facilities

There is a dedicated medical library in Southampton General Hospital where the School of Medicine is based. Also within the south academic block of the hospital there are a couple of IT

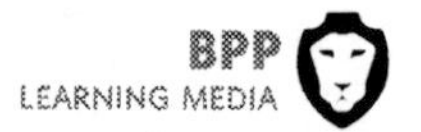

suites owned by the university. The medical school unfortunately lacks a common room at the hospital. Also in the hospital there is a large clinical skills departments used by both the hospital and the medical school.

Student support

The student support at Southampton is renowned. While every medical student has a dedicated personal tutor throughout their time at medical school there is also great pastoral tutor service catering for all students. New students will also be linked to a buddy in one of the upper years who will be there to answer any questions that they might have. There is also a lot of welfare support available from the university and students' union.

Medical societies

The medical society (Medsoc) is one of the biggest societies at the university and offers a lot to all of its members. Medsoc organise events throughout the year catering for all tastes including a toga party, scrubs crawl as well as hosting a huge Christmas ball. Medsoc membership also gets you discounts at bars and restaurants across town.

The medic's sports teams compete at high levels often dominating the intra-mural leagues and competing in leagues against other medical schools. Rugby, football and mixed hockey teams more than hold their own when competing against the university teams.

You will find that your halls mates not studying medicine will be envious of all the organised socials and sports teams that it is easy to get involved with and while they are sitting in their room watching Jeremy Kyle re-runs you are out trying new sports, getting involved with charities or hitting the streets of Southampton dressed as a smurf.

Further info: www.medsoc.susu.org

Finance

There are university bursaries and hardship funds available

Further info: www.som.soton.ac.uk/undergrad/money/

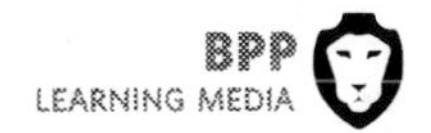

Student opinion

'Southampton is a fantastic place to be studying Medicine. The systems-based integrated course evokes interest from early on with patient contact from the first week. Within each system module normal function is taught alongside pathology in a clinically relevant way. Regular clinical symposia led by specialists cover all major diseases affecting each system in an informative and interesting way. At Southampton you feel like you are being actively taught by the experts and not just expected to go and learn everything yourself.'

The university

Accommodation	Non-campus
Further Info	www.susu.org/

Accommodation

All year 1 students are guaranteed accommodation in halls of residence (as long as the relevant criteria are met – see website for details). There are three main hall complexes in Southampton: Small Halls, Wessex Lane and Glen Eyre. Each of these complexes consists of several individual halls. There are other complexes outside Southampton, but medical students should not be placed in these.

There is a large variety in the size, character and facilities offered by different halls. The prices also vary. However, they all offer good quality accommodation in safe and friendly surroundings. Catering and self-catered options are available and all rooms have telephones, most with network points. All halls have access to laundrettes, and many have a mix of bars, fitness suites, computer suites, common rooms, rooms adapted for students with disabilities and secure bicycle storage.

Study facilities

There are five university libraries: four in Southampton, one in Winchester. The primary library is Hartley on the main campus.

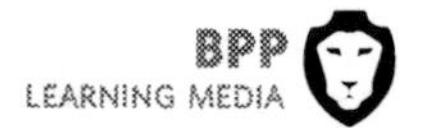

This facility along with the Health Services Library at the General Hospital, are the libraries which support the Medical and Science courses. Each library is well equipped with up-to-date IT equipment and an excellent library database system. Each campus has IT facilities. The medical course is highly dependent on IT, with all lecture notes, timetables, course information and teaching aids (including virtual patients) being on the medical school's MEDIS site.

University sports & students' union

£125 will get you one year's Sports & Recreation membership (Sport Rec) in the year 20011–2012: this is electronically added onto your student ID. This membership enables you to access to the university's excellent sports facilities, including the state of the art Jubilee Sports centre (with a 25-metre swimming pool and 160 fitness stations). Being a coastal city, all manner of maritime activities are catered for. Whatever sport you are into, you will find it at Southampton.

Further info: www.sportrec.soton.ac.uk

Southampton has an extremely active students' union. Based on campus, the union runs bars, a night club, cafés, a shop, travel centre and cinema among other facilities. The union organises and runs high quality events often featuring top performers. It is also the organisation which all societies, clubs and sports teams are affiliated to. The union aims to represent students, develop a sense of community, develop and maintain good relations with the university, other organisations and local community.

Student opinion

'Southampton as a city offers the best of both worlds: a big city with a small feel. It is a welcoming place, which one grows to love more and more. Combined with a fine university, and well structured medical course, this is an excellent place to study Medicine.'

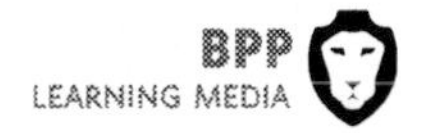

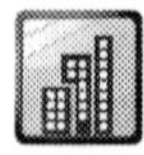 *The city*

Safety						Southampton is a relatively safe city with crime not being a huge problem
Nightlife						There are a good number of clubs in the city but by the time you enter the fifth year they may have become a little tedious
Transport						While parking is generally not too bad Southampton is proud to have the greatest density of traffic lights in the country
Cost of Living						Rent varies from £250–400 per month and beers can vary from 50p to £3.50 a pint depending on the night

Things to do

There is plenty of shopping to be done in the relatively new West Quay centre in the centre of town, with all the big high street brands and a massive John Lewis to be found there. Our newest asset is a big blue IKEA, perfect to get that much needed pot plant to complete your new room. Southampton Common, a massive green space stretching from the campus in the north of the city right down towards the middle of town is a great place for a jog, a summer BBQ or a cozy pint at the Cowherds. In terms of going out there are at least three main places to go: the union, the student dives of the cheerful and well meaning area of Portswood, and the town centre itself, where there's your usual selection of clubs and bars, many of which fit a student budget.

Looking slightly further afield for the more adventurous, the New Forest national park is only a few miles west of the city and great for weekend hiking / mountain biking / wild pony taming etc; the historic and very lovely Winchester is nearby, and you have great access to the Solent for all manner of watersports.

Places to Go		
Place	**Brief Description**	**Entry Fee/Opening Time**
Jesters	Legendary club not to be missed	From 9.00pm. Prices vary. Cheap
Cube	Student union club	From 9.00pm Fridays and Saturdays
Orange Rooms	Cool cocktail bar and club – often hosts great music nights	All day every day
Oceana	Superclub	Every night

Student opinion

'Southampton itself isn't a highlight of the experience of being at Southampton University. Saying that, it is a relatively cheap city to live in and has a large population of like-minded students, both at Southampton Uni, and at Solent Uni down the road. What's more, there are some very nice places close-by and connections to London are good (an hour and ten minutes from Parkway station to London Waterloo)...'

Student's view

Pre-clinical

'I had the view that the first two years would be a time of pure fun and games: having endured the ordeal of getting into medical school, I expected the pre-clinical years would be a case of doing the minimal amount of work possible. However, from quite early on, I realised that Medicine is a demanding course! Although the majority of teaching does not require compulsory attendance, most students choose to be present. If one attends everything, the timetable is pretty full from 9.00am–5.00pm Monday to Friday with lectures, tutorials and practical sessions. However, Wednesday afternoons are free and there are gaps in the timetable (something that changes every week). Sometimes one gets fed up at sitting in lecture theatres hour after hour.

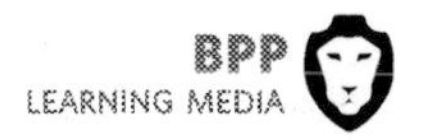

Keeping the long-term goal in sight aids this condition, and is helped in Southampton by the early weekly/fortnightly clinical exposure as part of the Medicine in Practice Unit (MIP). The course in Southampton has a lot of focus on sociology, ethical issues, and team-working (there is a whole inter professional learning unit). These along with the Student Selected Units do provide variety from the bread and butter science. It can be tough returning back to halls after a long day to find other non-medic flatmates sometimes still in bed, having had a day free from anything! However, the family of medics is a really close-knit one with a strong sense of community across the years. Medics do tend to spend a lot of social time together.

However, in the first two years, medical students are able to integrate well with other students from other courses, which provides good variation. Lectures are as much of a social tool as they are a teaching one. We may work the hardest, but also play the hardest, and there are plenty of opportunities to get rid of stress! It is important to get the right balance between work and play. I feel one must work hard enough to pass, but still have fun. I did not manage this initially, failing my Semester 1 exams and having to re-take that summer – something I would recommend against having to do! Exam time is particularly tough, as it is in any university. Something Southampton deserves praise for, is the superb student support available. There is always someone to talk to when things are not going so well personally or academically. One feels that the staff and administration really want students to be happy and succeed.'

Clinical

'A typical day in the clinical years involves a full day and an early start although this varies a lot between surgery and psych attachments. Being present at the Consultant ward rounds can often be a good teaching experience but also gains you valuable credit with your team. There are often good opportunities to help the junior doctors with any of the jobs they have to do and if you are lucky assist with some procedures. The rest of the day is best spent clerking the latest admissions and trying to find some interesting clinics to sit in on. Experiences vary hugely depending on which team you find yourself attached to.

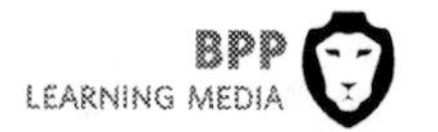

Opinions vary on the best way of going about learning during the clinical years but there can be no doubt that getting stuck in and becoming a part of the firm gains you the respect of the doctors and nurses and some extra bits of teaching.

Throughout the clinical years there is continual assessment. This varies from the observed history and examination in the third year to the structured mini CEX in the final year. Passing of these assessments are important for progression. The key exams are at the end of the third year and the end of the final year. The Intermediates at the end of the third year are used to determine the year quartiles and comprise OSCEs and short answer papers. The finals exams include MCQs, ethics papers, the writing of a discharge letter and of course OSCEs.'

Postgraduate

'Not coming from a science background made me less likely to sit back and hope previously gained credentials would see me through – I was forced, in a good way, to participate fully in all aspects of the course without complacency. The exams were fair – it was definitely a good thing to get on with OSCEs right from the first year, since I have heard how daunting these are for undergraduate medics when they are suddenly faced with them quite late on in their degrees. I would say to new first years: come prepared to learn, not prepared to know. As long as you keep asking questions you'll soon start to make the most of the very interactive nature of the first two years and get to understand things. In any case you will probably be better prepared than your undergrad peers for this part of the course (you will be joining up with first the BM5 third years in year 3, then the BM5 fifth years in year 4) having done significantly more clinical preparation over the preceding two years.'

Once you get in...

Once you get in, the first things to make sure are sorted are accommodation and finance. You should receive the appropriate information regarding accommodation. If you are required to enrol, make sure you do this.

The first week, like the first week at any university, may be a little scary especially if this is your first time away from home. The freedom and opportunities available can be a little overwhelming for some, and many people indulge excessively in certain liberties to their detriment! It is important to have fun, but also to be sensible!

The Best Thing	There is a really friendly feel to the medical school and you will get to know lots of fantastic people
The Worst Thing	When it rains in Southampton it really rains

Student top tips

- Southampton is right on the coast and is ideal for water sports so bring your goggles.
- The Isle of Wight is just a hop away.

Summary Table

Positives	Negatives
Really friendly atmosphere	Rain
Fourth year project gives a great change to experience research	Road congestion in rush hours
The solent is fantastic for sailing	Small city with limited nightlife
Early patient contact	
Really friendly atmosphere	

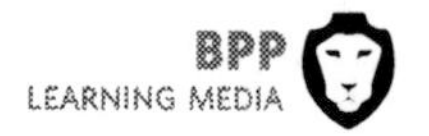

St. Andrews

The Bute Medical School
University of St Andrews
Bute Building
St Andrews
KY16 9TS

http://medicine.st-andrews.ac.uk

The third oldest in the English-speaking world and oldest in Scotland, St Andrews is a traditional university based in a beautiful, small town on the east coast of the country. It has a friendly, supportive atmosphere and vibrant social scene. Its medical school runs a three-year course which provides students with the essential scientific knowledge and skills necessary for future excellence in practice, with clinical training then being undertaken elsewhere. The school's staff are highly enthusiastic and often encourage students to pursue their own, unique interests in Medicine outside the course, with research opportunities available very early on. Overall, St Andrews is an excellent venue to begin a successful, enjoyable medical career.

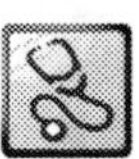

The medical course

Key facts

Course Type	Traditional 3 years pre-clinical	Degree Awarded	BSc (Hons) Medicine
Basic Entry Requirements	AAA	Entrance Exams	UKCAT
Year Size	Approx 160	Open Days	October to March
Admissions Website	http://medicine.st-andrews.ac.uk/		

Getting in – student tips

Evidence of appropriate personal qualities should be on a candidate's personal statement, especially that showing empathy,

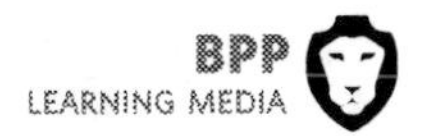

refined communication skills, the capacity to work with or lead a team, determination and an interest in academia. Additionally, the prospective student should demonstrate that they are aware of what a career in Medicine involves and any experiences of shadowing or volunteer work should also obviously be discussed. Finally, any appropriate non-academic achievements (such as sporting victories and positions of responsibility held) should be described.

The school is open to prospective students taking gap years after finishing school, although they should be in some way relevant to a future career in Medicine.

At the interview, half the panel are pre-clinical staff and half are clinical. Students are initially asked to spend ten minutes reading a short article on a medical topic. When the interview itself begins, questions focus on the candidate's understanding of the course at St Andrews and on any medical work experience they may have had. The interviewee is then quizzed on the article they read previously, with staff assessing their comprehension and communication skills.

Course details

Foundation / Pre-Med	NA	**Graduate**	NA
Student Population	Male: female ratio: 40:60	**Term Length**	Pre-clinical: 11–12 weeks Commencing: end of September
Erasmus / Foreign Exchange	NA	**Elective Period**	NA

Anatomy teaching

There are usually two one-hour anatomy lectures every week. A two-hour session in the dissection room then follows in which this material is reinforced. These sessions are attended in small groups and typically consist of a mixture of student dissection and teaching with the cadaver, prosections and models. Much dissection of the cadaver is purposefully left to students, as it

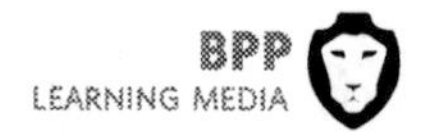

demands the practical application of lecture material, which in turn encourages the retention of this knowledge. Students are taught in these sessions by anatomists and medical demonstrators, the latter of which typically have a background in clinical practice and contextualise much of the purely anatomical material. Despite the traditional methods by which anatomy is taught at St Andrews, students only learn in any great detail that which is truly clinically relevant.

Pre-clinical/Years 1–3	
Topics	Teaching is grouped into several 'strands', which are taught throughout the three-year course. ***Year 1*** *First semester:* Introduction to Medicine *Second semester*: Musculoskeletal System ***Year 2*** *First semester*: Cardiovascular and Respiratory Systems *Second semester:* Renal, Gastrointestinal and Reproductive Systems ***Year 3*** *First semester*: Nervous and Endocrine Systems *Second semester:* Student Selected Component
Teaching	Lectures; small group tutorials, including patient scenarios; self-study assignments and GP, community and hospital attachments.
SSC Periods	There is one Student Selected Component in the second semester of the third year, where students work closely with a supervisor to answer a specific research question. Projects can involve laboratory work, reviewing the literature on a particular subject or even data collection in a clinical setting.
Exams	Each semester, there is a mid-semester and an end of semester assessment (both of which count towards a student's final grade). Assessments consist of short written answers, multiple-choice questions (not negatively marked) and extended matching questions. Students should not be greatly pushed for time.

The medical school

Work						Brief summary on volume of work
Facilities						Good standard and recently replaced by new facilities
Support						High quality support is always available from both the staff and fellow students
Feedback						Great feedback on exams

Facilities

Currently, the school is in a transition phase with a brand-new building with up-to-date facilities being scheduled for completion in 2010. The old buildings have several lecture theatres, a clinical skills lab, a large dissection room and an anatomy museum. A great deal of dissection is carried out at St Andrews, so the school owns a vast array of high quality prosections for students to view upon request. Two histology labs, a 24-hour access IT suite and several small tutorial rooms are shared with the School of Biology. The medical school is in the centre of town, with several places to eat and relax right outside.

Student support

St Andrews is a very friendly university and both staff and students are extremely willing to provide whatever help they can. Similar to many other major institutions, academic 'parents' in the upper years adopt 'sons' and 'daughters' from the first year. There is no formal allocation system in place, but students usually find it easy to seek out parents with similar interests early on during their time at the university. This relationship is considered highly important at St Andrews; academic 'families' meet regularly throughout the new student's first year and will often stay in contact for a long time thereafter. Everyone is also assigned a staff tutor, who is there to monitor his or her academic and personal progress throughout the entire three-year course and assist where necessary. Finally, the university's Student Support Services is a further resource, which is

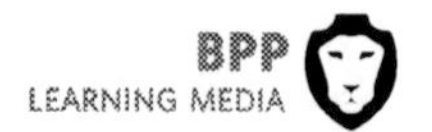

known to efficiently deal with most problems typically encountered by undergraduates and postgraduates alike. They can be seen to be highly active from the very first day of freshers' week.

Finance

The university has a Discretionary Fund, which typically awards £400-500 per year. There is also a childcare fund and a Young Student bursary (the latter only for student's receiving support from SAAS). Students studying certain subjects or with talent in sports or music are eligible for a number of scholarships and bursaries.

Further info: www.st-andrews.ac.uk/admissions/scholarships/

Student opinion

'The school has an atmosphere of friendliness and help is never hard to come by. Lecturers are highly enthusiastic about their subjects and many also participate eagerly in the school's social life. Each timetable is scheduled to allow a healthy balance between study and relaxation, ensuring that the student's enjoyment of the course and productivity are both maximised.'

The university

Accommodation	Non-campus
Further Info	www.yourunion.net

Accommodation

Halls of residence are spread throughout the town, with the closest to the medical school being right next-door and the furthest 25 minutes' walk away. All first years are guaranteed a place in halls. Moreover, each hall organises regular social events for its residents to enjoy.

Those in the second year or above may not be offered a place in halls and often live in private accommodation. This can be hard to come by in St Andrews, with a shortage of quality, private housing

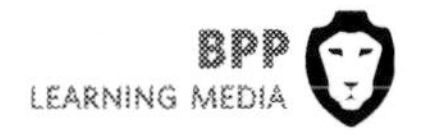

for students becoming increasingly evident although the university has now acknowledged this issue and is taking action against the deficit. Students should apply early to get the best selection of properties, however those who do not manage to find a place to live early on should not fret as new properties trickle onto the market right up until the start of term.

Study facilities

Medical students typically use the university's central library, as it is a quiet place to study, has numerous copies of each textbook referenced in the course, houses extensive IT facilities and is open until midnight most days. Additionally, there are a number of smaller, departmental libraries that are open to all students of the university. Medics find these useful during the exam periods, when the central library's resources are unable to adequately deal with the needs of the entire student population.

University sports & students' union

The union is at the centre of the town's nightlife. The 'Bop!', inexpensive dancing and drinks every Tuesday and Friday night, is where most pub crawls and other nights out eventually end up. This takes place in Venue 1, but there is also a smaller Venue 2 upstairs. Societies are free to book and use these as they please and there is generally at least one major event taking place in the union every night. The Bute Medical Society hosts most of its events either in one of these venues or in a lecture theatre at the school; at other times, medics frequent the union just like most other students. The union also has a bar with a large screen television, pool tables, extensive seating, a games room and a place to buy food (the latter is open only during the day).

Use of the sports centre costs between £35 and £100 depending on membership for a semester. The gym is relatively small and during peak hours can be difficult to use, but has a good selection of equipment. There are wide ranges of sports clubs authorised by the Athletic Union, including a number, which are still relatively obscure (including Ultimate Frisbee and 'Korfball'). There are no swimming facilities at the sports centre, however there is a cheap, clean, privately-owned pool towards the east of the town and the swimming club also has access to a number of other local venues.

Student opinion

'Life as a student at St Andrews is never dull, with the halls, union, medical school and societies working together to provide a constant stream of interesting and unique things to do, with everyone being able to find something they enjoy. The lengthy history of the university means that it has many well-established traditions that have taken place for decades (if not centuries!) and are still continued today. These include the infamous Raisin weekend, which never fails to disappoint and is enjoyed by all!'

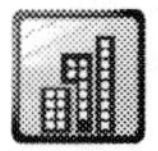

The city

Safety	⛨	⛨	⛨	⛨	⛨	Students are rarely reported victims of crime and police regularly patrol the streets
Nightlife	☾	☾	☾	☾		Vibrant, but lacks a clubbing scene
Transport	🚌	🚌	🚌	🚌	🚌	Most places are well within walking distance, but there are also local buses available. Parking isn't great for those with cars
Cost of Living	🐖	🐖	🐖			Accommodation can be expensive

Things to do

St Andrews is a small, quaint seaside town in which the majority of the population are students. A rich past has preceded that which exists today, demonstrated by the vast number of interesting historical buildings and sites that are littered throughout the town.

The many varied pubs and bars around St Andrews are where most of the student nightlife occurs, with 'The Raisin' being the establishment where most medics choose to congregate. Fans of clubs should think carefully before deciding to study at St Andrews, as there are none in the town (although certain pubs in St Andrews do organise transport to Dundee's more popular clubbing venues several times a week). Most students find the absence of clubs is more than compensated for by the amazing number of events put on by student organisations almost every night, including regular balls, fashion shows, music festivals, plays, ceilidhs, the 'Bop!' and much, much more.

The town is host to a variety of interesting, pleasant places to eat, drink and relax at a range of prices. These include 'Jannetas', a famous ice cream parlour opposite the medical school that is renowned for its taste and originality. During the summer months, the several beaches surrounding St Andrews are popular locations for students to unwind with friends. With regard to shopping, there is a selection of small businesses in St Andrews and some larger chain stores. When this isn't enough, Dundee's shopping malls are only 30 minutes away by bus.

Students feel very safe around the town, with minimal crime rates and police presence.

Places to Go		
Place	**Brief Description**	**Entry Fee/Opening Time**
The Victoria	Very popular pub near the union	£Free, Mon–Thurs, 9.00am–1.00am; Fri–Sat, 10.00am–1.00am; Sun, 9.00am–midnight
The 'Bop!'	Inexpensive dancing and drinks at the union	£Free with a beverage on Tuesday, 9.00pm–1.00am; £3.50 on Friday, 9.00pm–2.00am.
Jannetas	Renowned ice-cream parlour near the medical school	£Free, Mon–Sun, 9.00am–6.00pm
The Victoria	Very popular pub near the union	£Free, Mon–Thurs, 9.00am–1.00am; Fri–Sat, 10.00am–1.00am; Sun, 9.00am–midnight

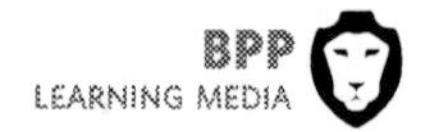

Student opinion

'St Andrews is small but host to a large, sociable student population. The streets are frequently packed with both undergraduates and postgraduates, and new students should prepare themselves to regularly come across numerous friends on every journey they make around the town. Although it lacks some of the luxuries of big cities, St Andrews is packed with things to do, friendly people to meet and new places to visit.'

Student's view

Pre-clinical

'A regular day for a first year medical student begins at 9.00 or 10.00am with one to three lectures lasting anywhere between 40 minutes and an hour. Lunch is from 1.00 to 2.00pm, and then in the afternoon there are usually one to two more lectures or alternatively a session in the dissection room, laboratory or clinical skills rooms. Students also occasionally have morning or afternoon attachments to GPs and hospitals to attend and a few self-study assignments that typically only take a few hours each week. As is common in other institutions, classes are never scheduled on Wednesday afternoons to allow time for sports. The schedule is more intense in the second year and the first semester of the third year, although in the second semester of the third year students have only a few clinical skills sessions each week to allow them time to complete their research dissertation. In my opinion, the overall balance between time for study and relaxation in the course is very well planned.

Personally, my choice to study Medicine at St Andrews was based mainly on the school's emphasis on gaining a respectable understanding of pre-clinical science, the pleasant, amicable feel to the place and the opportunity to move on to another institution and experience a different town or city for the clinical years of my medical training.

The highlights of my time at the medical school have been conducting ophthalmic research in India, my first ever Bute ball and taking

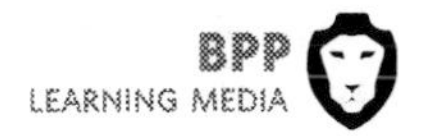

part in 'Raisin Monday' - where first year students pack into St Salvatore's quad clad in fancy dress and engage in a foam fight of epic proportions!'

Once you get in...

Firstly, the university will request you fill out a form which they will use to allocate you to suitable halls of residence. Be sure to get this back to them promptly as you may not get a place in halls if you miss the deadline.

The medical school will also ask you to complete a few tasks before term starts, all of which are discussed in detail on their user-friendly 'Flying Start' website for new students (http://medicine.st-andrews.ac.uk/flyingstart/index.html). Also included on the site are reminders of the essential items to bring with you and a frequently asked questions section.

Students hear little about what's on in freshers' week until they arrive, when stacks of programmes containing details of the hundreds of events on offer are suddenly piled onto them.

The Best Thing	Thorough coverage of all major pre-clinical subjects in a friendly, supportive atmosphere
The Worst Thing	The small size of the medical school, university and town can be frustrating for some

Student top tips

- Think carefully before purchasing any textbooks prior to arriving at the medical school, as certain stores in St Andrews offer great discounts if you buy them all together.
- Make sure to send in a photograph for your student ID prior to arriving at the university, as otherwise they will take a picture of you on the day you matriculate and you will be stuck with it for the next three years!
- If you are in halls and have a computer, buy an internet cable at home as stocks run out quick in the town during freshers' week.

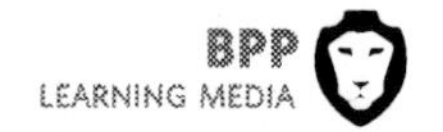

Summary Table

Positives	Negatives
Gain an excellent understanding of pre-clinical science	Lacks certain luxuries found in big cities, including a clubbing scene
Friendly, supportive atmosphere	Small size means can be hard to escape from university life if you want to
Vibrant social scene, with a wide range of different events constantly being organised	Can be difficult and expensive to get good accommodation
Promising research opportunities from early in the course	Some students find the course too heavily influenced by science
Staff are very enthusiastic and keen to help	GP and hospital attachments can be far away

Swansea

College of Medicine
Grove Building University of Wales Swansea
Singleton Park
Swansea
SA2 8PP

www.swan.ac.uk/medicine/

With the Gower Peninsula, Britain's first area of outstanding natural beauty and Rhosilli Bay just minutes away, the sunny seaside city of Swansea has everything to offer. Although still in its infancy, Swansea College of Medicine is growing annually in achievement and reputation, and has a graduation record second to none. Initially in partnership with Cardiff medical school, Swansea now stands alone and invites graduates of all disciplines to train using a clinical-case based learning week with thorough anatomy and clinical opportunities.

The newly developed curriculum and its delivery are specifically designed with graduates in mind and fully integrate the learning and teaching of medical knowledge, clinical and communication skills from day one. Teaching is delivered by a highly qualified team of clinical staff in newly refurbished labs and learning environments, utilising innovative and proven methods.

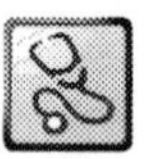 *The medical course*

Key facts

Course Type	Four-year postgraduate	Degree Awarded	MB ChB
Basic Entry Requirements	2:1 degree	Entrance Exams	GAMSAT
Year Size	Approx 70 places	Open Days	March and June
Admissions Website	www.swan.ac.uk/medicine/		

Getting in – student tips

The Swansea interview process has a large focus on personality. While you will need to perform at GAMSAT and have a 1st class or an upper 2.1 degree, interest will be in your personal statement and character. It is desirable that you have at least some experience of Biology or Chemistry at post-GCSE (or equivalent) or higher level, but this is not a limiting factor if you do not. Also you should also be able to demonstrate a proficiency in Mathematics and English language. You will need to show a commitment and interest in Medicine, supported by suitable work experience. Age is no factor at Swansea and in fact life experience and a real desire to study Medicine will stand you in good stead. Although each year is different, around 50% of all applicants will be interviewed and of those around 50% will be made offers. From the offers over 50% will accept a place at Swansea. Interviews are informal and seek to select the individuals who will thrive in a competitive and challenging environment. You will need to demonstrate preparedness, awareness of current affairs, self-confidence and knowledge of what a career in Medicine entails. Typically an interview panel will consist of one clinician and one member of teaching staff. Occasionally student members may also sit on the panel.

Course details

Foundation / Pre-Med	NA	**Graduate**	Graduate only
Student Population	Male: female ratio: 40:60	**Term Length**	Commencing: 1 September 10 weeks
Erasmus / Foreign Exchange	Not offered	**Elective Period**	Six-week period offered at the end of the year 3

Anatomy teaching

The anatomy facilities at Swansea College of Medicine are excellent and the teaching is led by a well-respected team of clinical anatomists with years of experience. An atomy teaching is over the full four years but will progress from traditional taught anatomy (years 1 and 2) into diagnostic reasoning where students will be expected

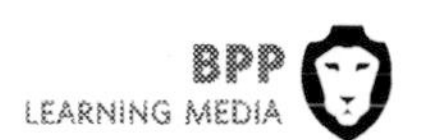

to look at scans and X-rays within the hospital environment (years 3 and 4).

Pre-clinical/Years 1–2	
Topics	***Year 1:*** Subjects are taught as clinical cases (delivered by clinicians) and provide the foundation to years 3 and 4. ***Year 2:*** As above but with a clear clinical focus.
Teaching	Teaching is mainly delivered by lectures, seminars, anatomy sessions and integrated clinical methods.
SSC Periods	Offered as a Family Case Study (year 1), an Oncology Case Study (year 2). Also Learning Opportunities in the Clinical Setting (LOCs) and Clinical Information Management will be offered in both years 1 and 2.
Exams	Examinations are by extended matching questions (EMQs) and are at the end of each term. The level and complexity of exams is high and of course there is the occasional 'fail' mark but generally speaking teaching is pitched at an adequate level and the results are very good.

Clinical/Years 3–5	
Topics	***Year 3/4:*** You will use the skills acquired in years 1 and 2 to analyse full sets of patient records in years 3 and 4. Teaching will focus on issues raised in the patient notes and will be predominantly based in the hospital setting.
Elective	At the end of year 3 you will go on a six-week elective – allowing students to explore an area of medicine (of particular interest) that would not normally be possible within the 'normal' curriculum.
SSC Periods	There will be two further Case Studies that are partly student selected in years 3 and 4, these will be a Chronic Disease Case Study and probably an audit (to be confirmed).
Exams	Examinations are by extended matching questions (EMQs) and are at the end of each term.

Hospital placements/academies

The School will be engaging with both hospitals and primary care services within:

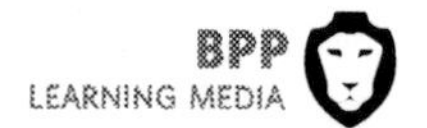

- Abertawe Bro-Morgannwg University NHS Local Health Board
- Hywel Dda Local Health Board

As well as with Public Health Wales

The programme will not include rotations as traditionally known. Students will gain knowledge required within the designated learning weeks; the clinical placements in years 3 and 4 will provide you with experience in each of the major specialties.

Hospitals and Travel Times from University	
Singleton (general)	On site
Morriston (infirmary)	20 minutes
Cefn Coed (psychiatric)	20 minutes

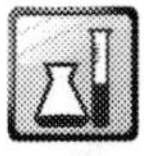

The medical school

Work						Good work life balance
Facilities						Modern and well maintained
Support						Personal tutor system and excellent pastoral support at every stage
Feedback						Prompt return and detailed feedback

Facilities

Medical students share the main library with the rest of the university, but do have devoted areas with a surplus of texts. The library staff are always willing to help and search for requested literature and there are post-grad and quiet study areas available. There are also two lecture theatres, an excellently equipped anatomy suite, a clinical skills suite with beds and bays, a recently refurbished IT suite, as well as a common room.

Student support

The medical school has a student-parent system in place, in which first years are assigned a set of two second year students (called 'parents') to look after them. There is a parents' social at the beginning of the year so the first years can meet their 'medical parents'. Generally this system works very well and the first years are well looked after by their peers. Also there is a staff tutor from faculty who will allocated to students, who will be able to guide and support students during their time at Swansea. Most tutors have a relaxed 'open door' policy about meeting their tutees. Other services on campus include a chaplaincy, medical and dental practices.

Finance

Several bursary schemes are offered.

Student opinion

'For me, Swansea medical school is perfectly equipped to provide excellent teaching and support during my training. The course is well constructed and provides a balanced fusion of scientific and clinical components from the outset. Financially, the first year is quite costly, however years 2 to 4 are subsidised by the NHS bursary system. It is advisable to consider your financial position in advance to avoid difficulties later. The MedSoc is well organised and renowned for its pragmatic approach – especially relating to its planned socials.'

The university

Accommodation	Nearly all medics will choose to live in private rented accommodation. The Uplands, Brynmill and Sketty are all popular areas of residence
Further Info	www.swan.ac.uk/accommodation

Accommodation

While accommodation is offered on campus to all first year medics, most students opt to take up private rented accommodation. After

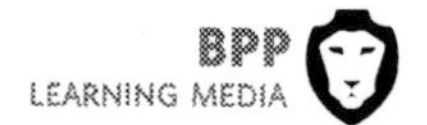

your first degree or time in employment most graduate entry students feel that living in halls with first year undergrads is not for them. Not only will it be difficult to find quiet time to study but the course terms may last longer than your residency in halls, so generally speaking living in halls is not ideal.

Study facilities

The main university library is open to all students and medics regularly use it to study and prepare for exams. It's well stocked and there are several quiet study areas and post grad areas located around the library. Opening hours are set around the undergrads and so during extended terms the library doesn't always offer suitable opening hours for medics, but the library in Singleton hospital is open 24/7 so there will always be somewhere to enjoy the unrelenting revision!

University sports & students' union

The SU in Swansea is entirely led by sabbatical students with a real passion and drive to develop the university. The whole team are easily accessible, located on campus and always happy to help. The SU holds several noted events each year and these are open to everyone including medics. The SU hosts countless societies from RAG through to the real ale society and all of these are on display at the freshers' week.

Finance

Further info: www.swan.ac.uk/sport/

Gym membership will cost £70/term or £180/year, which seems relatively expensive, but it is well equipped and just off campus so easy to get to. There is also a fantastic Olympic size pool, courts, pitches and classes for just about everything as well as qualified physiotherapists and masseurs' at hand.

Student opinion

'For me, Swansea University just like its medical school is a great place to be. It has the organisation of a university five times its size, yet it is quaint enough to instantly make you feel at home. The facilities at Swansea are surplus to requirement and ever developing, furthering its reputation. If you have concerns about whether Swansea University will have everything you need to allow you succeed in Medicine – then don't. It is an ideal setting and a conscientious choice for your training as a doctor.'

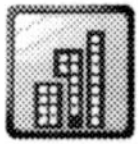

The city

Safety						Generally safe
Nightlife						Good mix of clubs and bars
Transport						Most placements are commutable
Cost of Living						Generally well-priced

Things to do

Swansea city has a rich cultural and social history. The city has all of the expected shops and stores, and you will easily find every service you'll need without travelling too far. Swansea city is student friendly and during term time it becomes incredibly lively. Wind Street is the best place to go out to socialise, as it has several clubs and countless popular bars most of which honour student cards for great discounts. The best thing about being a student in Swansea has to be having the city on your doorstep and the sandy beaches just minutes away. The worst thing... has to be the rain!

Places to Go		
Place	**Brief Description**	**Entry Fee/Opening Time**
Oceana	Recently developed super club	£Varies, 12.00pm–3.00am

Student opinion

'Swansea city is a really great place to live and learn. It has all of the essential facilities you'll need and is near to the university. Bus services are good and the train station has great service to the whole of the UK. Traffic and parking like most cities can at times be difficult. Swansea is not renowned for its nightlife but it does have a few good clubs and of course Cardiff is only a short train journey away. Swansea city is currently under planned development and has a lot of promise for the future.'

Student's view

Postgraduate

'Applying to medical school is in itself hard work. But for graduate applicants it is more difficult still as many of us will need to leave the security of employment, or maintain prolonged study with mounting debt. And so, choosing to become a doctor is a big commitment, which needs to be carefully considered. Swansea medical school has everything you need to fulfil your potential and maximise your training. Teaching is neatly packed into case-based learning weeks and it is supported by proactive clinical and anatomy sessions.

For me, Swansea medical school seemed unique to the other universities I had visited before. On the open day I was made to feel very welcome and instantly felt confident in the organisation and management of the school. I was thoroughly impressed by the student involvement in the open days and I knew that if I got an offer I would definitely accept it. I think that Swansea medical school has the right attitude about teaching and has a proven curricula based on the one used at Cardiff medical school. While the graduate entry programme is intense and holidays are short, it is possible (and very important) to maintain a healthy work-life balance. So far, highlights have to include LOCS, thorough anatomy teaching and the opportunity to represent my medical school as the medical society president.'

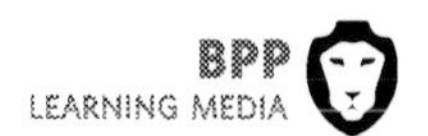

Once you get in...

Once you are made an offer, you will be invited to a 'meet and greet' in which you will have the opportunity to get to know your colleagues and the teaching staff. When you arrive at Swansea, you will be presented with a freshers' pack, full of key information about the university, the school of medicine, the MedSoc and details of your course. It will all be self explanatory and designed to give you a warm welcome to course. For the most keen amongst you, we will also make suggestions of text books and reading which may help your transition into medical school. Also in advance you will also receive a freshers' week timetable detailing your first week at medical school, which lectures you need to attend and where you will need to be – and don't worry, you'll also receive a map!

The Best Thing	The innovative course, the enthusiasm of the faculty and most importantly... the beach!
The Worst Thing	The consistency of assessment still needs to be improved, but this will come as the course matures

Student top tips

- Make sure you buy your MedSoc freshers' week tickets and membership in advance – it will save you money.
- Consider your living arrangements very carefully – nearly all medics choose to live in private rented accommodation – for very good reasons.
- Don't forget that while doing Medicine is about the best teaching and facilities available, it's also about spending four years of your life in an area, and where better to relax and unwind than on the sandy beaches or the Gower Peninsula.
- If you need any more information about the course or Swansea, please contact the school or if you want advice from a student the MedSoc we'll happily help where possible.

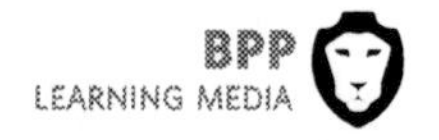

Summary Table

Positives	Negatives
Modern, innovative teaching methods	No proven track record of the new four-year course at Swansea
Beautiful area to live	Hilly, rainy, it's in Wales!
Proactive and busy MedSoc	Quite a small school – possibly limited by its size
Very good support during exams	Inconsistent levels of assessment

Warwick

Warwick Medical School
Gibbet Hill Road
Coventry
West Midlands
CV4 7AL

www2.warwick.ac.uk/fac/med/

The university is located on the south side of Coventry on the border of Warwickshire. Coventry is most famous for producing 70s ska legends The Specials, naked horse rider Lady Godiva and her voyeur Peeping Tom, and writer Philip Larkin. Coventry was the most damaged city in the UK after being bombed by the Luftwaffe in 1940 and as a result, most of the city was rebuilt. Coventry now boasts an impressive cathedral built in the 1960s, the first ever city based IKEA built in 2007, and the Ricoh (football) Arena where Take That recently performed as part of their Circus tour! Film buffs amongst you might recognise Coventry from *The Italian Job* (the bit with the mini coopers driving through sewer pipes in Turin), and it's very likely that you will spend your clinical placements at the George Eliot Hospital in Nuneaton (Nuneaton being home of George Eliot), or the Walsgrave Hospital (where part of TV medical series *Angels* was filmed). Warwick Medical School is the largest purely graduate entry course in the UK and began in 2000 under supervision of Leicester University. Its first students graduated in 2004 and it gained independent degree status from the GMC in 2007. Warwick University has consistently featured amongst the top 10 UK universities and the medical school was involved in the creation of a Centre of Excellence for Anatomy and Surgery, with the provision of plastinates from Gunther Von Hagens's lab in Germany.

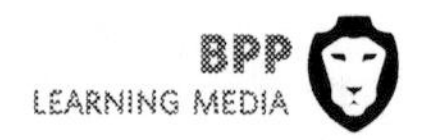

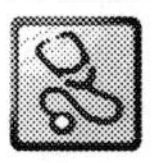

The medical course

Key facts

Course Type	Traditional – Postgraduate only	Degree Awarded	MBChB
Basic Entry Requirements	2:1 honours degree	Entrance Exams	UKCAT
Year Size	Approx 175	Open Days	February, June, September
Admissions Website	www2.warwick.ac.uk/fac/med/		

Getting in – student tips

WMS looks for, in addition to academic ability, a clear awareness of the demands of Medicine, interpersonal and communication skills, and significant work experience in a caring environment. As well as this Warwick looks for well-rounded individuals who are not only dedicated to Medicine and can cope with the course, but can also bring other qualities that will make them a better doctor.

WMS adopts and innovative admissions process designed to assess applicants across this broad range of criteria. Should an applicant's reference, personal statement and UKCAT score meet the suitable requirements you will then be invited to the selection centre.

Course details

Foundation / Pre-Med	No	Graduate	Yes
Student Population	Male: female ratio: 40:60	Term Length	Pre-clinical: 12 weeks Clinical: variable
Erasmus / Foreign Exchange	N/A	Elective Period	Year 3 – 8 weeks

Intercalation

Stage	N/A	Degree Awarded	N/A
Requirements	N/A	Subjects	N/A

Anatomy teaching

Anatomy is taught in a variety of innovative ways at Warwick Medical School. WMS students are taught the majority of anatomy using 'plastinated' prosections once a week. These sessions involve rotating between prosections with your teaching group and receiving short tutorials and Q&As with the models from clinical education fellows. The models are designed for teaching, can be touched and everything can be easily identified. The introduction of the plastinations in 2009 received a fantastic response and feedback showed that students felt the teaching was better than that they would have received with dissection.

Anatomy teaching is also supplemented with online teaching, integration with the core lecture material and small group tutorials on imaging and radiology.

Pre-clinical/Years 1–2	
Topics	***Year 1:*** Essentials of Medicine, Health in the Community, Gastrointestinal System, Health and Disease in Populations, Molecules and the Human Body, Histology and Embryology, Health Psychology, Infection and the Immune System, Musculoskeletal System, Cardiovascular System, Reproductive System, Mechanisms of Disease, Inter-professional Learning, Clinical Skills. ***Year 2:*** Values in Medicine, Introduction to the NHS, Mechanisms in Clinical Pharmacology, Urinary System, Human Lifespan, Neurobiology, Respiratory System, Clinical Skills.
Teaching	The majority of modules are taught entirely by traditional lectures and small group learning. Students are allocated a group at the beginning of the course and all group sessions are conducted within these groups. Group work comprises case studies, presentations, integration of modules and broadening of the subject matter covered in lectures. Some modules include patient interviews / examination, tutorials and seminars plus online learning.

SSC Periods	There are two Student Selected Components in Phase I of the course; these are the Clinical Applications Special Studies Module (CASSM) and the Special Studies Module (SSM).
Exams	End of Semester Assessments (ESAs) in January, June and December. ESAs are an integrated exam and assess all material covered in the course so far (ie ESA 1 covers semester 1, while ESA 2 can examine semester 1 and 2, and ESA 3 can examine all three semesters). ESAs are formed of a number of questions and the pass mark is given as a number of questions which must be passed to successfully progress to the next stage of the course. The exams are naturally difficult due to the accelerated nature of the course however the majority pass. ESAs are supplemented by Observed Structured Clinical Examinations (OSCEs) which cover anatomy, histology, clinical procedures/examinations and history taking.

Clinical/Years 3–4	
Topics	As Phase 1 is around 18 months long, and finishes part-way through year 2, Phase 2 falls out-of-sync with the standard academic year. It is therefore split into two rotations; Junior and Senior. *Junior Rotation (Year 2 to 3):* General medicine (2), general surgery, general practice, psychiatry, and orthopaedics and anaesthetics. *Senior Rotation (Year 3 to 4):* Elective, general medicine, general surgery, acute medical specialties (emergency medicine, critical care, acute medicine, and complementary therapies), child health, obstetrics and gynaecology.
SSC Periods	During Phase 2 students have the opportunity to complete a Professionalism Special Study Module (SSM) and can choose from one of the following five subjects: Clinical System Improvement, Leadership, Medical Education, Research, and Safe Practice. These take place during clinical placements and are completely voluntary. There are many opportunities to perform audits and undertake research during Phase 2, and often students are able to get involved with the current research of their consultant teachers.

Exams	At the end of each eight-week clinical placement students are graded by their consultants on their attendance, clinical competence, and attitude and behaviour. Some (but not all) clinical placements have assessments at the end. The format of these varies according to the specialty, but includes MCQ, EMQ, SAQ, and OSCE. The main summative assessment in Phase 2 is the Intermediate Clinical Examination (ICE) at the end of Junior Rotation. ICE comprises a clinical and a written component and must be passed in order to proceed on the course. The Final Professional Examination (FPE) takes place at the end of Senior Rotation and includes an extended form of the ICE clinical component and a written assessment covering the entire curriculum. Students who fail a component of ICE or FPE may have the opportunity to resit.

Hospital placements/academies

The Junior and Senior Rotations are split into eight-week clinical placements (or 'blocks'), during which pairs of students are attached to two consultants, usually a 'generalist' and a 'specialist'. Other students may be placed at the same site, but only one pair is attached to each consultant at a time, so teaching is nearly always on a 1:1 basis.

There are three main hospitals where students are placed for most blocks: University Hospital (or 'Walsgrave' – the old hospital's name), Warwick Hospital, and George Eliot Hospital. University Hospital is a 1,250-bed tertiary referral centre and the principal teaching hospital for Warwick Medical School. The other two hospitals are smaller general hospitals, each of around 350 beds.

Clinical time is spent in a variety of primary and secondary care settings depending on the placement. Students on General Clinical Education blocks (general medicine and general surgery) will spend most of their time on wards, in theatre, and attending out-patient clinics. Each site also provides a number of additional teaching sessions for medical students by senior clinicians. These take various forms, including bedside teaching, small group teaching, seminars, and formal lectures.

Undergraduate co-ordinators at each site ensure the smooth running of clinical placements, and are approachable should students encounter any problems. Facilities are good with the standard battery of libraries and IT suites at every hospital. Well-equipped clinical skills labs at University Hospital and George Eliot Hospital provide excellent training, and are a great resource for students to learn and perfect their practical procedures.

On-site accommodation can be provided for students who require it, such as those with on-call commitments or for students placed at Alexandra Hospital in Redditch. The standard of accommodation ranges from basic with communal facilities to modern with en-suite shower rooms.

Hospitals and Travel Time from University	
University Hospital	15 minutes
Warwick Hospital	20 minutes
George Eliot Hospital	30 minutes
Alexandra Hospital	40 minutes

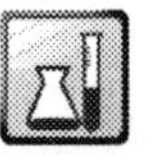

The medical school

Work	✚	✚	✚			Good work life balance
Facilities	☕	☕	☕	☕		Modern and well-equipped medical teaching centre. Good university library, but relatively small Medicine section
Support	👥	👥	👥	👥	👥	Student 'parents' scheme. Peer-mentoring programmes. Student welfare reps. Personal Tutors/Clinical Educational Supervisors
Feedback	📋	📋	📋	📋		Individual feedback on exam performance. 1:1 feedback for students who require it. Extra teaching provided

Facilities

The Medical Teaching Centre is the mainstay of medical student teaching in Phase 1. It is a modern building with a 200-seat lecture theatre, student common room, IT suite, and a number of tutorial rooms, each with computer and audio-visual equipment. Also on the same campus is the Medical School Building, which is home to the restaurant and coffee bar with comfy sofas and plasma TVs. The Biomedical Learning Grid is also located here; a small, but perfectly formed study space with computers, interactive smart boards, and a small collection of medical texts and reference books.

The main university library underwent a major facelift and now provides lots of different working environments from silent study to more relaxed social spaces that are coffee and mobile-friendly.

Student support

Students at Warwick are well catered for in terms of welfare and support. Each student is assigned to a member of Faculty who will be their Personal Tutor for the duration of Phase 1. In Phase 2 students are provided with a Clinical Educational Supervisor with whom they will meet regularly. In addition to the more formal pastoral support, there are also student-led initiatives that are extremely successful. These include the popular Mums and Dads scheme for first years, providing each new student with a second year 'parent', and the peer mentoring programme run by Phase 2 students to help second years prepare for their pre-clinical exams.

Outside of the medical school, the main university has a vast array of Student Support Services which are all freely accessible. A good place to start is at the students' union where the Student Advice Centre provides free, confidential, and informal information and advice about a whole range of issues. They can also signpost students towards more specialist services available from the university, such as the Counselling Service, Disability Services, Health Centre and Mental Health Co-ordinators, and chaplaincy.

Medical societies

There are many clubs and societies within the medical school and, where one doesn't exist, like-minded students have the opportunity to set up their own. The current list is a diverse mix of themes and interests, ranging from surgery to singing, from global health to getting fit.

Warwick Medical Society (MedSoc) is the largest society for medical students at Warwick. It is responsible for organising the infamous medics' social calendar as well as other extra-curricular activities and academic events. MedSoc aims to integrate all years of the medical school and works hard to help students achieve a healthy work-life balance.

Sport at Warwick is also a popular pastime. As well as dozens of university-wide clubs, there are a number of dedicated medics' sports teams, including men's and women's football, rugby, cricket, mixed hockey, and netball. Each team also participates in the annual National Association of Medical Schools (NAMS) tournament. Tournaments such as NAMS are really popular and provide a fantastic opportunity for students to meet other medics from all over the UK.

Many students also choose to get involved with one of the charitable societies, such as the Warwick branch of the national global health charity Medsin, or Students for Kids International Projects (SKIP). One of the newest charitable societies is The Green Wing, an environmental group set up by a group of students as part of Medsin's Healthy Planet campaign. As well as the many rewards of charitable work, students have in the past had the opportunity to spend a summer volunteering with SKIP projects in India and Sri Lanka.

Other popular societies include those that are health-related or have an academic focus, such as Marrow @ Warwick, Warwick MS Society, WMS Careers Society, and WMS Surgical Society. And importantly, for further enhancing that work-life balance there is also M-Body, a dance and exercise group, and Warwick Medical School Singers.

Finance

Further info: www2.warwick.ac.uk/fac/med/study/ugr/fees/

Student opinion

'Although it could be said that Warwick Medical School is still in its infancy, in this short time it has developed a modern approach to learning Medicine in which the curriculum is delivered by passionate and enthusiastic staff.'

The university

Accommodation	Campus and off-campus available
Further info	www.warwicksu.com/ www2.warwick.ac.uk/services/accommodation/

Accommodation

In the first year medics have a choice of applying for campus accommodation (Tocil) or off-campus with the university managed accommodation. There are limited spaces at Tocil halls and places are offered on a first come, first served basis, so the majority of medics will be placed up off-campus, despite the majority applying for halls. Students that apply through Warwick accommodation will be placed in a house of three to five students in Coventry, Leamington Spa or Earlsdon. The houses are made up of mostly medics with the odd PGCE or post-graduate student thrown in for good measure. Within Coventry or Earlsdon, the student areas are a short five to ten minutes by car from the medical school. These areas are also easily accessible by the brilliant public transport, and many students cycle or walk between their accommodation and the university. Leamington Spa, though much nicer, is a good 20-minute drive from the medical school and it is slightly more expensive. This doesn't however dissuade most medics from moving there in the second year.

Study facilities

The university offers a huge state of the art library which is used by medics as well as others students. The library offers quiet areas, as well as group study areas equipped with smart boards, white boards, projectors etc. There is also the essential coffee shop for

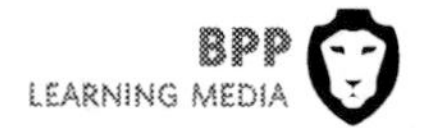

those late night sessions. The library is open 8.30am-12.00am, Monday to Sunday.

The university also has a 'Learning Grid', which is a 24 hours self study area, only closing on Christmas Day and providing an area where students can eat, drink and discuss while they study. The 'Learning Grid' also boasts many of the perks of the library, such as projectors and smart boards.

The medical school also has its own 'BioMed Grid', a much smaller version of the 'Learning Grid' which is specifically tailored towards Biology and medical students, situated at the medical school with plenty of books and models to aid our learning.

University sports & students' union

Membership of Warwick Sport is a flat annual rate of £49. Members can then get unlimited access to all university facilities (except the premium facilities such as the climbing wall etc) and the ability to join any university sports team. WMS students do not have Wednesday afternoons protected for sports like other universities, and therefore joining the main university teams can be difficult. There are plenty of medics teams available such as rugby, football, netball, mixed hockey, cricket and badminton. And if the sport you play is not there, start it up!

The students' union is located on the centre of campus and is one of the largest unions in the country. The union offers a shop, pub, hairdressers, banks, a bistro bar and restaurant, a bespoke sandwich and salad bar and a catering service offering hot and cold buffets, drinks receptions and wine tasting. As well as this the newly built Copper Rooms not only houses the many club nights the union offers but also showcases live music and comedy acts on a regular basis.

The students' union also provides a hub for student societies such as MedSoc, where all the daily running can go smoothly, with plenty of help from the friendly staff. If you want something done, they can, and will, do it.

Student opinion

'WMS is like a big family, as a smaller medical school we all know each other, and as everyone is postgraduate and that little bit older, everyone seems to be in a fantastic mindset. We are all here to get involved, work hard and play hard.'

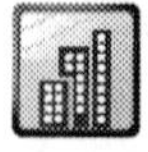

The city

Safety	🛡	🛡	🛡			Coventry is like any other city and generally safe in the right areas
Nightlife	☾	☾	☾	☾		There is a huge range of nightlife across the two student areas: Coventry and Leamington Spa
Transport	🚌	🚌	🚌			The buses are brilliant however a car is essential for Phase II of the course due to the distance between hospitals. And parking is a nightmare
Cost of Living	🐖	🐖	🐖			While rent can be cheap, taxis and nights out can be expensive travelling between Coventry and Leamington Spa for the various events

Things to do

Coventry itself is a large city; however the majority of shops and cafés are all within a small area of town. The 'Skydome', near to the town centre, boasts a cinema, ice rink, restaurants, pubs, clubs and possibly the largest IKEA you will ever see. The surrounding areas of Warwick, Leamington Spa and Stratford upon Avon also provide many opportunities for days out, from shopping on Leamington Spa's beautiful parade to traipsing around Warwick Castle, there's plenty to do when you have visitors.

For those that enjoy a drink, nights out tend to be either in Coventry or Leamington Spa, the majority taking place in the latter due to

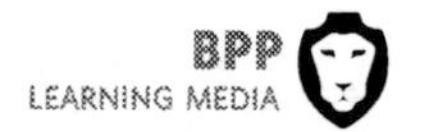

the vast amount of bars in such a small town. As medics have a rather hectic schedule, the majority of the nights out tend to fall on weekends and therefore miss the student nights that take place during the week. But, once again due to the nature of the course, nights out tend to be quite an affair, with entire cohorts venturing out to the same place after a week of hard work.

Places to go		
Place	**Brief Description**	**Entry Fee/Opening Time**
Kelseys	For that after club party (Leamington)	£Free, open til late
Evolve	One of the two big clubs in Leamington	£5. Thur–Sun 10.00pm–3.00am
Smack	The other big club in Leamington	£5. Tues, Fri–Sun 10.00pm–3.00am
Skydome	Various pubs and clubs to explore	£Free–£5. Various opening hours.

Student opinion

'The University of Warwick is on the fringe of Coventry giving an unfortunate lack of a 'big city' feel, although this is balanced in part by the very nice university campus. Most medical students choose to live in (Royal) Leamington Spa, which is a pretty, but relatively small Warwickshire spa town. If you've completed your first degree in a city and are looking to downsize (or city life just isn't your cup of tea) you should be very happy here. However Birmingham is not too far away!'

Student's view

Pre-clinical

'Phase 1 can be pretty tough, they don't call it "fast-track" and "intensive" for nothing. You spend most days working from 9.00am to 5.00pm, but it's also extremely fun. As an entirely postgraduate course most people have spent years getting here and there is a

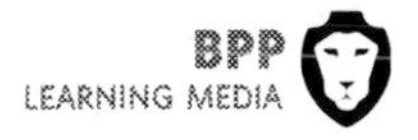

real sense of family and camaraderie. We are also lucky to have world class lecturers and innovative and progressive teaching. Staff are constantly encouraging feedback and the course is constantly evolving because of it.

The course itself is heavily focused towards theory and clinical relevance in the first 18 months before the clinical phase and there is a lot to learn. Most days consist of arriving at lectures for 8.00am or 9.00am and having two lectures, sandwiching a group session in the middle. This is usually repeated after lunch and you often don't leave until gone 5.00pm. The group sessions are fantastic. When joining WMS you are allocated a group of nine to ten students and spend all group sessions with them in Phase 1. You really become a team and learn to draw on each other's strengths, which is great preparation for when you get to the multi-professional environment of healthcare.

As it is a lot of hard work, it makes the extra-curricular aspect of being a medical student even more important. Social events put on by MedSoc and the various sports teams are always very popular, attracting a high proportion of students. The various societies and sports teams are a great way of meeting older students who are always willing to tutor and give a helping hand should exams loom! I would encourage any first year to get as involved as possible; it really makes your WMS experience. My highlights include seeing the Medics Rugby Team reach the final of the NAMS tournament, the induction week events, and the Summer Ball after the first year exams where everyone was in high spirits enjoying a well deserved party.'

Clinical

'Starting the clinical years was quite daunting because the wards were still a little unfamiliar, and as a student I was invariably in somebody's way all of the time! I found the best way to overcome this initial anxiety was to simply put in the hours and not shy away from those uncomfortable moments (despite really wanting to). This way I not only became more familiar with my surroundings, but also with the nurses and junior doctors who later played a pivotal role in maximising the usefulness of my time spent on the wards. The best thing about Phase 2 is that it allows you to gain

an appreciation for the first time of what you'll actually be doing when you qualify, and I found this particularly exciting.

There is less structure to the teaching in Phase 2 and the onus is much more on the student to take advantage of learning opportunities. Some formal teaching is provided during most placements, but this varies according the site of your placement. I found the standard of teaching from consultants to be excellent overall (although some were much better than others) and most of my consultants would provide 1:1 teaching at the bedside or in clinics. I believe that seeing patients regularly to take histories and perform examinations is by far the best way to practise new skills and gain confidence – and this pays dividends when it comes to clinical exams.

One unfortunate downside of this course being a fast-track graduate entry programme is that not all post-graduate specialties are explicitly covered by your clinical placements. In theory this could mean getting to Finals (FPE) without having completed a placement in cardiology for example – quite a worrying prospect! Therefore students are expected to be proactive during their clinical time to ensure they are receiving adequate exposure to a variety of specialties. In reality I found that this was quite difficult to achieve and so have needed to work independently to cover the gaps in my knowledge. I would emphasise to junior students or future applicants the importance of self-directed learning and the ability to meet your own learning needs with supplementary reading.'

Once you get in...

Expect a lot of paperwork. There will be plenty of forms to fill in before arrival including Criminal Record Bureau checks and Occupational Health forms. As well as this you can expect to find the usual university information: accommodation, freshers' week timetables and information on all the facilities and societies.

The medical school will also send you information about the induction week and first semester. A new reading list and list of 'Assumed Knowledge' has now been implemented after previous feedback. Due to the course taking students from a variety of disciplines, this gives students a chance to brush up on their gaps in knowledge before attending should they need to. MedSoc also send out a Student Guide, with their induction week events

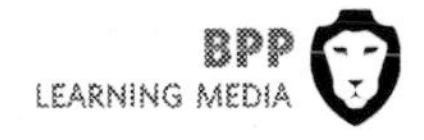

timetable, as well as their own spin on textbooks, modules and university life to help freshers get acquainted with Warwick before they arrive.

The Best Thing	Family atmosphere / Work hard-play hard attitude / Brilliant teaching
The Worst Thing	Very hard work / Can feel separated from the main university

Student top tips

- Make sure you join MedSoc in induction week and get involved in other societies and sports teams. Networking is key in the medical profession and it's never too early to start
- Take the first semester to acclimatise to the new course. You may need to adjust how you study, but also make sure you get to know the people and staff you will be spending the next four years with.
- Stay on top of things; it is very easy to fall behind.

Summary Table

Positives	Negatives
Innovative, world class anatomy teaching	Intensive course
Brilliant atmosphere and work ethic	May have to travel long distances between placements and the university
School is progressive and constantly evolving	Lack of integration with the main university
Excellent social life and plenty of extra-curricular activities available	Minimal time off
Students are well supported by staff	Parking

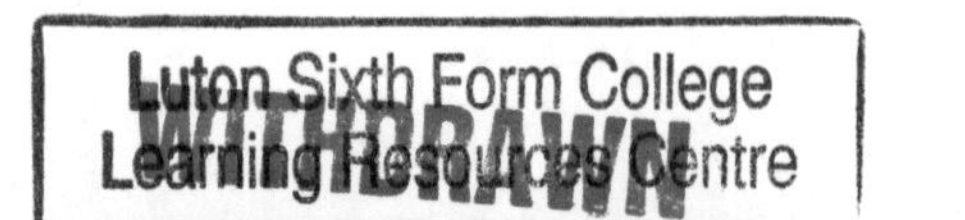

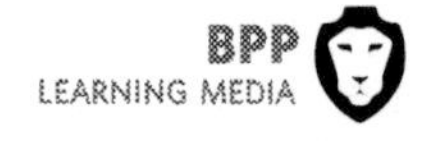

Chapter 35

Quick comparison table

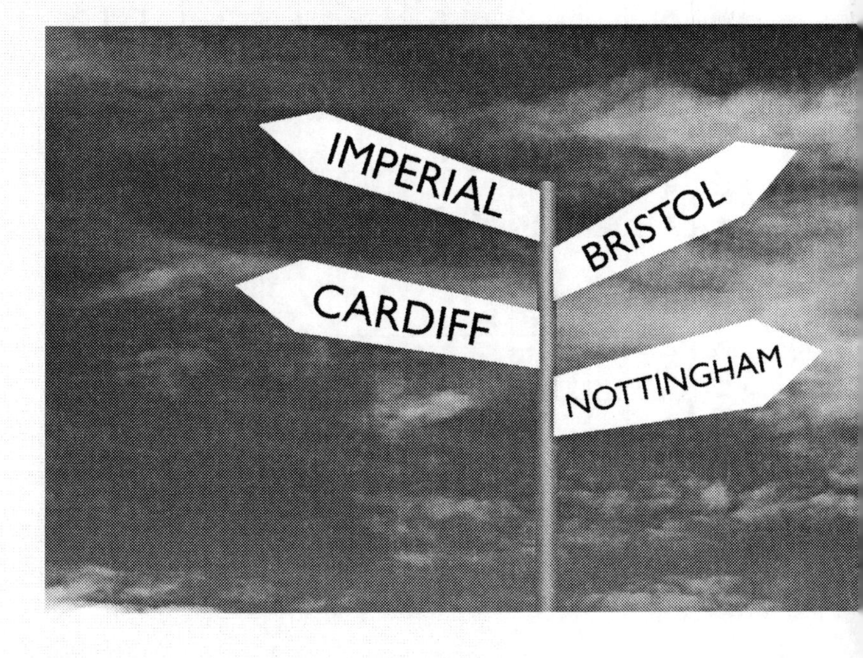

Quick comparison table

Med school	Page	Premed	GEM	Year size	Undergrad	Admission tests	Course type	Interview time	Interview length	Interview panel	Degree	Open days
3 Aberdeen		N/A	N/A	175	AAA	UKCAT	Traditional	Oct–March	20 minutes	2	MBChB	Sept
4 Belfast		N/A	N/A	270	AAA	UKCAT	Traditional	None			MB, BCh	April
5 Birmingham		N/A	Yes	300	AAA	None	Traditional	Oct–April	15 minutes	3	MBChB	Sept, June
6 Brighton and Sussex		N/A	N/A	140	AAA	UKCAT	Integrated	Nov–Feb	20 minutes	3	BMBS	July–Aug
7 Bristol		Yes	Yes	216	AAB	None	Traditional	Nov–March	20 minutes	2	MBChB	June, Sept
8 Cambridge		N/A	Yes	330	AAA	BMAT	Traditional	Dec	20-45 minutes	2	MB BChir	July
9 Cardiff		Yes	N/A	300	AAA	UKCAT	Traditional	Nov–March	20 minutes	3	MBChB	April, July
10 Dundee		Yes	Yes	160	AAA	UKCAT	Traditional	Jan–Feb	50 minutes	Stations	MBChB	June, Sept
11 Durham		N/A	N/A	100	AAA	UKCAT	Traditional	Nov–March	20 minutes	2	MBBS	By request
12 East Anglia		Yes	Yes	140	AAA	UKCAT	Integrated	Feb–May	50 minutes	Stations	MBBS	Oct–July
13 Edinburgh		N/A	N/A	218	AAA	UKCAT	Traditional	Nov–March	30 minutes	2	MBChB	June, Sept
14 Glasgow		N/A	Yes	220	AAA	UKCAT	PBL	Nov–March	15 minutes	2	MBChB	June, Sept
15 Hull York		N/A	N/A	140	AAA	UKCAT	PBL	Nov–Feb	20 minutes	2	MBBS	March, July, Oct
16 Keele		Yes	Yes	120	AAB	UKCAT	PBL	Nov–Feb	20 minutes	3	MBChB	June, Aug
17 Leeds		N/A	Yes	220	AAA	UKCAT	Integrated	Jan–March	20 minutes	3	MBChB	Throughout year

Med school	Page	Premed	GEM	Year size	Undergrad	Admission tests	Course type	Interview time	Interview length	Interview panel	Degree	Open days
18 Leicester		N/A	Yes	180	AAA	UKCAT	Traditional	Nov–March	15–20 minutes	2	MBChB	June–Oct
19 Liverpool		N/A	Yes	300	AAA	None	PBL	Nov	15 minutes	2	MBChB	Throughout year
20 London: Barts		N/A	Yes	280	AAA	UKCAT	PBL	Nov–March	15 minutes	2	MBBS	late Aug/ Sept
21 London: Imperial College		N/A	Yes	280	AAA	BMAT	Traditional	Jan-April	15–20 minutes	4 - 5	MBBS	June, July
22 London: King's College		Yes	Yes	300	AAA	UKCAT	Traditional	Nov-April	15-30 minutes	2	MBBS	On request
23 London: University College		N/A	Yes	330	AAA	BMAT	Traditional	April	30 minutes	3	MBBS	April
24 London: St George's		N/A	Yes	150	AAA	UKCAT GAMSAT	Integrated	Oct-March	15 minutes	3 - 4	MBBS	Throughout year
25 Manchester		Yes	No	350	AAA	UKCAT	PBL	Nov–March	60 minutes	3	MBChB	June
26 Newcastle		N/A	Yes	310	AAA	UKCAT	Traditional	Nov–March	20 minutes	2	MBBS	Aug
27 Nottingham		Yes	Yes	240	AAA	UKCAT GAMSAT	Traditional	Nov–March	30 minutes	2 - 4	BMBS	Throughout year
28 Oxford		N/A	Yes	150	AAA	UKCAT BMAT	Traditional	Dec	College-specific	2+	BM BCh	July

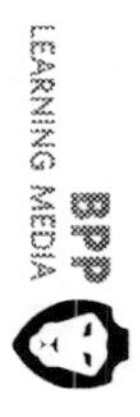

Med school	Page	Premed	GEM	Year size	Undergrad	Admission tests	Course type	Interview time	Interview length	Interview panel	Degree	Open days
29 Peninsula		N/A	N/A	215	AAA	UKCAT GAMSAT	PBL	Nov, Dec, March	15-20 minutes	3–4	BMBS	June, April
30 Sheffield		Yes	Yes	250	AAA	UKCAT	Traditional	Nov–March	20 minutes	3	MBChB	June, July, Sept
31 Southampton		Yes	Yes	175	AAA	UKCAT	Traditional	None			BM	Sept
32 St Andrews		N/A	N/A	160	AAA	UKCAT	Traditional	Nov–March	20 minutes	2+	BSc	Oct-March
33 Swansea		N/A	Only	70	N/A	GAMSAT	Post-graduate	Jan	20-30 minutes	2	MBChB	March, June
34 Warwick		N/A	Only	175	N/A	UKCAT	Post-graduate	March	One-day selection centre		MBChB	Feb, June, Sept

Appendix

Student organisations, further reading and glossary

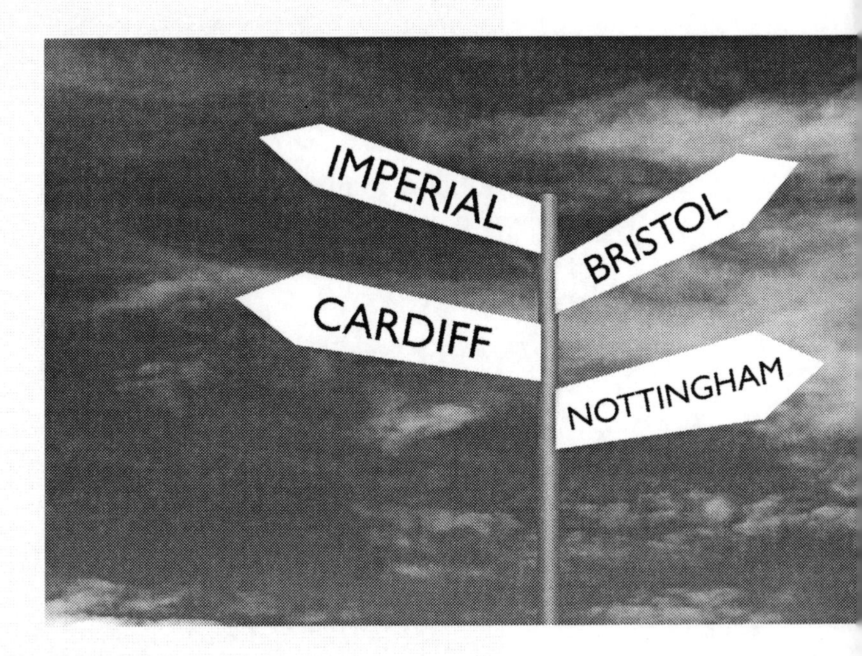

Student organisations

Below is a list of useful medical societies and student organisations. Many of the below offer prizes, lectures of interest and provide help and support to medical students.

BMJ

The British Medical Journal and Student BMJ are definitely worth reading prior to attending medical school interviews. The Student BMJ and its website offer news and information aimed specifically at medical students.

www.bmj.com

www.studentbmj.com

GMC

The General Medical Council is the governing body of UK doctors and is responsible for implementing changes to the medical school curriculum. Vital GMC publications include *Tomorrow's Doctors* and *Good Medical Practice*.

www.gmc-uk.org

RSM

The Royal Society of Medicine is located at Wimpole Street in London. The society offers a number of events for potential medical students including a day devoted to medical careers.

www.rsm.ac.uk

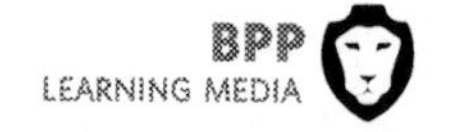

Further reading

Prospective students

BPP Learning Media offer a number of books to complement this guide for those who are considering a career in medicine.

Succeeding In Your Medical School Interview

Becoming A Doctor: Is Medicine Really The Career For You?

Succeeding In The Biomedical Admissions Test (BMAT)

Succeeding In The 2009 UK Clinical Aptitude Test (UKCAT)

Medicine Personal Statement

Books to get through the first year

While most universities provide first year medical students with a comprehensive reading list, we have offered our opinion on must buy textbooks. Medical libraries will stock an excellent selection of textbooks and it is recommended taking out library books early, as the library will be bare when exams begin.

Gray's Anatomy

Davidson's Medicine/Surgery or Kumar and Clarke: Clinical Medicine

Oxford Handbook Clinical Medicine

Clinically Oriented Anatomy

Human Histology

Rang & Dale Pharmacology

Essential Cell Biology

The Anatomy Colouring Book

Glossary

Anatomy	study of the structure of the body
Attachment	see rotation
Audit	process of studying and evaluating current hospital practices in order to improve results. Audits are a vital part of medical training and hospital life
Cardiology	study of the function of the heart and blood vessels
Consultant	senior doctor that has completed all specialist training
Dissection	a method used to teach anatomy by reducing a cadaver to reveal anatomical structures
Elective	period of study (usually eight weeks) spent in a medical setting anywhere in the world
Endocrinology	the study of hormones and their physiological effects on the body
Epidemiology	the study of how often diseases occur in different groups of people and why
Firm	a clinical teaching group usually consisting of Consultant, Registrars and junior doctors
Gastroenterology	study of the digestive system
2-in-1/GEM	term used for postgraduate medics who complete years 1 and 2 in one year on the post-graduate course
Histology	study of microscopic, cellular anatomy
History taking	see patient clerking
Intercalation	a year taken out of the medicine course to complete another degree.
Mess	doctors' common room area
Neurology	study of the brain and its functions
Nights	where you are expected to spend time in hospital through the night to manage acute patients.
Obstetrics and Gynaecology	study of maternal disease and womens' health

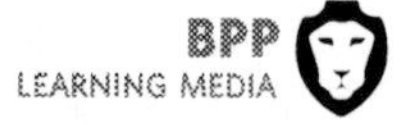

On-call	when you are expected to be available to come into hospital at short notice to manage acute patients
Orthopaedics	branch of Medicine concerned with muscles and bone
Paediatrics	branch of Medicine concerned with child health
Patient clerking	taking a history and / or performing an examination on a patient
Pharmacology	study of drugs and their effects on cells and the body
Pre-clinical	biomedical sciences teaching before beginning clinical teaching at medical school, usually lasting two to three years depending on university
Pre-med/Foundation	a year taken to complete the university equivalent of science A levels for students who apply without science A levels
Prosection	anatomy teaching from pre dissected and presented cadavers
Radiology	study and application of imaging technology such as X-rays
Rotation	a rotation is a period of time you will spend in one department
Surgery	use of manual tools and interventions to treat amenable injuries and diseases
Viva	an oral examination